Urbanising Cholera

New Perspectives in South Asian History 2

The New Perspectives in South Asian History series publishes monographs and other writings on early modern, modern and contemporary history. The volumes in the series cover new ground across a broad spectrum of subjects such as cultural, environmental, medical, military and political history, and the histories of 'marginalised' groups. It includes fresh perspectives on more familiar fields as well as interdisciplinary and original work from all parts of South Asia. It welcomes historical contributions from sociology, anthropology and cultural studies.

Urbanising Cholera

The Social Determinants of Its Re-emergence

RAJIB DASGUPTA

Orient BlackSwan

ORIENT BLACKSWAN PRIVATE LIMITED

Registered Office
3-6-752 Himayatnagar, Hyderabad 500 029 (A.P.), India
E-mail: centraloffice@orientblackswan.com

Other Offices
Bangalore, Bhopal, Bhubaneshwar, Chennai,
Ernakulam, Guwahati, Hyderabad, Jaipur, Kolkata,
Lucknow, Mumbai, New Delhi, Noida, Patna

First Published 2012

ISBN 978 81 250 4660 8

Typeset in Minion Pro 10/13 by
Jojy Philip, New Delhi 110 015

Printed at
Glorious Printers
Delhi

Published by
Orient Blackswan Private Limited
1/24 Asaf Ali Road, New Delhi 110 002
E-mail: delhi@orientblackswan.com

Contents

Tables

Figures

Figures

Preface

Most 'scientific' accounts of communicable diseases epidemiology characterise the men (and very few women) of medicine and science as the single, dominant hero—as 'a positively good man', to borrow Fyodor Dostoevsky's expression. The germ, on the other hand, is the villain of the piece—to be cracked (in the laboratory) and controlled (in the conventional germ theory approach, through vaccines). Accounts with greater social sensitivity (coming largely from historians and anthropologists) have dealt with a wider range of epidemiological nuances that affect common women and men in myriad ways. The present study, by a former public health officer, is an insider–practitioner's view that places the common people's concerns and coping strategies at centre stage.

There is a dearth of social-epidemiological accounts of cholera with a focus on the urban poor. The literature on social determinants has dealt in the main with chronic, non-communicable diseases. Detailed analyses of the social determinants of a single disease (cholera) are not very common. The present work incorporates recent epidemiological methodological approaches, such as eco-social approaches and spatial epidemiology, and brings to the fore the transformation of cholera from an 'old-world' epidemic to an endemic entity (with a propensity for focal outbreaks) in contemporary megacities. The focus in this in-depth situational analysis of Delhi is on the vulnerability of the urban poor to waterborne infections, and on the unfinished agenda of water and sanitation.

This work draws, in part, upon my doctoral thesis for the Centre of Social Medicine and Community Health (CSMCH), Jawaharlal Nehru University, for which I express profound gratitude to Dr Imrana Qadeer and Dr Ritu Priya.

Major revisions were undertaken during my tenure at the Johns Hopkins School of Public Health as a Fulbright Nehru Senior Research Fellow. I gratefully acknowledge the support and encouragement of Professors Robert E. Black and Joanne Katz.

I am thankful to my colleagues and to staff at the Documentation Unit, CSMCH, for their support.

I acknowledge the help and support of all the officials and fieldworkers of the Municipal Corporation of Delhi (MCD) and the respondents who provided information on the ground situation and helped me develop an understanding of the field situation. The MCD was trifurcated into three municipal bodies in April 2012.

I am also indebted to the Delhi Jal Board, Infectious Diseases Hospital and the National Centre for Disease Control (formerly National Institute of Communicable Diseases). I thank the staff members of the several libraries that I accessed during the course of this study. Special mention may be made of the Welch Medical Library, the National Medical Library, and the libraries of the All India Institute of Medical Sciences, the National Institute of Health and Family Welfare, the Institute of Economic Growth and Jawaharlal Nehru University.

Words are inadequate to express my feelings towards my parents, who have been instrumental in providing encouragement for this piece of work, specially during the incubation period. I am deeply indebted to my parents-in-law for their words of cheer and support.

Finally, I acknowledge the endless help I got from Dr Purnamita Dasgupta, my wife. She has made major contributions to this work based on her knowledge and expertise as an environmental economist. She has enriched the thesis as an in-house statistician and critic. Equally important, it would have been impossible to complete this large volume of work without a caring, understanding and encouraging partner. Rajdeep deserves special mention for cheerfully supporting his father's academic pursuits through his own little sacrifices.

Abbreviations

ADB	Asian Development Bank
CDC	Centers for Disease Control
CFR	case fatality rate
CGWA	Central Ground Water Authority
CMDA	Calcutta Metropolitan Development Authority
CNG	compressed natural gas
CPCB	Central Pollution Control Board
CSDH	Commission on Social Determinants of Health
CSE	Conservancy and Sanitation Engineering (Department)
CT	cholera toxin
DCB	Delhi Cantonment Board
DDA	Delhi Development Authority
DIT	Delhi Improvement Trust
DJB	Delhi Jal Board
DMC	Delhi Municipal Committee
DUEIIP	Delhi Urban Environment and Infrastructure Improvement Project
DWSSDU	Delhi Water Supply and Sewage Disposal Undertaking
ESI	Employees' State Insurance
EWS	economically weaker sections

FAR	floor area ratio
GE	gastroenteritis
GSDP	gross state domestic product
HIG	high-income groups
HUDCO	Housing and Urban Development Corporation
ICDDR,B	International Centre for Diarrhoeal Diseases Research, Bangladesh
IDH	Infectious Diseases Hospital
IPP	India Population Project
ITRC	Industrial Toxicology Research Centre
JJR	Jhuggi-Jhonpri Relocation (scheme)
JNNURM	Jawaharlal Nehru National Urban Renewal Mission
LIG	low-income groups
lpcd	litres per capita day
MCD	Municipal Corporation of Delhi
mcm	million cubic metres
M&CW	Maternity & Child Welfare (Centre)
MDG	Millennium Development Goals
MGD	million gallons per day
MPD	Master Plan of Delhi
MPN	most probable number
NBO	National Buildings Organisation
NCR	National Capital Region
NCTD	National Capital Territory of Delhi
NDMC	New Delhi Municipal Committee
NEERI	National Environmental Engineering and Research Institute
NGO	Non-governmental Organisation

NICD	National Institute of Communicable Diseases
NICED	National Institute of Cholera and Enteric Diseases
NSS	National Sample Survey
NUHM	National Urban Health Mission
NUSP	National Urban Sanitation Policy
ORS	oral rehydration solution
ORT	oral rehydration therapy
PIL	public interest litigation
RMP	registered medical practitioner
RP	Regional Plan (Delhi)
RSBY	Rashtriya Swasth Bima Yojana
RWA	residents' welfare association
SLF	sanitary landfill
SPHC	selective primary health care
STP	sewage treatment plant
TB	tuberculosis
TCPO	Town and Country Planning Organisation
UBS	Urban Basic Services (Department)
VHAI	Voluntary Health Association of India
WDR	*World Development Report*
WHO	World Health Organization

1 Cholera

An Emerging Urban Health Issue

To a doctor, cholera is a disease caused by *Vibrio cholerae*. The 'causation of the disease, however, involves a lot more than just the bacteria. The bacteria thrive and spread in certain conditions. The urban milieu particularly for the urban poor and infrastructurally disadvantaged provides ambient conditions for the bacteria to thrive and be transmitted. Processes such as urbanisation, migration, planning and provisioning of infrastructure are thus at the core of the incidence of cholera. While some of these issues are understood at the macro (or city) level, others require dissection at the micro level—at the level of settlements and households. The recurring mantra of the urban health paradigm is: does location matter?

THE BRAVE NEW ERA OF SOCIAL DETERMINANTS

The social determinants of health, a wide and complex field of enquiry, encompass social class, caste, gender, ethnicity, education, infrastructure and access to public health services, to name a few. Life course epidemiology, along with the social determinants framework, highlights the idea that socio-economic position is a powerful predictor of health.[1] Such analyses pose methodological challenges, requiring datasets that often necessitate repeat measures of exposures and/or outcomes.[2] They offer an opportunity to examine and understand dynamic processes. While, in one sense, the social determinants approach is as old as public health itself, the brave new era ushered in by the World Health Organization (WHO) Commission on

Social Determinants of Health (CSDH) has provided the opportunity for this approach to emerge "from the underground". Social action needs to be based on a variety of types of evidence, including historical evidence. The emphasis is on identifying the "causes of the causes". That is what this book sets out to do for cholera in the context of a megacity (Delhi) where a large proportion of the population are "urban poor", and live and work in conditions of deprivation.

The "proximal–distal" discourse pervades the social determinants of health perspective.[3] Distal factors (largely) include state policy, priority and practice, while proximal physical, behavioural and biological exposures trigger specific pathogenic processes in a susceptible host. Susceptibility would be determined by a range of factors—macro, such as nutrition, and micro, such as genetic variants. Moving beyond this framework, it has been argued that societal distributions and determinants of disease need to take into account political economy and political ecology; thus, "power—both power over and power to do"—is crucial in exposure to health hazards. Since, in real-life situations, the different levels exist simultaneously (not sequentially), the proximal/distal framework may create disjunctive levels rather than connecting them. Examination of the problem of cholera as an urban health issue requires this sensitivity, and thereby an adequate breadth of canvas. The present account of cholera brings to the fore the transformation of cholera from an "old-world", highly fatal epidemic disease to a milder disease, an endemic entity (with a propensity for focal outbreaks) in contemporary megacities, clustered in locales where the urban poor reside. The social determinants of this acute, communicable disease operate at multiple levels, mired in local economics and politics.

REVIVAL OF SOCIAL EPIDEMIOLOGY

While in one sense epidemiology is almost as old as medicine itself, in another sense it is a very young discipline.[4] Hippocrates spoke of infectious disease in terms that are of relevance to today's epidemiologists. Put simply, the essential purpose of epidemiology has been to identify things in people and their surroundings that affect the occurrence of diseases, focusing on human populations and relying considerably on non-experimental situations and observations.[5] Wade Hampton Frost considered epidemiology as essentially an inductive science, concerned not merely with describing the distribution of disease but, equally importantly, fitting it into a consistent philosophy.[6] As a scientific discipline matures, he pointed out, "a desire develops among scientists in the field to express the phenomena they are studying in mathematical terms. If the deduction from the mathematical model corresponds to the observations, the underlying hypothesis is strengthened, resulting in a better understanding of the phenomenon."

Classically, epidemiologists developed hypotheses and tested them classifying individuals with health problems into groups that appeared to have common aetiological features. Epidemiologists are now concerned not so much with the acquisition of new knowledge about the origin of diseases, as with applying existing knowledge about the causes of diseases to understand patterns that diseases exhibit in a local area or community. The emphasis of the reasoning process was classically deductive rather than inductive. The latter (with the increasing application of qualitative approaches) attempts to utilise information from a set of observations to derive principles that have greater generality.[7]

Until the 1970s, epidemiologists were mostly physicians; their interests focused on the incidence patterns of diseases. There was no movement to pursue the development of a theory of epidemiological investigation. The physicians collaborated with statisticians, who provided expertise in making observations on large populations as well as in data analysis. The statistical approach in public health research began with the work of the French physician Louis in his paper on bloodletting, in which he demonstrated that there was little merit in that therapy. Though this was rejected by the French Academy of Medicine, the application of numerical methods to studying disease at the population level gained acceptance with the work of sanitary physicians such as Farr and Guy in England, who were both students of Louis. Farr established that understanding the population perspective was crucial for the analysis of disease aetiologies.[8] The influence of statistical thinking in epidemiology has increasingly been growing strong.[9] Statistical hypothesis testing as a mode of analysis has, however, been criticised as offering less insight into epidemiological data than alternative methods that emphasise the estimation of interpretable measures. The history of epidemiology is conventionally grouped into three main eras (see Table 1.1).

Table 1.1: Eras and Paradigms in Epidemiology[10]

	Era	Paradigm	Analytical approach	Preventive approach
I	Sanitary statistics	Miasmatic theory	Demonstration of clustering and patterns of morbidity and mortality	Drainage, sewage and sanitation
II	Infectious diseases epidemiology	Germ theory	Laboratory isolation of pathogenic organisms	Interruption of disease transmission through technological intervention on a mass scale, including drugs and vaccines
III	Chronic diseases epidemiology	Causality due to exposures other than infection	Determining risk ratio of exposure to outcome at individual level	Controlling risk factors by modifying lifestyle

The Hippocratic School of ancient Greece was the earliest proponent of the idea that environmental factors could influence the occurrence of diseases. British sanitarians like Chadwick and Smith reinforced the environmentalist approach, providing the impetus for solving public health problems through sanitary reforms. In the first half of the nineteenth century, two landmark studies were undertaken by Villerme in France and Snow in England. Villerme's epidemiological studies on the mortality patterns of different communities in Paris established for the first time that poverty was a major cause of disease and death. This work influenced further research in different countries (Alison in Scotland, Engels in England and Virchow in Germany) that emphasised the role of social and economic factors in disease aetiology.[11]

In 1849, John Snow (while investigating cholera in London) observed that cholera rates were particularly high in areas supplied with water by Lambeth Company compared to areas supplied by Vauxhall Company. This study marked the beginning of modern observational epidemiology. Snow's studies confirmed his earlier hypothesis that cholera was a communicable disease and that the mode of transmission was polluted drinking water. He applied statistical measures to count and compare the number of cholera deaths in different London districts with different water supplies. Thus, he established through epidemiological study that cholera was probably transmitted through contaminated water, much before the discovery of *Vibrio cholerae*.

The foundation of the London Epidemiological Society in 1850 indicates that the discipline was in existence by the mid-nineteenth century. It is interesting that the society was initially proposed to study anti-cholera activities—and was thus to be named the Epidemic Medical Society—and also to explore issues that today would be considered as health services research.[12] The term "epidemiologist" was apparently not used until the 1860s, and the profession as such emerged only in the early part of the twentieth century.

The decline of communicable diseases in the global North and the rise in the relative importance of non-communicable diseases led to the development of a new epidemiological paradigm in the mid-twentieth century. This involved the recognition of the role of multiple causes, and also led to the development and application of new techniques of study design and tools of analysis.[13] Risk factor epidemiology thus emerged as a strong discipline from the 1950s, entailing the use of statistical tools to identify factors having a damaging or protective effect on health, i.e., risk factors. High-risk behaviours are increasingly being held responsible for a number of diseases, including personal and household-level factors in the aetiology of diarrhoeal diseases. The notion of risk factor was not used by the earliest epidemiologists, who relied on simple but powerful associations between environment and disease. With the discovery of specific, causal microbiological agents of prevalent communicable diseases, there was optimism about overcoming the challenges. However, epidemiologists recognised that this oversimplified approach ignored complex realities. There were efforts to develop alternative approaches to epidemiology that re-emphasised the interplay of multiple factors in disease epidemiology.

Modern epidemiology models complex relationships among risks. The notion of the "web of causation" first emerged in 1960. This approach sought to move beyond germ theory, and advocated replacing single-agent germ theories of disease by more complex models of host, agent and environment. Social determinants of health were also included in the web. Epidemiological thought was influenced during this period by two more events—the discovery of the double helix structure of DNA in 1953, and the growing use of computers to store and analyse large datasets, especially using complex statistical techniques.

Risk factor epidemiology provided insights into disease processes, but was based on narrow definitions of individual risks with little emphasis on social and environmental factors. The discipline of epidemiology was often reduced to the role of identifying, measuring, ranking and predicting risk factors related to individual behaviours and practices. Though specific risk factors may appear to operate at the individual level, exposure and susceptibility may occur due to a wide range of political, economic and social factors.[14] Scholars grappling with multi-causality evolved the notion of the web of causation to reflect these complexities.

A web theory only expresses complexity, and does not expose causality. It was critiqued by epidemiologists who asked the question, "Has anyone seen the spider?"[15] The belief that population patterns of health and disease can be explained by a web of interconnected risk and preventive factors has become a central theme of epidemiology, and is embedded in statistical techniques of multivariate analysis. Its corollary is that epidemiology's role in improving public health rests upon its ability to identify and predict the results of breaking selected strands of this causal web.

Molecular biology and genetics are increasingly acquiring a major space due to their therapeutic, preventive and profit potentials. Just as the occurrence of diseases within a population can be studied at multiple levels—populations, individuals, organs, tissues, cells and molecules—causality can also be studied at these different levels—socio-economic factors, lifestyle, the organ burden of a carcinogen and DNA adducts. The date on which DNA sequencing of the human genome was announced—26 June 2000—is hailed as a landmark in the history of human knowledge. Smith and Ebrahim raise the question of whether, "viewed through DNA-tinted spectacles", epidemiology was to be considered merely as a discipline with a glorious past.[16] The challenge before epidemiology, wrote the authors, was to shift the focus from mere description to explanation (gene expression).

It is against this backdrop that the emergent era of epidemiology has been termed eco-epidemiology, on the track of ecologism.[17] Noting that exclusive focus on risk factors at the individual level within populations will not serve the purpose of holistic public health goals, Susser and Susser advocate the need to be concerned with causal pathways at the societal level, and with pathogenesis and causality at the molecular level. A fully adequate causal model of public health must therefore be able to explain the disease at the ecological level. In contrast with the universalism of the natural sciences, the ecologism of the biological sciences entails localisation and attention to the bounds that limit generalisations about biological, human and social systems. Ecological constructs try to address the true complexity of the biological world.

The theoretical conclusions drawn from certain empirical observations in the past can now be considered wrong; yet their empirical basis at the population level remains irrevocable. These observed relationships (classically in miasmatic theory) were behind the positive public health effects of strategies based on dealing with these relationships. Those who thought cholera was airborne miasma were as likely to demand appropriate sanitary reform as those who saw it as a contagious disease.[18] Snow recognised this, accepting that anti-contagionist theories of cholera causation were "in a hygienic sense as useful as . . . the real truth".[19] Thus, miasma, as opposed to simple contagionist theories of cholera, prompted interventions that reduced the severity of subsequent cholera outbreaks. John Snow was right for the right reason; this is what marks his relevance to epidemiological understanding and public health measures.

Pearce points out that any meaningful analysis of the causes of disease in populations should integrate the individual–biological and population levels of analysis without collapsing one into the other or denying the existence of either.[20] He argues that the top–down approach (that stems in part from the demographic tradition) starts at the population level in order to ascertain the main factors that influence health status within the population. It therefore implicitly uses a structural model of causation rather than a behavioural model or a biomedical model. Causation is to be seen as resulting from mechanisms that are internal to the population under study and that operate dialectically, rather than involving associations between externally related independent objects. Since the goal of epidemiological studies is to understand and prevent the causation of disease in populations, studies should start at the population level and address the major determinants of health or disease at this level by exploring the structure of population.

Populations are not collections of individuals that are conveniently grouped for the purposes of study. Every population has its own history, culture, organisation and economic and social divisions that influence how and why people are exposed to particular risks, and how they behave and react to these risks. It is therefore essential to understand the historical and social context and to emphasise the importance of diversity and local factors, rather than searching for universal relationships. Studying these phenomena will require researching factors including environment and group variables beyond individual-level variables. It is within this emerging frame of social epidemiology, one that is more contextual and holistic and also uses statistics wherever necessary, that the present book proposes to examine the disease profile of cholera in the fast urbanising city of Delhi.

THE TRAVAILS OF CONTEMPORARY URBANISATION

Classical cholera (caused by *Vibrio cholerae*, classical biotype) was primarily a rural disease. The emergence of the El Tor biotype (beginning in the 1960s) coincided with a period of accelerated urbanisation in many developing countries, and the infection entrenched itself largely among the urban poor.

The causative factors behind urbanisation have varied from time to time. Ramachandran observes that in the prehistoric period, urbanisation was synonymous with the origin and rise of civilisation itself, and was thus essentially a cultural process.[21] In the historical period, urbanisation was linked to the rise and fall of kingdoms, dynasties and empires—a political process. In recent times, urbanisation has been associated primarily with industrialisation and economic development, and is seen therefore as essentially an economic process.

The historical process of urbanisation in developing countries is different from that in advanced industrial societies.[22] The rapid growth of cities and urbanisation in developing countries has been explained by two major hypotheses: (a) unusually rapid rates of population growth vis-à-vis limited farm acreage, forcing landless labour into cities ("push factors"); and (*b*) various economic forces attracting migrants into the cities ("pull factors"). Pull factors include domestic terms of trade squeezing agriculture; the diffusion of technology from advanced economies favouring the setting up of large-scale urban industries; and foreign capital inflow into urban infrastructure, housing, power, transportation and large-scale manufacturing. Pull factors are applicable to both migrations within the country and illegal ones across borders.[23] These have resulted in a process of rapid industrialisation and the concomitant rise in demand for labour. The literature on new urban economics therefore views cities as market responses to opportunities for production and incomes.[24] Further, at the current time, the impact of information and communication technology on human settlement has manifested itself in what is called a "divided city", where new landscapes of innovation, economic development, cultural exchanges, political dynamics and social inequalities within cities and urban regions are emerging.[25]

Safa explains that differences in patterns of urbanisation are due primarily to the late entry of Third World countries in the global capitalist economy and their dependence on advanced economies for capital, technology and export markets.[26] This dependency started during the colonial period, and resulted in undermining traditional modes of production, precipitating major changes in the organisation and structure of production and distribution, and therefore in the labour force. Urbanisation has been viewed as a reflection of the overall socio-economic development of a society, and consequently its attainment has been regarded as a critical determinant in progress.[27]

Economists have viewed the problem of development in the Third World in terms of a division of the economy into dual sectors—a modern, expansive capitalist sector with large-scale production and orientation towards export, and a traditional, subsistence sector for the domestic market.[28] The failure to integrate these two sectors has been assumed to be a major deterrent in these countries' trajectory of growth and development. The dual sector approach has been criticised.[29] Rather than an impediment in the expansion of a modern capitalist economy, the informal sector has been considered to be the major means of survival of those not directly employed by the formal modern sectors. Most of the urban poor in Third World cities across the world work in small-scale enterprises requiring a low level of skill and capital investment, and often utilise the labour of unpaid family members to cut down on production costs. Because of its labour-absorptive capacities, the informal sector is capable of sustaining large numbers of urban poor at low standards of living and infrastructure. They inhabit squatter settlements built with their own labour and often do not get access to basic facilities, including water supply, sanitation, electricity, transport, education and health services. Squatter settlements are a survival strategy of the urban poor; at times the focal point of political unrest, they also constitute a "subsidy" by cutting down on the need for providing urban infrastructure and low-cost housing to the poor. Contrary to earlier notions of the discreteness of formal and informal economies, their interdependence is now increasingly recognised: the formal sector is dependent on the informal for cheap labour, goods and services, and the informal sector depends upon the formal for its clientele and as the source of new income-generating activities. Whereas earlier the informal sector was considered a residual one, it is now regarded as dynamic, continuously reconstituting itself to meet the challenges of the "modern" sector.[30]

During the 1980s and 1990s, poverty became increasingly concentrated in urban settlements for economic and demographic reasons.[31] Structural adjustment policies introduced in the Third World further accentuated this problem owing to rising food prices, declining real wages and redundancy in the formal labour market, and reduced public expenditure on basic services and infrastructure.[32] Globally, the urban poor are estimated to have grown at a faster rate than the numbers of rural people.[33] In 1980, there were twice as many poor rural households as poor urban ones; by 2000, more than half of the absolute poor were considered to be located in urban areas. It is also of concern that in many parts of the developing world, urban poverty has been growing faster than rural poverty due to macroeconomic adjustment, inefficiencies in the urban economy and misapplication of public resources. While examining the sustainability of the cities of developing countries, one trend has been to emphasise the basic problem of rapidly increasing numbers, both due to intrinsic growth and due to extrinsic migration, predominantly of the rural poor.

However, this is not the uniform pattern across all countries. The critical factors underlying urban change in Third World nations are changes in their economic and employment base. In nations with weaker economies, population movements are oriented towards destinations where employment (and, to a less extent, educational) opportunities are located.[34] Cities like Dhaka, Lagos, Lima, Manila, Rangoon and Sao Paulo accounted for significant proportions of industry and contributions to national gross domestic product (GDP),which in turn is linked to the rapid growth of population in these urban centres. The movement of people to these cities that attract large numbers of migrants is also because the uncertainties of survival here are less.

A high percentage of population that is urban always accompanies sustained economic growth.[35] India's economic growth has been modest but sustained; one would thus expect a similar pattern in its urbanisation. The urban population grew at an average annual compound rate of 2.26 per cent during 1901–81, 1.74 times the 1.30 per cent growth rate of the total population. The urban growth rate was zero or negligible until 1921. Then it accelerated rapidly during 1931–41 and 1941–51. There has been a greater correlation between real income growth and urbanisation in the later decades than was visible in the earlier decades for most of the twentieth century in India.[36] Nationally, the 1960s and 1970s represented the most rapid phase of urbanisation.[37] Given this pace of urban migration, it was inevitable that pressure on services and housing would increase. El Tor cholera appeared in India in 1964.

For people with low incomes, living on cheap land adjacent to employment opportunities is a rational choice, notwithstanding the risks. These vulnerable communities lose their homes, belongings, sources of income and previous social networks when they relocate.[38] In contrast to rural communities, the urban context is marked by loss of kinship-based networks, making coping with stress all the more difficult.[39] Risks include diseases associated with contaminated water and food, poor drainage and garbage collection, vectors, overcrowding and poor ventilation. The quality of environment has been deteriorating in many Third World countries About 30 to 45 per cent of the urban centres in India consist of slums and squatter colonies; 99 per cent of the housing shortage of 24.7 million at the end of the 10th Plan was among the economically weaker sections (EWS) and low-income groups (LIG) sectors.[40]

Hardoy and Satterthwaite point out that most of the new housing and new neighbourhoods in Third World cities are organised and built outside the legal framework.[41] In these cities, an estimated 30 to 60 per cent of the population, across countries, live in houses and colonies that are developed illegally; also, 70–95 per cent of all new housing colonies are built illegally. Residents of these colonies are naturally subject to exploitation by landowners, business interests and the police. Poor people make such constructions with great ingenuity in matters of design and construction materials that are suited to local needs, local climatic conditions and local resources. In sharp contrast, the official (legal) standards and specifications, generally derived from western models, often do not take care of such felt needs.

The colonial legacy in urban planning and architecture is conspicuous in Third World cities across continents. The colonial mindset and form of administration have influenced the contemporary city, its institutions, laws and regulations, and particularly the attitudes of those governing it towards the poor. The *cordon sanitaire* (quarantine line) segregated Europeans from epidemics and the diseases of poverty. In keeping with that mindset, most urban planning and state investment in water supply, sanitation, drainage and roads take place in high- and middle-income localities that, overall, house a minority of the population. Hospitals and health services also follow the pattern of serving the elite. The spatial distribution of medical institutions in a city follows predictable patterns in favour of privileged sections of the society. Medical research during the colonial period paid attention to diseases that affected the rulers and troops (like malaria and sleeping sickness), rather than those that ravaged the native population.[42]

Urban settlements develop in a way that groups capitalist enterprises in a cost-effective spatial configuration.[43] Environmental health problems faced by the urban poor often result from the spatial juxtaposition of industrial/livelihood and residential functions, marked by competition for land, high population densities and residential settlements in hazardous areas. Most people are attracted to cities by opportunities of work. The externalities of urban production are unfortunately borne disproportionately by the poor. Cheap housing areas and industries often tend to be located close to each other on lands not designated for these purposes. In the absence of strict regulations, this proximity can cause special environmental problems, the Bhopal gas tragedy being a case in point.

URBAN POVERTY AND ENVIRONMENTAL HEALTH CONCERNS

It is predicted that by 2025, 80 per cent of the global urban population will belong to the smaller and larger urban centres of developing countries. This needs to be viewed against the backdrop of the fact that, overall, 50 per cent of the world's population will be urban. It has been estimated that 35 per cent of India's population will reside in urban areas by 2020; the urban population will account for up to 50 to 75 per cent of the total population increase—creating unprecedented demands, but at the same time offering a "demographic gift".[44]

The *World Development Report (WDR)* in 1990 estimated that about a quarter of the world's urban population lived in absolute poverty—and many more lived in substandard conditions.[45] The poorer sections are hit the hardest as environment and infrastructural services deteriorate. As a consequence of their lack of access to basic services, the urban poor are the most vulnerable to natural and man-made environmental hazards, including health hazards. The *WDR* defined poverty as the inability to attain a minimum standard of living as measured by household incomes and expenditure.[46] Ownership or access to physical facilities is often used as a proxy for measuring poverty, particularly where data on income is weak. The WDR stressed that in order to ensure that growth is consistent with poverty reduction, access to these basic services is essential.[47]

An estimated 30–70 per cent of urban populations in developing countries are living in conditions of extreme poverty. The deteriorating environment has disproportionate health impacts on the urban poor. At the same time, there is an urgent need to recognise that the social dimensions of poverty have not translated adequately into approaches to environment and public health. Neighbourhood factors play significant roles in the case of child health compared to individual household characteristics like parental education, income and feeding practices. Thus, while a poor household struggles to get its own facilities, the benefits may elude the health of its children if the surrounding environment is poor, as is so often the case in underdeveloped countries.

Baker's report on "endemic colic" in Devonshire (lead poisoning), published in 1767, was one of the earliest published environmental epidemiology studies. Environment was considered exogenous to disease and health. Environment includes not only physical, chemical and biological agents but also social, political, cultural, engineering and architectural factors.[48] Exposure to environmental agents is frequently determined by social factors—where one lives, works, socialises or buys food. That the social, political and economic context is integral to most environmental epidemiological problems has not been fully appreciated. Environmental exposure is also largely involuntary. The environmental health problems of developing countries are wide-ranging and far-reaching. Poor collection and disposal of solid and liquid wastes, unsafe and inadequate drinking water, deforestation and indoor pollution due to unclean fuels are some of the critical problems that will be the challenges of the current millennium. In most low-income communities, the pollutant of primary concern is human excreta.

The WHO has classified diseases associated with water into the following groups:[49]

- Waterborne diseases: caused by the consumption of water contaminated by pathogenic viruses or bacteria from human or animal faeces or urine. Acute diarrhoeal diseases including cholera are important waterborne diseases in the developing country context.
- Water-washed diseases: caused by infection arising from lack of personal hygiene due to inadequacy of water
- Water-based and water-related diseases: caused by ingestion of intermediate hosts or insect vectors

Prevention of waterborne and water-based diseases requires improvements in the quality of water; the prevalence of water-washed diseases in a community indicates the need for improving the total quantity of water that an affected population can access. Maintaining adequate and safe water sources is of paramount importance for public health. The older agenda of providing sanitation services to all urban households remains an unfinished one. The new agenda, meanwhile, demands that urban wastewater be safely managed and that the quality of vital water resources be protected. The urban sanitation sector faces a dual environmental health challenge. The underprivileged urban poor are concentrated in settlements that are subject to insanitary conditions, hazardous emissions and accident risks, and therefore are in acute need of improvements in these services. It is often the case that these are the very segments that are conveniently overlooked during the development process. Provision of sanitation services, including sewerage, has failed to keep pace with population growth in urban areas. The health consequences of the service shortfalls are enormous and fall most heavily on the urban poor, though not necessarily sparing the privileged sections.

The WHO identifies poor sanitation, contaminated drinking water and lack of food hygiene as the key problem areas in the context of diarrhoeal diseases in developing countries. Diarrhoeal diseases are the second leading cause of death among under-5 children, with two billion cases annually and 1.5 million deaths.[50] Diarrhoeal death rates are typically about 60 per cent lower among children living in households with adequate water and sanitation facilities than among those in households without such facilities.

An increasing share of urban sanitation services is being provided by sewerage, especially in middle-income countries. User contributions, however, have been low, and public subsidies on these household services have benefited primarily the middle class and the rich. This has left few public resources to be spent on sewage treatment and safe disposal, raising concerns about the quality of the water environment. The costs of water resources degradation can be seen in many respects. The majority of rivers in the cities and towns of developing countries are little more than open, stinking sewers. Apart from degrading the aesthetic attributes of the city, they constitute a reservoir for a large number of waterborne diseases. The outbreak of cholera in Peru in 1991 was traced to inadequate urban sanitation and water contamination. The presence of typhoid in Santiago for over three decades has been attributed to the pollution of irrigation waters by untreated metropolitan discharges.

The term "Fourth World" has been used to describe an urban sub-proletariat marked by inadequate housing, sanitation, clothing and food; lack of support from politicians and unions; limited information, education and voice; and systematic exclusion from the exercising of rights that other people take for granted.[51] From the economic point of view, they are a "burden", and from the health point of view, a "danger". As policies and programmes seek to prevent malnutrition, supply safe water, provide shelter and environmental services, and provide health care and education, deprivation should be stated in terms of these factors as well as in terms of income.[52]

Though "health risks inside the home", i.e., behavioural factors and practices, are often highlighted as key determinants of diarrhoeal diseases, dangers in the neighbourhood in which poorer households are located are no less critical.[53] The deficiencies impact on each other. The most critical neighbourhood factors are:

- Dangerous sites: large clusters of illegal housing are often located on steep hillsides, floodplains or desert land. They may also be located on unhealthy and polluted land sites; around solid waste dumps, beside open drains and sewers or around industrial areas. Such sites are often the only locations where the poor can build or rent accommodation. Industrial areas provide employment. They are thus rational residential choices for the poor for reasons of survival.
- No collection of household garbage: about 30 to 50 per cent of solid waste generated in these urban areas remains uncollected and accumulates in the neighbourhood. This results in the proliferation of disease vectors and also constitutes a fire risk.
- Inadequate site infrastructure: particularly lack of transport and health services.

Many of the health problems of the urban poor in Third World cities are related to water. The main constraints related to access to an adequate quantity of safe water include:

- Quality: either frankly contaminated or of unreliable quality
- Available quantity
- Cost: the poor may pay up to 10 times the price of piped supply, and up to 15–20 per cent of their household income[54]
- The number of households served per public standpost (hydrant)
- About two-thirds of households have no access to proper disposal facilities for wastewater[55]

The expectation that improvements in water supply and excreta disposal facilities would play a major role in controlling diarrhoea in developing countries formed the motivating force for the International Water Supply and Sanitation Decade (1981–90). In this context, Esrey et al. reviewed the findings of 67 studies from 28 countries on the effectiveness of water supply and excreta disposal improvements in reducing diarrhoea rates in young children in developing countries.[56] The median reduction in diarrhoea morbidity rates was 22 per cent from all studies and 27 per cent from the better-designed ones. The study concluded that improvements in water quality had less of an impact than improvements in water availability or excreta disposal.

J. Briscoe, in a 1984 study, focused on assessing the impact of any single intervention, given the complexity of transmission routes of diarrhoeal diseases.[57] He cautioned that where multiple routes were involved in disease transmission, one had to be careful while assessing the impact of an intervention to eliminate any one of these transmission routes. Where dose–response relationships between the ingestion of a pathogen and the incidence of disease are non-linear, the reduction in incidence due to the elimination of a particular transmission route may be an incorrect indicator for measuring the importance of that particular route. Improvements in the bacteriological quality of drinking water have played a central role in most discussions on eliminating or reducing the incidence of diarrhoea. This view has been strengthened by the experience in Europe and North America in the nineteenth century, where improvements in drinking water quality played a central role in controlling diarrhoea and cholera. Improvements in drinking water quality are also relatively easier to monitor, and bacteriological examination is less expensive than, say, the monitoring of food quality or person-to-person contact.

Microbiological data collected on each of the possible transmission routes of cholera in Matlab, Bangladesh, established that most transmission was through drinking water. Because of the existence of secondary transmission routes such as contaminated water during bathing, and because the dose–response relationship was approximately log-linear, the elimination of the main route was not reflected in large reductions in the incidence of diarrhoea. However, Briscoe pointed out that it would be erroneous to conclude that improvements in drinking water are not an important intervention strategy for controlling cholera. Rather, it has to be understood that interventions to eliminate the secondary routes of transmission would have dramatic effects on the incidence of cholera if prior improvements in drinking water quality were achieved.

Esrey et al. review 144 studies to examine the impact of improved water supply and sanitation on the incidence of diarrhoea and other waterborne diseases, including schistosomiasis, dracunculiasis and hookworm infestation.[58] These diseases are widespread in developing countries and illustrate the variety of mechanisms through which water and sanitation can protect the health of the people. The review concludes that it is difficult to distinguish between health improvements due to improvements in water quality and those due to improvements in water quantity. While considering diarrhoeal diseases, therefore, the reduction in morbidity due to improvements in water supply clubs both the quality and the quantity aspects. Further, out of 15 studies that examined the effects of increased amounts of water specifically and independently of water quality, all but one reported a positive impact on reducing morbidity from diarrhoeal disease. The paper concludes that interventions that improve water quantity and excreta disposal along with better hygiene practices produce a greater impact than improvements in water quality. This is particularly true of highly contaminated environments with high diarrhoea rates.

Cairncross reviews the progress made during the International Water Supply and Sanitation Decade (1981–90).[59] He observes that problems regarding water supply systems are generally regarded as technical and economic, with little consideration of social or institutional aspects. Water supply in developing countries has hardly ever been addressed from the users' point of view. Investment in water is generally a function of three forces, in isolation or in combination—accelerating urbanisation, political pressure or international aid. Globally, by the late 1970s, the rate of water supply provision could hardly keep pace with population growth. Sanitation was even more neglected. Urban sanitation was usually understood to mean sewerage. Therefore, the majority of low-income families were actually excluded, as providing sanitation services was found to be neither "feasible" nor "affordable". Storm water drainage and solid waste disposal, which constitute basic environmental health interventions, were conspicuous by their neglect. In many new project areas, the issue was who would benefit from the improved water supply. Often, new and old water systems coexisted and communities did not prefer to use the new sources.

The issue of whether water supply and sanitation could be combined in a single programme has also been examined. In the context of low-income groups of households in developing economies, improved water supply means a tap in the street—an infrastructure in the public domain. Sanitation implies a toilet with an on-site disposal system—a part of the owner's house or his land, at his expense, and not infrequently with his own hands. Administrators considered both water supply and sanitation as an issue of laying pipelines beneath the street. However, an agency that could implement one of these efficiently was unlikely to be suited to the other. Hygiene education, a critical component, could neither be delivered by these agencies nor was envisaged in these programmes.[60]

There are examples of self-help initiatives in the construction of water supply systems in many African nations. It has also been suggested by several international agencies that governments tend to avoid being providers of these services. However, by and large, governments do provide for the well-off and privileged sections of society. If local communities invest in local infrastructure, it would also imply local control; often, politicians, technocrats and experts with their own models of urban development are reluctant to accept such shifts of patronage.

INDIA URBANISES, AND FAST

The colonial period in India witnessed urban stagnation everywhere, except in administrative centres including cantonments and railway towns. The post-independence period (since 1947) has been notable for its rapid urbanisation. The major changes that have occurred include:

- Influx of refugees and their settlement/rehabilitation, primarily in urban areas in northern India, and to a lesser extent in the east
- Construction of new industrial cities and industrial townships near existing cities
- Stagnation and, in some cases, the decline of small towns
- Massive increase in squatters and the proliferation of slums in major cities

- Emergence of a rural–urban fringe
- Introduction of city planning and general improvement in city amenities

In India (and China), a large proportion of the urban population resides in cities with populations of 500,000 and above.[61] In 2001, 68.7 per cent of the total urban population was living in Class I cities (defined as cities having a population of over 100,000). The shares of medium and small towns in the total population stood at 21.9 per cent and 9.4 per cent, respectively.

Rural–urban migration even in metropolitan cities (except Mumbai) has contributed less than 35 per cent of the total population growth.[62] Migrants in search of urban employment do not account for a significant percentage of urban labour force growth. Gugler points out that, for developing countries, rural–urban differentials in natural growth rates are not significantly different, in contrast to those of developed countries.[63] Mitra and Murayama, however, argue that for India, though urban birth and death rates are lower than the rural figures, urban rates of natural increase are only marginally lower than rural rates.[64] It is hypothesised that the increasing participation of women in the labour market is another factor contributing to labour force growth.[65]

Apart from the forces of rural–urban migration and natural growth of population, the reclassification of areas as "urban" over time is a significant factor in the increase of urban population. Rural areas adjacent to cities or towns are more rapidly reclassified as "urban" than relatively remote rural areas that are also growing rapidly. The "development pole" theory explains how economic activities get concentrated in a limited number of cities to maximise the advantages of interdependence of industries in terms of input–output linkages, availability of infrastructure and marketing.[66] Therefore, groups of industries cluster around a "core", and growth impulses are transmitted through both forward and backward linkages. As the income levels of these areas are high, they create higher demands for other products and services leading to further overall growth of these centres. Adjoining semi-urban and/or rural areas also get involved in this process, giving rise to further urban agglomerations.

Rural-to-urban migration rates are generally higher than the urban-to-urban rates. The exceptional cases are Delhi (for females), Madras (now Chennai), Bangalore (now Bengaluru) and Jaipur. Sundaram observes that, with the exception of Bombay (now Mumbai), inter-state and intra-state migrants from rural areas account for less than a third of the total decadal increase in the population of these cities.[67] Economic factors emerge as the most important cause of rural male migration in about 50 per cent of cases.[68] Among females, economic factors account for less than 10 per cent of migration. The distinction between economic and non-economic factors is not very clear. Persons who have migrated for non-employment reasons (like education or marriage) may also subsequently enter the urban labour market.

Against the backdrop of increasing rural-to-urban migration, the supply of labour in the urban segment grows further. With employment opportunities in the high-productivity sector being limited, most migrant groups get residually absorbed into low-productivity activities. Two key factors that play a role in this process are the poor asset base and the lack of specific skills among population groups migrating in search of employment. As a result, a large proportion of these activities are in the tertiary sector; rural-to-urban labour migration raises the share of the services (tertiary) sector in the total workforce.

Short-duration migrants have been defined as those whose duration of residence at the destination is less than one year. Their unemployment rates are relatively higher; the rates decline sharply with an increase in the duration of residence, more so among male migrants. Among long-duration migrants (duration of residence equal to or more than five years) unemployment rates are lower than those of the city population (for both sexes). Mitra cautions against the notion that the large share of tertiary activities in the total workforce is a measure of the excess supply of labour in urban centres.[69] Though there is a positive association between the rural-to-urban migration rate and the share of tertiary activities, it is to be noted that the skill levels required may be lacking in the migrants. The natural growth of urban population, and not just rural migrants, contributes to a large extent in sustaining the growth of the tertiary sectors.

Among the largest Indian cities, the population of Delhi grew fastest during 1961–81; Calcutta (now Kolkata), the largest of the four metros, grew the slowest. Some commentators divide India into five regions—

north, east, south, west and central, dominated by Delhi, Kolkata, Chennai, Mumbai and Kanpur, respectively.[70] From 1931–61, the eastern region dominated by Kolkata was the most primate of the five regions. The western region has remained the second most primate region. Delhi's domination of the northern region has increased over the decades. The central region has remained the least primate of all the regions.

In India, among the 12 million-plus cities, Lucknow, Kolkata and Kanpur were experiencing net out-migration in 1981, while Bengaluru and Delhi were growing rapidly. Most of the rapidly growing cities in the 1970s had populations of less than 500,000 in 1971, and were typically single-industry cities, centres of raw material extraction, or state capitals. Many of them were located away from densely populated areas. Cities close to Mumbai (Nasik and Khopoli) and Kolkata (Asansol and Durgapur) grew more rapidly than these metropolitan cities. These single-industry cities and centres of raw material extraction were also essentially dominated by public sector enterprises. By the turn of the century, some of them had begun to decline with the industries going sick, resulting in out-migration.

The proportion of the urban population living in slum areas grew during 1981–91, while the share of the population living in poverty declined. Thus, it must be realised that the lack of access to basic services is really a welfare issue. Concern for poverty has always been at the centre of Indian socio-economic thinking. The Perspective Plan of 1961–75 had the removal of poverty as a major objective. All subsequent planning in the Indian economy has focused on poverty removal as a key objective of the development process.

In absolute terms, the number of urban agglomerations increased from 1,827 in 1901 to 5,161 in 2001. During this period, the urban population grew by 14 times, while the national population grew by 4.5 times. Nevertheless, India is urbanising at a slower rate compared to most other developing countries. For a large proportion of the urban population, access to housing, safe water and sanitation is grossly inadequate. For example, as noted earlier, the National Housing Policy 2007 records that, of the housing shortage of 24.7 million at the end of the 10th Plan, 99 per cent pertained to the EWS and LIG sectors.[71]

SLUMS: WHY AND HOW

The rapid growth of urban poor in cities is almost synonymous with the growth of slums. The definition of a "slum" varies widely. Ordinarily, a slum refers to mudstructures, overcrowded or dilapidated dwelling units. The Slum Areas (Improvement and Clearance) Act came into force in Delhi in 1956, and was later extended to 11 other states. Under this act, the slum is defined as areas with buildings

- that are in any respect unfit for human habitation
- that, by reason of dilapidation, overcrowding, faulty arrangements and design of such buildings, narrowness or faulty arrangement of streets, lack of ventilation, light or sanitation facilities
- or any combination of these factors, are detrimental to safety, health or morale.

The Bharat Sevak Samaj used the following definition of "slum" in Delhi:

> The term "slum" should be applied to those parts of the city which may (on the face of it) be considered unfit for human habitation either because the structures therein are old, dilapidated, grossly congested and out of repairs, or because it is impossible to preserve sanitation for want of sanitary facilities including ventilation, drainage, water supply, etc., or because the sites themselves are unhealthy.[72]

Katras (slum tenements) refer to a group of single-room tenements that are constructed generally in rows within a compound or enclosure having a single common entrance. *Bastis*, on the other hand, are clusters of *kutcha* [temporary] dwellings built on open land, often unauthorised. More recently, slums have been defined as "a compact settlement of at least 20 households with a collection of poorly built tenements, mostly of temporary nature, crowded together usually with inadequate sanitary and drinking water facilities in unhygienic conditions."[73] The 1961 census also adopted a similar definition, including "such dwellings which on account of such over-crowding, dilapidation and lack of ventilation are detrimental to safety, health and social morale". The Madras Corporation used this definition as well. The Calcutta Municipal Council Act of 1980 defined slums as "an area of land not less than 700 square metres occupied by, or for the purposes of, any collection of huts or other structures used or intended to be used for human habitation".[74] Taxes are collected from these registered slums. The Bombay Municipal Corporation uses a three-tier definition of slums:

- *Chawls:* areas with permanent, multi-storeyed buildings built long ago according to the then prevailing standards, but currently in a deteriorated condition
- *Patrachawls:* areas with semi-permanent structures—both authorised and unauthorised, often built of tin (*patra*) sheets
- *Zopadpattis:* squatter settlements, shanty towns or hutment colonies[75]

The Environmental Improvement Programme of Urban Slums began in 1972, and the slum was defined by it in greater detail.[76] Slums were defined as any area where such dwellings predominate, which, by reason of dilapidation, overcrowding, faulty arrangement of the design of buildings, narrowness or faulty arrangement of streets, lack of ventilation, light or sanitation facilities, inadequacy of open spaces and community facilities, or any combination of these factors, are detrimental to safety, health or morale. While this part of the definition was a continuation of the previous versions, certain criteria were added in order that a slum might be selected for improvement. The most important of these was that at least two-thirds of the families in a slum should earn incomes of less than Rs 250 per month.

Most of these definitions are not adequate for application and leave a lot of room for variation. Further, none of these definitions seeks to define the basic minimum criteria for the dwelling units of the poor in an urban setting. The loose nature of the definitions is an impediment to the estimation of slum populations and, therefore, to the subsequent formulation of plans for their improvement.

The highest incidence of slums in India is found in Mumbai, Kolkata, Delhi, Chennai, Kanpur, Nagpur and Lucknow, ranging from 30 to 40 percent of the city populations. In the cases of Jaipur and Lucknow, there are variations in the estimates by the National Buildings Organisation (NBO) and the Town and Country Planning Organisation (TCPO):the NBO figures refer to the urban agglomeration, while the TCPO estimate refers to the metropolitan corporation only. The National Sample Survey (NSS) estimates are rather low, as the "undeclared slums" are not included. The 1981 census data also suffers from two major deficiencies on account of which the figures are really underestimates. The first is that the information on slum population is provided by the municipal authorities and not through any surveys. Second, information on slum population is not available for each and every slum pocket.

It is important to understand why and how slums grow and the numbers of population groups inhabiting these settlements expand. Three possible situations have been considered:[77]

- Economic opportunities and infrastructure facilities lead to the concentration of population in urban centres. This pushes up land value and rents. A large proportion of the population therefore cannot afford to live in dwelling units of reasonable standard. Economies of agglomeration and the absence of planning lead to the creation of megapolises with low quality of life. The older dwelling units get overcrowded and basic amenities become inadequate to cater to increased demands, giving rise to "*pucca* slums"; these dwelling units were not slums at the time of their construction. In such situations, it is not just the poor, informal sector workers, but also formal sector workers with incomes much above the poverty line who reside in these settlements.
- Individuals may also avail of poor-quality housing so as to use their limited savings for consumption of other consumer durables.
- The residual absorption of labour in low-productivity informal activities generates low income in relation to the high cost of living in cities. This does not really allow such workers to have an above-poverty-line level of living. Earnings insufficient to meet urgent consumption requirements like food and clothing leave little scope for investment in better-quality housing. The existing dwelling units and basic amenities also get overused, leading to congestion and the rapid expansion of slums.

Industrialisation and commercialisation lead to increasing inequality in the urban sector during the initial stages of industrialisation. The level of inequality declines only at a later stage, when the share of wages in total income increases substantially.[78] This inequality in the initial phases also leads to unequal access to land and housing in the cities. While poor households may be expected to live in slums, all slum dwellers may not necessarily be poor.

A 10-year prospective study (1994–2004) in a large slum area of Delhi noted a huge burden of communicable diseases as well as an increasing load of non-communicable diseases, the classic double burden of developing countries.[79] An editorial on urban health problems in slums published in the *National Medical Journal of India* made the following assertions:

> Understanding public health needs in urban areas requires a different conceptual framework. Traditionally, it is understood that alleviation of poverty is the most important precursor of improving general health. But in urban areas, the marginal increase in income for the poor, in itself, does not assure better living conditions due to wide disparities, which make decent accommodation, and clean water and air unaffordable. Moreover, certain necessities, which existed as free goods in rural settings, are commodities in urban areas such as drinking water, cooking fuel, housing space, etc. The poor are typically driven to the margins of the urban space, where living conditions are the most degraded and of little economic value.
>
> The relative difference in income and wealth is much starker in urban areas. The higher purchasing power of the rich leads to the escalation of the prices of food and healthcare goods, making them unaffordable to the poor. The rich also consume more than their fair share of public goods, for example, water, infrastructure, electricity, which are often subsidized by the state. Urban policies and laws look upon migration (particularly of the poor) as the root of the problem. They respond by imposing penalties on the poor in different ways, such as by denying them the right to housing, refusing them a ration card or neglecting to create adequate infrastructure for their use. As a result, slums become the focal points of punitive action, which aggravates the deprivation caused by economic uncertainty faced by those dependent on casual wage labour.[80]

CONCLUSION

The present inquiry has three main objectives. First, it traces the transformation of cholera from an "old-world" epidemic into an endemic entity (with a propensity for focal outbreaks) in contemporary megacities. Second, it focuses on the vulnerability of the urban poor to waterborne infections, and draws attention to the unfinished agenda of water and sanitation. Third, it takes a social determinants approach to understanding an acute communicable disease at multiple levels—an approach that has hither to been applied by western scholars largely to understanding and explaining non-communicable diseases.

The subsequent chapters of the book deal with the following themes. Chapter II provides a detailed description of the process of planning for public health in Delhi.It focuses on the rapid post-independence expansion and growth of Delhi and the social inequities that have emerged in two key determinants—access to water and sanitation services. In Chapter 3, the successive pandemics of cholera are traced in the context of northern India, including Punjab and Delhi, where cholera spread initially largely on account of its importation through trade routes. The trajectory of cholera in the region is traced to the current (seventh) pandemic. A detailed analysis of time trends is offered, along with a discussion of the threat of a potential eighth pandemic owing to a new strain (O139) being introduced in 1993–94.

Chapter 4 deconstructs the 1988 cholera epidemic and examines its significance as one of the politically most sensitive public health events in contemporary times. Going beyond academic literature and NGO reports, it analyses official documents and collates a large range of information, synthesising these materials into a coherent story. Chapter 5 undertakes an analysis of the spatial distribution of cholera cases within Delhi, making a case for "area effects" as an epidemiological approach.

Finally, Chapter 6 is an in-depth study of 300 households (100 each from three infrastructurally disadvantaged settlements) where primary data was collected to examine the role of behavioural factors. Based on statistical arguments, this chapter argues that behavioural factors lose their significance when pitted against much stronger infrastructural determinants, access to which is a function largely of planned provision; these in turn are determined to a major extent by the legal status of the settlements.

NOTES

1. Anne-Marie Nybo Anderson, "Life-Course and Social Epidemiology, the Biological Fig Leaf and Bob Dylan", *International Journal of Epidemiology* 36, no. 3, 2007, 540–41.

2. Bianca L. De Stavola et al., "Statistical Issues in Life Course Epidemiology", *American Journal of Epidemiology* 163, no. 1, 2006, 84–96; Y. Ben-Shlomo, "Rising to the Challenges and Opportunities of Life Course Epidemiology", *International Journal of Epidemiology* 36, no. 3, 2007, 481–83.
3. Nancy Krieger, "Proximal, Distal and the Politics of Causation: What's Level Got to Do with It?" *American Journal of Public Health 98*, no. 2, 2008, 221–30.
4. G. Pappas, I. J. Kiriaze and M. E. Falagas, "Insights into Infectious Disease in the Era of Hippocrates", *International Journal of Infectious Diseases* 12, no. 4, 2008, 347–50.
5. Raymond S. Greenberg et al., *Medical Epidemiology*, 3rd ed. (New York: McGraw Hill, 2001), 3.
6. Wade Hampton Frost, "Epidemiology", in *Papers of Wade Hampton Frost*, ed. M. D. K. E. Maxcy (New York: The Commonwealth Fund, 1941), 493–542.
7. Leon Gordis, *Epidemiology* (Philadelphia: Saunders, 2009), 4.
8. David E. Lilienfeld and Paul D. Stolley, *Foundations of Epidemiology*, 3rd ed. (New York: Oxford University Press, 1994), 27.
9. Philip H. Kass and Ellen B. Gold, "Modern Epidemiologic Study Designs", in *Handbook of Epidemiology*, ed. W. Ahrens and I. Pigeot (Berlin: Springer, 2005), 322–23.
10. M. Susser and E. Susser, "Choosing a Future for Epidemiology—Parts I and II", *American Journal of Public Health* 86, no. 5, 1996, 668–77.
11. J. C. Smith, "The Basic Sciences of Public Health: The Theory and Practice of Modern Epidemiology and the Population Perspective on Health and Diseases", Centre of Social Medicine and Community Health, School of Social Sciences, Jawaharlal Nehru University, New Delhi, 1996.
12. George Davey Smith and Shah Ebrahim, "Epidemiology—Is It Time to Call It a Day?" *International Journal of Epidemiology* 30, no. 1, 2001, 1–11.
13. N. Pearce, "Traditional Epidemiology, Modern Epidemiology, and Public Health", *American Journal of Public Health* 86, no. 5, 1996, 678–83.
14. Pearce, "Traditional Epidemiology".
15. Nancy Krieger, "Epidemiology and the Web of Causation: Has Anyone Seen the Spider?" *Social Science & Medicine* 39, no. 7, 1994, 887–903.
16. Smith and Ebrahim, "Epidemiology—Is It Time to Call It a Day?"
17. Susser and Susser, "Choosing a Future for Epidemiology".
18. Smith and Ebrahim, "Epidemiology—Is It Time to Call It a Day?"
19. John Snow, "On the Pathology and Mode of Communication of Cholera", *London Medical Gazette* 44, 1849, 745–52 and 923–29.
20. Pearce, "Traditional Epidemiology".

21. R. Ramachandran, *Urbanisation and Urban Systems in India* (Delhi: Oxford University Press, 2001), xv–xvi.
22. Helen I. Safa, *Towards a Political Economy of Urbanisation in Third World Countries* (Delhi: Oxford University Press, 1982), 42.
23. Pranati Dutta, "Push-Pull Factors of Undocumented Migration from Bangladesh to West Bengal: A Perception Study", *Qualitative Report* 9, no. 2, 2004, 335–58.
24. Dutta, "Push-Pull Factors".
25. United Nations Centre for Human Settlements (UN-HABITAT), *Cities in a Globalizing World. Global Report on Human Settlements 2001* (London: Earthscan, 2001).
26. Safa, *Towards a Political Economy of Urbanisation.*
27. Amie Peck and Adam Tickell, "Neoliberalizing Space", *Antipode* 34, no. 3, 2002, 380–404.
28. David Bell, "The Hospitable City: Social Relations in Commercial Spaces", *Progress in Human Geography* 31, no. 1, 2007, 7–22.
29. K. Hart, "Informal Income Opportunities and Urban Employment in Ghana", *Journal of Modern African Studies* 11, no. 1, 1973, 61–89; Lakshman Yapa, "What Causes Poverty? A Postmodern View", *Annals of the Association of American Geographers* 86, no. 4, 1996, 707–28; R. Souza and V. Tokman, "The Informal Urban Sector in Latin America", *International Labour Review* 114 no. 3, 1976, 355–66.
30. Hart, "Informal Income Opportunities"; Yapa, "What Causes Poverty?"; Souza and Tokman, "The Informal Urban Sector in Latin America".
31. Ellen Wratten, "Conceptualising Urban Poverty", *Environment and Urbanization* 7, no. 1, 1995, 11–36.
32. O. Caroline et al., "Urban Poverty in the Context of Structural Adjustment: Recent Evidence and Policy Responses", TWU Discussion Paper No. 4, Urban Development Division, World Bank, Washington, D.C., 1993.
33. World Bank, "Urban Policy and Economic Development: An Agenda for the 1990s", World Bank Policy Paper, World Bank, Washington, D.C., 1991.
34. Matthew Gandy, "Rethinking Urban Metabolism: Water, Space and the Modern City", *City* 8, no. 3, 2004, 363–79.
35. Pranati Dutta, "Urbanisation in India", Paper presented at the European Population Conference, Liverpool, 21–24 June 2006. http://www.scribd.com/doc/27348441/Urbanization-in-India (accessed 21 August 2009).
36. Dutta, "Urbanisation in India".
37. Shekhar Mukherji, "Linkage between Migration, Urbanisation and Regional

Disparities in India: Required Planning Strategies", IIPS Research Monograph, International Institute for Population Sciences, Mumbai, 2001.

38. Paul R. Amato and Jiping Zuo, "Rural Poverty, Urban Poverty, and Psychological Well-Being", *Sociological Quarterly* 33, no. 2, 1992, 229–40.
39. Walter W. Powell and Laurel Smith-Doerr, "Networks and Economic Life", in *The Handbook of Economic Sociology*, ed. Neil J. Smelser and Richard Swedberg (Princeton: Princeton University Press, 1994), 368–402.
40. Ministry of Urban Development, *Report of the National Commission on Urbanisation* (New Delhi: Government of India, 1988); Ministry of Housing and Urban Poverty Alleviation, *National Urban Housing and Habitat Policy* (New Delhi: Government of India, 2007).
41. Jorge E. Hardoy and David Satterthwaite, "Shelter, Infrastructure and Services in Third World Cities", *Habitat International* 10, no. 3, 1986, 245–84.
42. Melvin E. Page and Penny M. Sonnenburg, *Colonialism: An International, Social, Cultural and Political Encyclopaedia* (Santa Barbara: ABC-CLIO, 2003), 380.
43. Wratten, "Conceptualising Urban Poverty".
44. Planning Commission, *Report of the Committee on India Vision 2020* (New Delhi: Government of India, 2002). A "demographic gift" signifies the initially favourable effect of falling fertility rates on the age dependency ratio.
45. World Bank, *World Development Report 1990* (New York: Oxford University Press, 1990).
46. World Bank, *World Development Report 1990* .
47. Ibid.
48. Kenneth J. Rothman and Sander Greenland, *Modern Epidemiology*, 2nd ed. (Hagerstown: Lippincott-Raven Publishers, 1988).
49. World Health Organization (WHO), *Our Planet, Our Health: Report of the WHO Commission on Health and Environment* (Geneva: WHO, 1992).
50. WHO, "Diarrhoeal Disease Factsheet N330", 2009, http://www.who.int/mediacentre/factsheets/fs330/en/index.html (accessed 4 April 2010).
51. I. Tabibzadeh, A. Rossi-Espagnet and R. Maxwell, "Spotlight on the Cities: Improving Urban Health in Developing Countries", World Health Organization, Geneva, 1989.
52. D. A. Cohen et al., "Neighborhood Conditions and Health", *American Journal of Public Health* 93, no. 3, 2003, 467–71.
53. A. F. Trevett, R. C. Carter and S. F. Tyrrel, "The Importance of Domestic Water Quality Management in the Context of Faecal-Oral Disease Transmission", *Journal of Water and Health* 3, no. 3, 2005, 259–70.
54. United Nations Educational, Scientific and Cultural Organization (UNESCO), "2003: International Year of Freshwater". http://www.wateryear2003.org/en/

ev.php-URL_ID=5970&URL_DO=DO_TOPIC&URL_SECTION=201.html (accessed 7 October 2006).

55. G. D. Rose, "Community-Based Technologies for Domestic Wastewater Treatment and Reuse: Options for Urban Agriculture", CFP Report Series, Report 27, NC Division of Pollution Prevention and Environmental Assistance, North Carolina, 1999.
56. S. A. Esrey, R. G. Feachem and J. M. Hughes, "Interventions for the Control of Diarrhoeal Diseases among Young Children: Improving Water Supplies and Excretion Disposal Facilities", *Bulletin of the WHO* 63, no. 4, 1985, 757–72.
57. J. Briscoe, "Technology and Child Survival: The Example of Sanitary Engineering", *Population and Development Review* 10, Suppl., 1984, 237–53.
58. Esrey et al., "Interventions for the Control of Diarrhoeal Diseases".
59. Sandy Cairncross, "Water Supply and Sanitation: An Agenda for Research", *Journal of Tropical Medicine and Hygiene* 92, no. 5, 1989, 301–14.
60. Cairncross, "Water Supply and Sanitation".
61. United Nations, *World Urbanization Prospects: The 2009 Revision* (New York: United Nations Department of Economic and Social Affairs, 2010).
62. Arup Mitra and Mayumi Murayama, "Rural to Urban Migration: A District Level Analysis for India", 2008, http://ideas.repec.org/p/jet/dpaper/dpaper137.html (accessed 11 June 2010).
63. Josef Gugler, "Over-Urbanisation Reconsidered", *Economic Development and Cultural Change* 31, no. 1, 1982, 173–89.
64. Mitra and Murayama, "Rural to Urban Migration".
65. Arup Mitra, "Women in the Informal Sector: Perpetuation of Meagre Earnings", *Development and Change* 36, no. 2, 2005, 291–316.
66. Niles M. Hansen, "Development Pole Theory in a Regional Context", *International Review for Social Sciences* 20, no. 4, 2007, 709–27.
67. K. Sundaram, "Agriculture-Industry Interrelations: Issues of Migration", in *The Balance between Industry and Agriculture in Economic Development,* Proceedings of the Eighth World Congress of the International Economic Association, Delhi, India, vol. 3: *Manpower and Transfers*, ed. S. Chakravarty (London: Macmillan, 1989), 177–206.
68. Mitra, "Women in the Informal Sector".
69. Brent Edelman and Arup Mitra, "Slum Dwellers' Access to Basic Amenities: The Role of Political Contacts, Its Determinants and Adverse Effects", *Review of Urban and Regional Development Studies* 18, no. 1, 2006, 25–40.
70. Arjun Adlakha, "Population Trends: India", 1997, http://www.census.gov/ipc/prod/ib-9701.pdf (accessed 23 February 2002).

71. Ministry of Housing and Urban Poverty Alleviation, *National Urban Housing and Habitat Policy*, 3.
72. Bharat Sevak Samaj, "Slums of Old Delhi", 1958, http://openlibrary.org/works/OL11148815W/Slums_of_Old_Delhi (accessed 12 May 2001).
73. Ministry of Housing and Urban Poverty Alleviation, "Report of the Committee on Slum Statistics/Census", National Buildings Organisation, Government of India, New Delhi, 2007, 7.
74. Nitai Kundu, "The Case of Kolkata, India", 2003, http://www.ucl.ac.uk/dpu-projects/Global_Report/pdfs/Kolkata.pdf (accessed 12 August 2004).
75. Neelima Risbud, "The Case of Mumbai, India", http://www.ucl.ac.uk/dpu-projects/Global_Report/pdfs/Mumbai.pdf (accessed March 2012).
76. Neelima Risbud, "Typology of Slums and Land Tenure in Indian Cities", National Workshop on Land Tenure Issues in Slum Free Planning, http://www.ucl.ac.uk/dpu-projects/Global_Report/pdfs/Mumbai.pdf (accessed 4 March 2012).
77. Edelman and Mitra, "Slum Dwellers' Access to Basic Amenities".
78. Simon Kuznets, "Modern Economic Growth: Findings and Reflections", *American Economic Review* 63, no. 3, 1973, 247–58.
79. Renuka Saha et al., "Changing Profile of Disease Contributing to Mortality in a Resettlement Colony of Delhi", *National Medical Journal of India* 20, no. 3, 2007, 125–27.
80. Neha Madhiwalla, "Healthcare in Urban Slums in India", *National Medical Journal of India* 20, no. 3, 2007, 113–14.

2

Urban Basic Services in Delhi

Evolution and Crises

Compared to other Indian million-plus metropolises, Delhi has experienced the highest demographic growth over the last few decades. In the 1951 census, Delhi recorded a decadal growth rate of 90 per cent owing to the Partition (in 1947).[1] The decadal growth rate declined to 52.44 per cent in 1961, and thereafter declined steadily to 46.31 per cent in the 2001 census, when the provisional population was 13,782,976. Despite a slowdown in the growth rate, such demographic expansion has obvious implications for town planning, as demands for urban services have been escalating. Delhi was the first Indian city where new ideas of town planning were launched after independence, and where the first master plan was implemented in 1962. The city has grown from a small entity named Shahjahanabad to what is today the National Capital Territory of Delhi (NCTD).

An outline of this history provides a framework essential for understanding the trajectory along which the provision of basic services has evolved over the years, in the specific context of waterborne diseases and the access of vulnerable populations to urban services.Most migrant labour increasingly belongs to the informal sector, and constitutes the urban poor. The health status and health indicators of these communities, which reflect the consequences of living in unhealthy conditions, are increasingly recognised as a matter of concern. The law tends to discriminate between better-off and poorer urban communities based on the legality of their places of residence, which has a critical bearing on access or deprivation with regard to basic infrastructure. Vulnerability in urban spaces is thus a function of institutional discrimination—a central idea pursued through the course of this book.

URBAN PLANNING IN DELHI: A BRIEF HISTORY

Delhi has been a capital through many centuries and under different emperors. The Rajputs had their capital in Delhi in the eleventh and twelfth centuries. From the thirteenth century, various Sultans ruled Delhi and developed their capitals at locations in the vicinity of the Qutub Minar. The capital shifted twice to Agra; once during the last Sultanate dynasty, and then again in the time of Akbar.

Delhi regained its importance as the capital when Shahjahanabad was built up as a walled city around the Red Fort by Shahjahan. The foundation of Shahjahanabad was laid in 1638. The new capital (which was shifted to Delhi from Agra owing to "excessive heat . . . unfit for the residence of a monarch"[2]) was named after the emperor himself, Shah-Jahan-abad. While the royal family and those connected with the court had their residence inside the fort, the general population lived outside, on the fringes of the town.[3] The British took over the city from the Marathas in 1803, starting a new chapter in the planned development of infrastructure for the inhabitants of Delhi. Civic services were started with the setting up of water supply, public toilets, sanitation services and dispensaries.

BEGINNINGS OF THE MODERN SERVICES

Following the Mutiny of 1857, the British developed the Civil Lines area and moved away from the walled city. The purpose of setting up the Delhi Municipal Commission was primarily to ensure civic amenities for the Civil Lines area (the seat of government and the residence of the elite), and to some extent for the walled city as well. The Delhi Municipal Commission came into being in 1862 to cater to the needs of about 121,000 inhabitants spread over only 2 square miles. The first meeting of the commission was held on 23 April 1863. The local body evolved over time—it cares now for an estimated 15 million people spread across nearly 1,483 sq km.

The year 1863 saw a series of "firsts"—the setting up of sanitation and conservancy systems, public latrines, a Unani dispensary in Sadar Bazar and the registration of births and deaths. Fire services began in 1867 with one fire engine stationed at the Kotwali. Water from some of the wells was found unfit for human consumption, and a proposal to set up a waterworks was initiated in 1869. Meanwhile, potable water began to be supplied through water carts during 1871–72. Street lighting was introduced with the provision of lanterns and lampposts. The first mass planting of 1,600 saplings was undertaken in 1875. The same year also witnessed the decentralisation of services and the representation of the community; the *ilaka* (area or neighbourhood) system was introduced to supervise conservancy activities. Each ilaka was supervised by a three-member committee.[4]

DELHI MUNICIPAL COMMITTEE

The Delhi Municipal Commission was classified as a class I committee in 1881 and became the Delhi Municipal Committee (DMC). It consisted of 21 nominated members, of whom six were government servants. The remaining members were non-officials comprising three Europeans, six Hindus and six Muslims. Elections were held for the first time in 1885. The elected committee consisted of four government officials, five nominated members, and 12 elected members representing the 12 wards. The total budgetary outlay in 1862 was Rs 94,512; octroi was the main source of income, generating Rs 82,000. Of this, 50 per cent was spent on the police establishment; one-sixth of the share was also diverted to military expenditure, leaving precious little for civic services.

House tax was introduced from 1 January 1902, which yielded an income of Rs 83,327 from 45,558 properties. The initial proposal for house tax was mooted in 1878 (a good 10 years after it had been introduced in Lucknow), but it met with great opposition. By 1902, owners were not so adamant in opposing it, as the burden was to be borne principally by the large numbers of tenants.[5] The total income in 1902–03 was Rs 624,000, and expenditure was Rs 925,000. The other sources of fund collection were octroi, animals, wheel tax, tolls, cattle pounds and hackney carriage.

The walled city was expanding meanwhile, and its population had spilled over into Paharganj and other suburbs. In 1881 and later during 1905, there were popular demands for systematic and planned extension of the "native" areas. The municipal committee, however, did little on this count.

NEW DELHI: TWICE-BORN

The constitution of the committee was changed in 1912 when Delhi Province was created. The number of ex-officio and elected members was brought down to three and 11, respectively. The number of nominated members was raised to 11, undermining the democratic nature of the body. In the same year, the government decided to build a new capital city in Delhi (where the capital was to be relocated from Calcutta). Following the setting up of the temporary capital of the Government of India in Civil Lines, the Notified Area Committee of Delhi came into existence on 16 January 1913. The Delhi Town Planning Committee consisted of Edwin Lutyens and his team of architects and engineers from England, who conceived of the new capital as a garden city after the then prevailing model in Europe. New Delhi was meant exclusively to be a capital city, and was kept separated from Old Delhi by placing vast *maidans* (green belts) between the two Delhis.[6] Simultaneously, there were plans to reconstruct the Pahargunj area of Old Delhi, which had become highly congested by this time; the plan was later abandoned due to resource constraints. Land meant for the expansion of Old Delhi was later "somehow" taken over to serve New Delhi.[7]

With the expansion of Delhi, more local bodies came into being. The District Board for Rural Areas was set up in 1883 for the nearly 300 villages surrounding the city. Notified area committees were set up at Najafgarh (in 1910), Mehrauli (1910), Narela (1919), Shahdara (1916) and the Red Fort Area (1924). In 1921–22, the constitution was again revised and the city was divided into 12 wards. Each ward elected members—one Hindu and one Muslim. Meanwhile, the Imperial Delhi Municipal Committee was renamed the New Delhi Municipal Committee (NDMC) in 1926–27.

The founding of New Delhi resulted in a rapid increase in population; an estimated 28 per cent addition took place during 1916–26. This is significant when viewed against the backdrop of a declining national trend in the 1921 census. The deteriorating urban ecology of Delhi due to the increasing "congestion of people in houses and of houses on land" as well as the existence of slums was noted by Hume in 1936 in his Report on Relief of Congestion in Delhi. Legg quotes from one of Hume's letters, written in 1936: "Old Delhi has waited for over 20 years for the Government to take pity on its squalor and slums while they poured out their gold on the Imperial New Capital."[8] The Delhi Improvement Trust (DIT) was set up in March 1937, principally on the recommendation of Hume's report. The development of extension areas and slum clearance were its major activities, primarily to "sanitise" Old Delhi. In 13 years, however, it managed to re-house only 300 families. The problem of increasing numbers of urban poor and fresh rural–urban migrants remained largely unsolved, and squatter settlements/slums started coming up in the fringe areas of New Delhi.[9] Rising infant mortality and deaths due to tuberculosis (TB) were attributed by the chief health officer to the housing crisis.[10]

Following independence in 1947, New Delhi was born again. The massive migration caused by Partition was reflected in the 1951 census. A decadal growth rate of 106 per cent was recorded for urban Delhi. The Ministry of Rehabilitation was responsible for providing housing to the Punjabi immigrants. A large number of colonies were built in a very short time, including Lajpat Nagar, Kailash Colony, Kalkaji and Malviya Nagar in south Delhi, Moti Nagar and Kirti Nagar in west Delhi, around Kingsway Camp in north Delhi and Gandhi Nagar in east Delhi. The South Delhi Municipal Committee (established in 1954) and the West Delhi Municipal Committee (1955) were formed with the sole purpose of taking care of the civic problems of the refugees. The Punjabi migrants, whose literacy levels were higher than those of the resident population of Delhi, were predominantly urban, middleclass and educated.[11] To provide basic infrastructural services, three more statutory bodies were formed. These were the Delhi Joint Water and Sewage Board (1926), the Delhi State Electricity Board (1951) and the Delhi Transport Authority (1952). The Municipal Corporation of Delhi (MCD) was created to cater to a growing, increasingly ambitious city.

MUNICIPAL CORPORATION OF DELHI

The Delhi Municipal Corporation Act 66 of 1957 was passed by the Parliament on 28 December 1957. Pending the establishment of the corporation under the notification issued by the Ministry of Home Affairs on 15 February 1958, the Government of India appointed, as an interim measure, a Commissioner of Local Authorities to take over the management of all the local bodies, to be later merged in the corporation. The first session was held in March 1958, and the Municipal Corporation of Delhi (MCD) came into being on 7 April 1958 as a result of the amalgamation of nine out of 11 local bodies and the Delhi District Board. The Delhi Cantonment Board (DCB) and NDMC continued to function as independent bodies. The three statutory bodies providing water, electricity and transport were placed under the overall control of MCD. Later, in 1971, the Delhi Transport Corporation was established by a central ordinance.

Initially, there were 34 wards in the MCD with 80 elected members. The entire area was divided into six zones. Decentralisation began in 1963 with the formation of zonal committees to take care of local matters. The number of elected members was raised to 100 in 1967. The DMC Act of 1957 was revised and amended in 1993. Currently, the municipal corporation consists of 272 elected members. The alderman system was also done away with, while the term of the house was increased from four to five years. The house also had representatives from among the elected members of Parliament (Delhi constituencies) and members of the Delhi assembly.

To carry out its day-to-day administration and to settle local problems, the MCD is currently divided into 12 zones, and the administration has been decentralised. These zones are: Central, City, Civil Lines, Karol Bagh, Najafgarh, Narela, Rohini, Sadar Pahargunj, Shahdara (North), Shahdara (South), South and West. Old Delhi falls within the City and Sadar Pahargunj Zones. Najafgarh, Narela and parts of the South Zone are primarily rural areas, except for some urban agglomerations.

DDA: MASTER PLANS OR PLANNING FOR THE MASTERS

At the end of 1955, the Delhi Development (Provisional) Authority was set up to initiate the process of planned development of Delhi. At about the same time, the Town Planning Organisation was set up in the Ministry of

Health to prepare the master plan. The first Master Plan of Delhi (MPD-I) was based on a detailed study of Greater Delhi and its residents by Rao and Desai, and was sponsored by the Planning Commission. The Delhi Development Authority (DDA) was set up by an Act of Parliament, and was to function as the sole development agency of Delhi. The MPD-I was basically a land management plan to channelise the growth of Delhi. It had projected a population of five million by 1981, and had set "urbanisable limits" for 1981, which were to be enclosed by a green belt 1 km wide to restrict further urbanisation.[12] Detailed planning was carried out for the renewal of different types of areas, including squatter settlements, adopting different strategies for areas with different qualities.

The review of MPD-I by the Town and Country Planning Organisation (TCPO) in 1972–73 noted that the housing deficit was 380,000 in 1970, up from 150,000 in 1961. The slum population was estimated at one million. The review noted that extensive unauthorised construction and commercial activities had infiltrated residential areas. The ridge and the green belt had been compromised, and little care had been taken to minimise environmental pollution. Population density was increasing in Old Delhi as well. The review commented that there was a preoccupation with higher-income residential areas and the beautification of Delhi, while low-cost housing was being neglected. Advocating better management, the review commented that development was taking place "in response more to pressures than according to programmes".[13]

Following the review, slum clearance was taken up as a priority. The MCD, which had been handling this job since 1930, was divested of the responsibility. The task was handed over to DDA in February 1974. In the next couple of years, which also coincided with the Emergency (1975–77), 27 resettlement colonies were set up for relocating populations from slums in different parts of the city. All-round development was envisaged for these colonies, with roads, parks, dispensaries and community centres. Industrial areas were also set up in the neighbourhood. The DDA constructed a total of 235,000 dwellings for low-income groups in the resettlement colonies during 1971–81, most of them during the Emergency.

Despite the laudable ideals, resettlement colonies suffered from basic public health and engineering deficiencies. They were located on peripheral, low-lying wastelands with poor drainage and outfall. These squatter resettlement colonies were site-cum-services schemes. The Delhi Improvement Trust had initially fixed the size of the individual plots at 89 square yards. The DDA master plan reduced it to 80 square yards, and later to 55 square yards. The final plot size that was allocated was 25 square yards. The DIT had conceived of houses with one to three rooms, a cooking verandah, a bathing platform and a courtyard. This housing standard was reduced to one small room, a cooking space and a small open space for the 25-square-yard plots. Neither the DIT nor the DDA planned for the provision of adequate safe water and waste disposal. Community latrines were constructed for these resettlement colonies; one latrine seat was provided for 20–50 persons.In practice, the standard deteriorated to one seat for upto 150 persons.[14]

During the two decades 1971–90, the housing stock of Delhi increased by almost one million. Of this, 75 per cent consisted of permanent dwelling units and the rest were semi-permanent and temporary units or slums. The DDA contributed 64 per cent of the permanent units. The real beneficiaries were, in most cases, communities belonging to the middle- and higher-income groups. The rate of resettlement slowed down for several reasons:[15]

- Change in priority in the national planning paradigm from slum clearance (and resettlement) to slum improvement
- The unpleasant memory of the Emergency
- The intrinsic deficiencies of the resettlement colonies—long distances from former places of work, poor road and transport services and underdeveloped physical and social infrastructure within the colonies
- The influence of vested interests—"slum lords, underworld dons and politicians"

V. Nath predicted the scenario through the decade 1991–2001 as follows:[16]

- Growth of population—upto 14 million by 2001
- Further growth of industries and consequent pollution, as the government elected in 1993 was "interested in encouraging further growth of industries and relaxing anti-pollution control over them"
- Proliferation of slums and unauthorised colonies—on account of

increases in jobs in the industrial and service sectors, and the promise of regularisation of unauthorised colonies and provision of electricity connections to all slums dwellers

- Air and water pollution and traffic congestion
- Increase in shortage of water and electricity
- Ribbon development along the highways

All these forecasts have proved right, as the decade of the 1990s has shown. Unauthorised settlements increased sharply, and the relocation of slums began again in the late 1990s. Pollution, both vehicular and industrial, continued to increase. The Supreme Court, acting on several public interest litigations, passed judgements ordering polluting industries located in non-conforming areas to be shut down or relocated. The judgement was implemented and a number of industries closed down. This created unemployment on the one hand, but reduced the pollution load on the other. Vehicular air pollution was also reduced after most diesel transport vehicles switched to compressed natural gas (CNG). While the pollution issue was tackled largely through judicial activism, water and energy shortages continue to be major challenges for the government.

Delhi was a union territory till 1993, when it was conferred statehood with limited powers. The new state was called the National Capital Territory of Delhi (NCTD). The NCTD is spread over an area of 1,484 sq km, and is bound by the states of Haryana and Uttar Pradesh. The NCTD is cared for by three local bodies—the MCD, the NDMC and the DCB. Among these, the MCD caters to the bulk of Delhi's population (about 90 per cent). As per the 2001 census, the population of Delhi is 13,782,976. The MCD is among the largest municipal bodies in the world in terms of the population served, and second only to Tokyo with respect to the area covered.[17] It covers 1,397.3 sq km and includes 238 villages. The NDMC serves 2.38 per cent of the city area, while the DCB serves a smaller population spread over 2.89 per cent of Delhi's area.

DEVELOPMENTS IN THE NEW MILLENNIUM

The 1980s were a decade of rethinking. Two major causes were identified for the failure of MPD-I:[18]

- Extensive in-migration into Delhi, with the great majority of the migrants being poor
- Freezing of all land for urban development in the union territory by the government

The DDA alone had the right to acquire and develop land for residential, commercial and industrial or other uses. The number of squatter households had increased seven-fold between 1961 and 1991, from 40,000 to 300,000. There were large deficits between demand and supply as far as housing and infrastructure were concerned.[19] Targets were claimed to have been achieved in two sectors—water (121 per cent) and electricity (100 per cent). The review observed that the basic requirement of water had been calculated at a lower standard of 50 litres per capita day (lpcd), and recommended that it be raised to 80 lpcd. The target for providing sewerage facilities remained at a dismal low of 35 per cent. The principal unsewered areas were Shahjahanabad (and parts of its extension into Pahargunj and Karol Bagh), unauthorised colonies and slums.[20] Another major failure of MPD-I was the poor performance with regard to shifting non-conforming (including highly polluting and hazardous) industrial units or markets from their old locations to new ones, as recommended in MPD-I itself. Worse still, new units continued to mushroom, often in densely populated residential areas.

The Regional Plan 2001 (RP) was adopted in January 1989. It envisaged developing the national capital region encompassing the states of Delhi, Uttar Pradesh (Meerut, Bulandshahr and Ghaziabad districts), Haryana (Faridabad, Gurgaon, Rohtak and Sonepat districts) and Rajasthan (Alwar district). A revised Master Plan of Delhi (MPD-II) was prepared by the central government in conformity with the objectives, strategies and policies of the RP. This came into effect on 1August 1990. Both plans targeted the regulation of the growth of commercial activities and of the population in the Delhi urban agglomeration by diverting the growth to priority towns within the national capital region. The two plans, however, had different projections for the population of Delhi. The MPD-II projected a population of 12.8 million for Delhi by 2001, while the RP projected 13.2 million. The census of 2001 put the population at 13,782,976.

The MPD-II continued to be essentially a land use plan for residential, industrial, commercial and other uses. It specified in great detail the floor area ratios (FAR) for different uses and for residential plots of different sizes located along roads of different widths. The MPD-II also recognised that some of the policies of MPD-I were "unrealistic and need to be changed".[20] The most important policy changes recommended were:

- Permission of non-residential activities on residential premises
- Significantly high FARs in view of the high price of land

The MPD-II estimated that 24,000 industrial units (about 50 per cent of the existing units) in non-conforming areas needed to be relocated. During the MPD-II period, industries increased by another 75 per cent, and an equal proportion (50 per cent) of industries were still located in non-conforming areas. Some of these imbalances were to a certain extent rectified by the intervention of the courts. A fairly large number of industries closed down during the drive following the courts' orders, though many of them later reopened. The MPD-II and the RP were terminated in 2001.

A collaborative project of the Ministry of Environment and Forests ofthe Government of India and the Planning Department of the Government of the National Capital Territory of Delhi, the Delhi Urban Environment and Infrastructure Improvement Project (DUEIIP) examined the inadequacies in different sectors of infrastructure in Delhi at the end of MPD-II and RP.[21] The project sought to estimate infrastructure requirements for 2021, with a particular focus on environmental health. The DUEIIP report of 2001 "refutes the contention" that DDA was the major provider of formal housing in Delhi. Between 1957 (when DDA was formed) and 2000, Delhi's population had increased from three million to about 14 million. The increase consisted of about 5.5 million people in the high-income groups (HIG) plus economically weaker sections (EWS), and another 5.5 million people in the "poverty group". The report pointed out that during this period, one million dwelling units had been provided by the DDA; the private sector (both formal and informal) provided another one million units. The shortfall in housing stood at 277,253 units in 1997 and was projected to be 342,000 units by 2002. The report argued that had there been a housing policy in place, this situation would not have arisen. The DUEIIP report went on to espouse the cause of the private sector, which it said could build at "six times the rate of the public sector". The principal cause of the failure of DDA, as identified by the report, was the lack of sharing of powers between the Government of India and the Government of Delhi, and the fact that the "majority of the citizens of the national capital are not in control of their own destiny"![22] The recently released National Housing Policy focuses on the state's role as an "enabler" and a "facilitator", and emphasises the role of private–public partnerships in improving access to land, construction and maintenance.

CHANGING DEMOGRAPHICS

The first census in Delhi was conducted in 1833; there were 119,860 people in the city, excluding the palace residents. The censuses of 1843, 1845 and 1853 registered populations of 131,000, 137,000 and 151,000, respectively. There was a sharp drop in population during the Mutiny of 1857. The population began to increase again from 1860—more in the suburbs than within the city walls. The famine years of 1861, 1867, 1877 and 1898 witnessed "distress migration" from areas as distant as Rajasthan. The number of men living in the suburbs in the 1870s was far higher than the number of women, in contrast to the city where the ratio was more even. The difference was most marked in the age group 15–45 years. While 5 per cent of the males were literate in the suburbs, as many as 25 per cent were literate in the city area. Most males in the city were employed in manufacturing and trading, while others were clerks and professional workers. In contrast, in the suburbs, as many as 50 per cent were labourers and others were petty shopkeepers; only one in 80 was in the service sector.

Following the Mutiny, population density increased sharply subsequent to the decision to locate the cantonment within the city and have a wide open space around the fort. The census of 1846 recorded 25,000 houses in the walled city, a number that increased to 38,000 in 1853. The 1881 census found only 17,498 houses, including the suburbs. There was increased building activity in the 1880s and 1890s. By the 1880s, there were demands from time to time to demolish the wall to expand the growing city, but this was opposed by the army. The rate of immigration slowed down; two-thirds of the immigrants continued to be males. There was an increase in the number of rented dwelling units and squatters on public land. The notion of residing in healthier and more open suburban houses evolved as a concept only at the turn of the century. By the 1890s, Delhi had become the commercial capital of the Punjab. It had also grown into a major military station. The shifting of the capital of India to Delhi from Calcutta in 1912 further boosted the growth of population.

By 1941, the population of Delhi had increased to 900,000. The 1951 census recorded the population at 1,744,000, indicating the largest ever decadal growth of around 90 per cent, in the aftermath of the Partition (Table 2.1).

Table 2.1: Population and Migration in Delhi, 1951–1991[23]

Year	*Population ('000s)*	*Net decadal increase ('000s)*	*Per cent*	*Total no. of immigrants ('000s)*	*Per cent of immigrants in the decadal increase of population*
1951	1,744				
1961	2,659	915	52.3	544	56.5
1971	4,066	1,407	52.9	525	37.3
1981	6,220	2,154	53.0	1,229	57.0
1991	9,421	3,201	51.5	n/a	n/a

Migrants contributed more than half the increase in the population during 1951–61, after the Partition. More importantly, during 1971–81, there was a boom in the growth of industries. The land mafia was also born and institutionalised to a great extent in this period. One estimate puts the origins of migrants as follows—83.9 per cent from rural areas, 15.8 per cent from small and medium towns and a minuscule 0.3 per cent from other million-plus cities.[24]

The 2001 census recorded the population of Delhi at 13,782,976. The decadal growth rate was 46.31 per cent, signifying a slowdown from the previous decade. The national growth rate (provisional) was 21.34 per cent. The population of Delhi accounted for 1.34 per cent of the total population in the country and ranked 18th among the states in the 2001 census.

Table 2.2: Population Density of Delhi[25]

Civic Body	Density of Population (persons/sq km)		
	1981	*1991*	*2001*
NDMC	6,388	7,050	10,310
DCB	1,982	2,197	3,208
MCD (urban)	13,547	13,464	19,706
MCD (rural)	476	1,190	1,740
MCD (total)	4,195	6,459	9,450
Delhi (urban)	9,745	12,361	18,086
Delhi (rural)	507	1,190	1,740
Delhi (total)	4,194	6,352	9,294

The rapid growth of population and a comparison of the population densities will give an indication of the degree of urbanisation (Table 2.2). A few densely populated urban areas in the MCD were redesignated as rural during the late 1980s. This explains the increase in the density of population in rural areas between 1981 and 1991, and the slight fall in density in urban areas. The population density for Delhi was 9,294 persons per sq km in the 2001 census, more than double that of 1981. The annual estimates of the population of Delhi by the Office of the Registrar General of India are presented in Table 2.3.

Table 2.3: Annual Estimates of Population[26]

Year	*As of 1 March*	*As of 1 July*	*As of 1 October*
1991	9,420,600	9,538,300	9,615,100
1992	9,756,500	9,858,900	9,958,000
1993	10,104,500	10,223,200	10,313,100
1994	10,468,400	10,587,700	10,680,900
1995	10,837,900	10,965,200	11,061,700
1996	11,224,400	11,355,500	11,454,800
1997	11,622,300	11,758,100	11,860,900
1998	12,034,400	12,117500	12,281,400
1999	12,461,000	12,606,500	12,716,800
2000	12,902,700	13,053,400	13,167,600
2001	13,360,100	–	–

Delhi ranks among the worst states in terms of female population per thousand males (see Figure 2.1). However, one has to be careful in interpreting this statistic, since there are significant numbers of single males migrating to Delhi for employment.

Figure 2.1: Sex Ratio in Delhi[27]

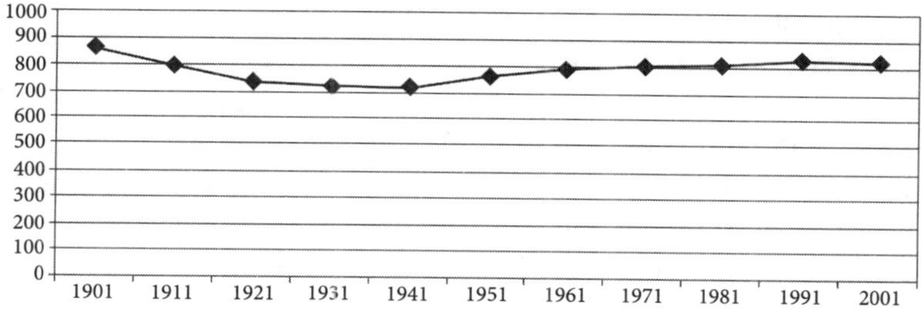

The sex ratio has declined throughout the century, and has never regained the 1901 level of 862 females per 1,000 males. There was a systematic decline till 1941 (when it stood at 715); the year 1951 saw a turnaround. Between 1951 and 1991, there was a steady increase from 768 to 827. The 2001 census recorded a fall in the sex ratio from the 1991 level in a contiguous block of north Indian states and union territories—Himachal Pradesh (from 976 to 970), Punjab (from 882 to 874), Chandigarh (from 790 to 773), Haryana (from 865 to 861) and Delhi (from 827 to 821). A similar pattern of declining sex ratios may be noted in another contiguous block of western Indian states and union territories—Gujarat (from 934 to 921), Daman & Diu (from 969 to 709), Dadra & Nagar Haveli (from 952 to 811), Maharashtra (from 934 to 922) and Goa (from 967 to 960).

Within Delhi, variations were observed in the sex ratio across nine revenue districts in the 2001 census. The lowest of 783 was noted in New Delhi, which has only 1.25 per cent of the total population. The highest was 851 in the north-east district, which has 12.80 per cent of the population. Between 1991 and 2001, the sex ratio increased only in the north and north-east districts, while all other districts registered a fall.

Analysis of sectoral growth in the gross state domestic product (GSDP) indicates that the primary sector, comprising agriculture, livestock, forestry, fishing, mining and quarrying, and also the secondary sector comprising manufacturing, electricity, gas, water supply and construction, are both on the decline. The tertiary sector, comprising trade, hotels, restaurants, transport, storage, communication, finance, insurance, real estate, business services and public administration, has emerged as the major contributor in the economy of Delhi. Between 1993–94 and 2000–01, the contribution of the primary sector to GSDP declined from 3.92 per cent to 1.40 per cent. By 2006–07 it had decreased to 0.81 per cent. The secondary sector declined from 25.61 per cent in 1993–94 to about 20.75 per cent in 2006–07. The contribution of the tertiary sector increased from 70.47 per cent in 1993–94 to 78.44 per cent in 2006–07. This trend has been attributed to rapid urbanisation, decline in agriculture and allied activities and substantial increase in the growth of the services sector. The closure of polluting industrial units has contributed further to the decline in the secondary sector.[28]

In real terms, the GSDP for Delhi registered an annual compound growth rate of 8.41 per cent between 1993–94 and 2000–01. During 2000–01, at constant prices, the annual growth rate of GSDP was 4.5 per cent as compared to the all-India growth rate of 4 per cent. At constant prices (1993–94), from 1993–94 to 2000–01, per capita income in Delhi grew at an annual compound growth rate of 4.45 per cent, as compared to the national rate of 4.20 per cent.

In the agriculture and allied activities sector, the decline in real terms has been associated with the ban imposed by the Delhi High Court in 1994 on the slaughtering of animals in the slaughterhouse, and with the output of floriculture being much less during 1999–2000. Mining and quarrying are minor economic activities in Delhi, partly due to the topography. Further, such activities have been curtailed because of the ban on the quarrying and extraction of Badarpur stone within Delhi. The manufacturing sector played a substantial role till 1995, when the court ordered a major chunk of big industrial units causing pollution to be closed. Again in 1999, under the orders of the Supreme Court, several additional units were closed for the purpose of controlling environmental pollution. As a result, there has been a decline in the contribution to GSDP from the manufacturing sector. Within the secondary sector, however, the contribution from the construction sector has been growing consistently. In the tertiary sector, trade, hotels and restaurants have been major contributors, accounting annually for approximately one-fifth of the GSDP of Delhi. Transport, storage and communication constitute another sector that has been growing consistently. Financing, insurance, real estate and business services have also been major contributors to the economy. In 1993–94, this sector contributed one-fourth of the total GSDP, rising to about one-third by 2000–01. The community, social and personal services sector has been growing over the period at an annual compound growth rate of 18.4 per cent. However, a major part of this growth is explained by the increase in public administration services.

SETTLEMENT PATTERNS: UNSETTLING TRUTHS

Delhi exhibits great diversity in its settlement patterns. The NDMC corresponds to the area that was developed when the capital of India first shifted from Calcutta to Delhi. In the post-independence period, it witnessed a further boost in its development. Institutions and state-owned residences form the bulk of the NDMC. The DCB caters exclusively to military installations, offices and residences. Both these local bodies are therefore planned areas, well provided for in terms of infrastructure. Most of the resident populations are socio-economically and politically well empowered. These two local bodies account for only about 5 per cent of the area and about 10 per cent of the population of Delhi. In contrast, the Municipal Corporation of Delhi (MCD) caters to 90 per cent of the resident population of Delhi spread over 85 per cent of the total area. It is in the MCD areas that Delhi has "expanded"—with new colonies being set up or allotted by the Delhi Development Authority, and unauthorised settlements mushrooming as well.

Delhi is estimated to be growing at a rate of about 1,000 persons per day and about 350,000 per year. Of these, 225,000 are accounted for by intrinsic growth, and the rest by migration. Provision of housing to this growing body of population is an enormous task. The DDA was set up in 1957 with the principal objective of developing land and providing housing. Between 1957 and 2001, the population of Delhi increased from three million to about 14 million, i.e., by 11 million. About half of this population lives in housing provided by the DDA. The DDA offers a wide range of housing, from houses meant for the high-income groups (HIG), to houses for the economically weaker sections, including resettlement colonies. The other half (more than five million people) are poor and live in substandard housing.

The different settlement types in Delhi include:

- Planned colonies
- Unauthorised colonies
- Regularised colonies (which were unauthorised to begin with)
- Slums/*jhuggi-jhonpri* (JJ) clusters
- Resettlement colonies
- Urbanised villages
- Villages (rural)

Despite Delhi's claims to historically being a planned city, only a quarter of its population lives in planned colonies (Table 2.4).

Table 2.4: Settlements and Population[29]

Type of Settlement	*Population (in millions)*	*Percentage*
JJ clusters	2.07	14.83
Slum designated areas	2.66	19.08
Unauthorised colonies	0.74	5.30
Resettlement colonies	1.76	12.71
Rural villages	0.74	5.30
Regularised-unauthorised colonies	1.77	12.72
Urban villages	0.88	6.36
Planned colonies	3.31	23.69
Total	13.96	100

Planned Areas

The planned areas include the area under the NDMC, which corresponds to the capital built by Lutyens and his team and other parts of New Delhi. These are the areas where infrastructure facilities have been developed in a planned manner and services are available to the residents. The older settlements in the walled city and Old Delhi have also been integrated into the planning process, and civic infrastructure has been made available to populations living in these areas. Planned colonies have been added in MCD areas over time, with proper services. They were generally developed by the DDA and later handed over to MCD for maintenance and provision of day-to-day services.

Resettlement Colonies

By definition, these are essentially planned areas, constructed by the state to relocate the slum population. The first such effort was made in 1961. Squatter settlements were removed from government and private lands and two-room tenements were provided to 3,560 households. The policy later changed to providing partially developed plots, the size of which was initially fixed at 80 square yards. The plot size was reduced over the years to 40 square yards, then 25, and finally to 12.5 square yards.

Slum clearance work received a major thrust in 1974; the responsibility was transferred from the MCD to the DDA by the Government of India. The DDA took it up as a mission during the Emergency years—1975 to 1977. Twenty-six resettlement colonies were constructed in the peripheries of the city during this period and 197,000 squatter households were relocated. A plan scheme was initiated in 1979–80 to provide and improve basic civic amenities in all 44 resettlement colonies, in which about 240,000 households were resettled. The resettlement colonies were site-cum-services schemes. Each family was provided a plot of 25 square yards. These colonies were provided with roads, parks, public toilets, shops, schools, dispensaries and community centres. Industrial areas were also earmarked in nearby areas to provide employment. The emphasis was on "resettlement" and not just "relocation". Despite these guiding principles, there were several major deficiencies in the resettlement colonies:[30]

- The colonies were located on low-lying wasteland, often along drains and ditches that were essentially unsuitable for human habitation.
- Resettlement colonies were set up in the trans-Yamuna area without developing an adequate drainage system as recommended in the master plan.
- The area of individual plots was lowered from the initial 89 square yards (recommended by the DIT) to 25 square yards (allotted by the DDA), leading to serious compromises in public health standards.
- Adequate water supply and proper waste disposal system were not provided for.

- The minimum standard for public latrines was fixed at one seat for 20–50 persons; in actual practice, it worked out to one seat per 150 persons. Open defecation, particularly by children, is a common practice.
- Parks almost invariably deteriorated into dumping areas for solid wastes and wastewater.
- The remote location of the resettlement colonies implied that the communities were far away or cut off from their previous employment and facilities, including health institutions/services.

Over time, the resettlement colonies have become densely populated, far in excess of what had originally been envisaged. In addition to the intrinsic growth of the relocated families, there are large bodies of tenants in the houses that often stand three to four storeys high. Further, squatter settlements have mushroomed around all the resettlement colonies. Unauthorised construction and small household industries have become major problems. In some of these colonies, sewers were constructed later, but the housing units did not have the space for constructing toilets. Some of the households have, however, encroached on the common space and constructed toilets that open directly into the open drains, with the attendant complications. Open spaces in many resettlement colonies have been encroached upon by squatters.

In 1992, the DDA introduced the revised resettlement policy. This had two major premises:

- No fresh encroachments would be permitted on public land.
- Encroachments previous to 30 January 1990 would not be removed without providing alternatives.

Since the mid-1990s, there has been a new spurt in relocating slum clusters. Clusters are relocated in only those cases where land is required to be made available to the landowning agency for "public interest projects". The landowning agency has to make a specific request to this effect, and should also be ready to bear the cost partially. A sum of Rs 44,000 is required to relocate one slum household—of which Rs29,000 is contributed by the landowning agency, Rs10,000 by the Delhi government for provision of services, and Rs 5,000 by the beneficiary. The services are provided by the Slum and JJ Department of the MCD.

Unauthorised Colonies

Unauthorised colonies (informal colonies) are built by promoters, builders and the land mafia on land that is generally not meant for human habitation as per the master plan. This is due to the demand for housing (or for land for housing purposes), since housing has not been made available at an affordable cost to significant numbers of the population. These segments have had no option but to settle in such illegal colonies in the hope that they will be "regularised" over time. The promoters are generally local landlords, property dealers or politicians and often various combinations of these—forming thereby the "land mafia".

Unauthorised colonies typically come up around villages in the peripheries of the city. The promoters generally belong to the dominant caste/s or groups of the village. In most instances, the designated land use was either agricultural or fallow land. The customers for these lands are typically individuals from the low- and middle-income groups, of whom a sizeable proportion are employed in formal or informal services. The complicity of the local police, MCD and DDA officials comes into play during the construction of the dwelling units; without such complicity, the physical structure cannot be built, since each of these agencies has a surveillance mechanism for checking illegal and unauthorised construction.

Unauthorised colonies, being illegal entities, do not qualify for any services, including piped water supply, sewerage, sanitation and electricity. People generally access electricity by illegal means, but do not have options for piped water and sewerage. Not all of these residents are poor; in fact, a large spectrum of socio-economic groups is represented in the unauthorised colonies. These colonies are regularised periodically, following which they become eligible for the provision of basic services, for which developmental charges are levied.

Jhuggi-Jhonpri (JJ) Clusters

Jhuggi-jhonpri clusters or squatter settlements are encroachments on public or private lands, and are illegal settlements. They are essentially kutcha dwelling units (huts); many families in JJ clusters manage to climb the economic ladder and construct pucca dwelling units over time. Jhuggi-jhonpri clusters are notified under the Slum Improvement and Clearance Areas Act of 1956, and become eligible for benefits under this act. They are not entitled to any individualised services, but are provided with community-level services like public hydrants, tankers, latrine blocks, street lighting, *dhalaos* (dustbins) for collection of domestic wastes, paved pathways and drains.[31] They are also eligible for relocation/resettlement schemes that are periodically implemented. It is important to distinguish JJ clusters from JJ colonies, which are actually resettlement colonies from the 1960s.

About 25 per cent of Delhi's population resides in these JJ clusters—three million in 1997. There were 1,100 clusters with about 600,000 jhuggis in 1997. Of these, 713 clusters were located on 1,838 acres of land owned by DDA alone or jointly with other agencies. Eighty-seven clusters were situated on about 146 acres of land belonging to the Land and Development Office. The remaining clusters were located on land owned by the railways, other government agencies and private owners. About a third of the clusters have less than 100 jhuggis, and another one-third have between 100 and 500 jhuggis. The rest are bigger, with 5 per cent of the clusters having from 1,001 to 1,500 jhuggis and another 6per cent having more than 1,500 jhuggis.[32] The key issues and deficiencies in the provision of services in these clusters, as identified by the DUEIIP report, are as follows:[33]

- Standard norms for basic services too low
- Inadequate environmental services infrastructure
- Ineffective delivery and service maintenance
- Inadequate social support systems, particularly health centres and schools
- Lack of coordination and consultations between authorities, non-governmental organisations (NGOs) and communities

Villages

Delhi has 165 villages, and its rural areas comprised 147,488 hectares of land in 2007–08, of which the total cropped area was 32,434 hectares. The "rural" villages still have agriculture as their principal means of livelihood. Parts of the village have diversified into other economic activities like manufacturing industries and agro- and food-based industries. Villages where land (including agricultural land) was taken up for the expansion of the city are known as "urbanised villages". They are surrounded by planned city areas. The landowners are paid suitable compensation as per the prevailing rates. The compensation money is generally invested in setting up industries within the villages, or in real estate, where houses or dwelling units are constructed with the specific purpose of sale or rent. The quality of houses built depends upon the socio-economic group of tenants that the village attracts, and is a function of the location of the village within Delhi. An important feature of these villages—both rural and urbanised—is that municipal bye-laws are not enforceable within village limits, also called the *laldora*. Few regulations are enforced in terms of the buildings constructed or the industries set up in such areas.

SOLID AND LIQUID WASTE MANAGEMENT

Solid Waste

Munasinghe distinguishes between three types of urban solid wastes:[34]

- Municipal solid wastes, including paper, plastics, glass, metals, street sweepings and general refuse from households, commercial and institutional establishments. In some countries, sludge from sewage and water treatment plants isco-disposed with municipal solid wastes.
- Hazardous and industrial wastes. These include heavy metals, dioxins and polycyclic aromatic hydrocarbons. The major characteristics of this group include their toxicity for humans, ignitability, infectiousness and potential for effecting ecological damage.
- Waste generated by health care services and hospitals. This is considered separately as clinical or biomedical waste. This includes pharmaceutical, pathological and infectious wastes such as syringes, needles, chemicals (aerosols/disinfectants) and low-level radioactive wastes (xrays, radiation vials).

For the disposal of solid wastes, there are two main alternatives, incineration and sanitary landfills. Each of these has its advantages and disadvantages. Incineration can cause air pollution, and is a more expensive and complicated alternative. However, it is useful for reducing the bulk of the waste and disposing of toxic or hazardous waste. Sanitary landfills are more appropriate for handling non-combustible wastes and the ashes from incineration. For most municipal solid wastes, landfills are the appropriate method of disposal. No matter which of these methods is adopted, ensuring environmentally safe disposal requires direct involvement by governments in planning and regulation, because disposal involves large externalities and economies of scale that make competitive provision nonviable. However, for collection of urban solid wastes, contracts with private parties are both feasible and are being practised in developing countries. Till date, 50 to 70 per cent of solid wastes in developing countries are collected by municipal sanitation departments.

Delhi produces the highest percapita solid waste, 0.475 kg/day, among the Indian class I cities.[35] The Central Pollution Control Board (CPCB) conducted a two-year survey of the management of solid wastes by the two civic agencies, the NDMC and the MCD.[36] It was found that there was no significant change for the better over the years in the overall management of solid wastes within the city. Further, the landfill sites were found to be grossly polluted in terms of the land, water and air environment at these sites. Table 2.5 presents the comparative picture on solid waste collection across different Indian cities.

Table 2.5: Solid Waste Generation and Collection in Major Indian Cities[37]

City	*Collection Efficiency (per cent)*
Ahmedabad	90
Bengaluru	68.1
Bhopal	93.5
Coimbatore	64.6
Mumbai	96.6
Indore	83.3
Delhi	75
Lucknow	83
Chennai	90
Pune	70
Surat	96

Delhi's solid waste collection efficiency is among the lowest compared to the major Indian cities. All other metros and major cities have collection rates of 80 per cent. The low percentage in Delhi has serious implications in the context of waterborne diseases, particularly if uncollected waste is not stored in proper bins and percolates to contaminate groundwater.

The Conservancy and Sanitation Engineering Department (CSE) of the MCD is responsible for the collection and disposal of solid waste, street sweeping and cleaning of open drains. The CSE maintains 332 major nullahs carrying sewage, and 2,900 km of drains. Further, there are 1,583 septic tanks, mainly in resettlement colonies. In addition, there are four sanitary landfill sites (in use) for disposal of garbage, at Ghazipur, Bhalaswa, Sanjay Gandhi Transport Nagar and Okhla.

The current daily generation of municipal solid waste is about 8,000 metric tonnes, and the average composition is 38.6 per cent biodegradable, 34.7 per cent silt and 26.6 per cent recyclable. Thirty-five sweepers are employed per 10,000 persons, which is a higher rate than in the other metro cities in India. The three urban local bodies have 773 trucks of 4-tonne capacity. At two trips per truck, it is possible to dispose of all the solid waste daily.[38] Gross managerial inefficiencies and poor maintenance of vehicles remain principal obstacles to the proper collection and disposal of solid waste. Further, no services are provided for unauthorised colonies that account for about 20 per cent of the population. It is, therefore, obvious that the solid waste generated in those colonies is not reflected in the official statistics. Disposal of solid waste is being "carried out by land filling in an unscientific manner at four disposal sites".[39] Biomedical and industrial wastes also reach these landfill sites to a significant extent. All this implies contamination of groundwater with organic matter and chemicals. Only 300 metric tonnes of waste are composted daily, against an installed capacity of 800 metric tonnes.[40]

Liquid Waste

Munasinghe outlines three essential steps in a water management programme in the context of solid waste collection and disposal:[41]

- First, there must be source reduction (or waste minimisation) to reduce the amount and toxicity of wastes through changes in design, technology or input mix; this measure finds a place as part of a pollution prevention strategy.

- Second, waste reuse, recycling and recovery would reduce the load.
- Finally, there must be mechanisms for appropriate collection and disposal of remaining wastes.

In addition to water supply, the Delhi Jal Board (DJB) is responsible for safe disposal of liquid waste, including maintenance of the sewage treatment plants (STP) and about 3,000 km of underground sewers. Fifty-five per cent of the urban population is served by the sewer system. Several more sewers are under construction. The current total capacity is 512 million gallons per day (MGD). Most of the trunk sewers are heavily silted and non-functional at places due to poor maintenance. Sewage therefore cannot reach the STPs. The Delhi Jal Board claimed in June 2000 that 1,332 million litres per day (MLD) was being treated, amounting to 85 per cent of the capacity. A study by the CPCB is quoted by the DUEIIP report of 2001, stating that despite the DJB's claims, only 950 MLD (60 per cent of the installed capacity) of sewage was reaching the STP and being treated.

An analysis of the sanitary situation of the poorer localities of Delhi is interesting. Outfall sewers exist in 10 resettlement colonies (22 per cent). Out of 108 urban villages under MCD, sewerage exists in just 69 villages (64 per cent). The Eighth Five-Year Plan laid stress on completing work on sewerage in both resettlement colonies and urban villages. The situation in JJ colonies and in the resettlement colonies developed by the DDA is indeed serious. The sullage flows in open surface drains, which ultimately reach the Yamuna river. Out of the 17 drains, five drains carry 95 per cent of the pollution load. These were previously meant to be rainwater drains but, due to the lack of sewage systems, sullage/sewage is also being discharged into them.

SUPPLYING WATER

In the early nineteenth century, the prevalent water-related diseases in Delhi were cholera, malaria and Delhi Sore.[42] Public health considerations gained importance as the military presence in the city increased.

The diseases were considered to be caused by waterborne contagion, transmitted through running water, brackish well water and waterlogged pools. The dried-up Ali Mardan canal was reopened to provide drinking water in 1821. Water was overexploited, particularly for irrigation; the canal dried up in about two decades. The availability of water from this source led to the neglect of wells and, in 1843, as many as 555 of the 607 wells in the city were found to be brackish. By 1867, the canal was restored but the wells continued to decline. Freshwater was additionally accessed from the springs in the ridge and from Jhandewalan.

Waterworks and the Water Board

In 1867, the Punjab sanitary commissioner suggested building a waterworks to tap the Yamuna water. Planning for the waterworks began in 1869. In 1889, construction began with a loan, 12 years after the Lahore waterworks scheme was completed successfully and became operational. The water supply wells were located at Chandrawal village on the banks of the Yamuna. The residents were shifted out and resettled at New Chandrawal village. The walled city was supplied first, followed by the western suburbs and finally Civil Lines. When the canal's supplies became erratic and scanty, there were applications for private connections. In 1892, the municipality banned the Chamars (untouchables) from using the public standposts, but the resolution was later withdrawn. Safe water from the waterworks led to a reduction in the incidence of cholera, typhoid and "Delhi Boil" (cutaneous leishmaniasis). The consumption of piped water increased with more house connections.

The Joint Water Board was set up in 1925 by the Delhi municipality and the New Delhi municipality. Larger proportions of water were being diverted to the notified area, New Delhi and the Cantonment. The Delhi municipality refused to pay. The new capital continued to gain in importance. The most developed municipal service, the water supply system, was used to serve the "new" at the cost of the "old". To meet the growing requirements of the expanding city, waterworks were constructed and expanded at Chandrawal, Wazirabad and Okhla. Ranney wells and tubewells were also commissioned and sunk.

In 1957, the water board was replaced by the Delhi Water Supply and Sewage Disposal Undertaking (DWSSDU) of the MCD. The undertaking had sole responsibility for the management of the water supply and liquid wastes of Delhi, including the sewage treatment plants. It supplied water in bulk to the NDMC and Cantonment areas; in MCD areas, supply was through a network of reservoirs, pumping stations and distribution mains. The DWSSDU was reconstituted as the Delhi Jal Board in 1998, and thus converted from a semi-autonomous undertaking to a department of the Government of Delhi.

Surface Water Sources

At present, the surface water sources in Delhi are the river Yamuna, the Upper Ganga Canal and the Western Yamuna Canal (Table 2.6).

Table 2.6: Surface Water Sources in Delhi[43]

Source	*Tapped at*	*Treated at*
River Yamuna	Wazirabad	Chandrawal plant
Upper Ganga Canal	Murad Nagar, UP	Bhagirathi plant
Western Yamuna Canal	Bawana, Haiderpur	Haiderpur plant

Delhi has a fixed share of raw water in the Yamuna and in the Ganga canal. There is not much scope for further harnessing freshwater from any of these sources. During the summer months, efforts are made to harness additional supplies from neighbouring states. The installed capacity of the major water treatment plants are: Chandrawal, 90 MGD; Wazirabad, 120 MGD; Haiderpur, 200 MGD; Bhagirathi, 100 MGD; Nangloi, 40 MGD; and Sonia Vihar, 140 MGD.

Ranney wells and tubewells add another 100 MGD. The total installed capacity is thus 790 MGD, but the actual production is constrained owing to reduced raw water supply to the Sonia Vihar and Nangloi plants. Table 2.7 presents the physico-chemical, bacteriological and biological parameters of the raw water being tapped from the Western Yamuna Canal at the water treatment plant at Haiderpur. This provides an indication of the quality of raw water.

Table 2.7: Parameters of Raw Water: Western Yamuna Canal, Haiderpur[44]

I. Physico-chemical	
Colour	Hazy
Odour	Earthy
pH value	7.8
Turbidity	65 NTU
Electrical conductivity	280 mho
Chlorides	6.0 mg/l
Nitrites	0.004 mg/l
Ammonia	0.04 mg/l
Dissolved oxygen	6.4 mg/l
Oxygen absorption (3 minutes)	0.36 mg/l
pH, alkalinity	Nil
Total alkalinity	68 mg/l
Chlorine demand	1.1 mg/l
Residual alumina	–
Total hardness	86 mg/l
Cyanides as CM	Absent
Nitrates	0.88 mg/l
Fluorides	0.1 mg/l
II. Bacteriological Coliform/100 ml (MPN) 11 X 105	
III. Biological 2,500 members/1,000 ml	

Note: NTU: nephelometric turbidity units; MPN: most probable number.

Yamuna River Corridor

The 25 km stretch of the Yamuna extending from Wazirabad to Okhla has been considered "perhaps the most threatened riverine ecosystem in world".[45] Delhi has three distinct geomorphic units—rocky tracts, alluvial uplands and riverine zones. The riverine zones are characterised by floodplains (3,100 hectares), seasonal pools (40 hectares) and marshy areas (110 hectares). The river is regulated in the Delhi stretch with three barrages—the Wazirabad barrage, the Yamuna barrage and the Okhla barrage—to control the flow of the river for the major part of the year, except during the floods. The inputs and outflows in the Delhi stretch of the river are summarised as follows:

Inputs	*Outflows*
Release from Wazirabad barrage	Release from Okhla barrage
Runoff generated from Delhi area	Water for two power plants
Sewage falling into the river	Release into Agra canal
Evapotranspirational losses	

Sewage generated in Delhi is carried by 17 major drains, with outfall into the river in the Wazirabad–Okhla stretch. The CPCB puts the average daily production of sewage in Delhi at 2,100 million litres. Till March 2008, the installed capacities of the sewage treatment plants were 512 MGD.

The water balance profile indicates a peak flow in July (2.3×10^9 million cubic metres) and reaches normal flow in October. Of the total water, 81 per cent enters the Delhi area during the three monsoon months. Soil moisture studies have indicated a negative balance for nine months, implying reduction of groundwater levels in the area. Soil moisture is, however, positive during the monsoon, when a large amount of water is available that is more than sufficient for saturating the floodplain aquifers. The maximum lean-season depth of the water table was found to be 3 metres in the floodplain and neighbouring areas. Recharge of groundwater during the monsoon leads to an increase in the groundwater level from 3 metres to 2.28 metres.

Kumar and Babu tested water quality at Palla, where the river enters Delhi from Haryana; this represents the raw water quality for Delhi's water supply.[46] Total coliforms/100 ml were 5,766.16, and faecal coliforms/100 ml were 1,904.69. Water quality was also tested at Nizamuddin to assess the impact of untreated wastewater discharge into the river. The number of total coliforms/100 ml was found to be 154,764.50 and the number of faecal coliforms/100 ml, 148,454.50—a three-fold rise in total coliforms and an 80-fold rise in faecal coliforms, implying discharge of enormous amounts of untreated sewage with adverse implications for downstream residents.

Groundwater Sources

Groundwater is harnessed through Ranney wells and tubewells. The tubewells sunk by the DJB are deep-bore and are fitted with chlorinators. Ranney wells are first sunk vertically deep into the ground. The boring is then done radically in different directions. This enables the groundwater to flow into the main bore under its natural pressure. Water is chlorinated before distribution. According to estimates made by the Central Ground Water Authority (CGWA), the total annual groundwater recharge potential in Delhi is as follows:[47]

- Rooftop rainwater harvesting: 6 million cubic metres (mcm)
- Check dams in ridge areas: 2 mcm
- Dewatering and refilling of Yamuna floodplain: 78 mcm
- Bhatti mines excavated pits/mine areas: limited additional scope for recharging
- Storage tanks: negligible
- Najafgarh *jheel*/drain: 10 mcm

Natural recharge of groundwater has decreased due to the shrinkage of open area as a consequence of increased construction. Groundwater levels have also registered a marked decline. Unplanned disposal of solid and liquid wastes has simultaneously caused deterioration in the quality of groundwater. Given a per capita demand of 363 lpcd, and a total water demand of 4.8 mcm per day, groundwater plays a major role in fulfilling the demand for water, especially in areas without piped supply. There are about 100,000 groundwater extraction structures registered with the CGWA, though about 400,000 such installations are estimated to be in use. In view of the demand–supply position, newer techniques such as rooftop rainwater harvesting are being promoted by CGWA to augment groundwater storage by such artificial recharge methods. The CGWA is being supported by the DJB and various NGOs in its efforts.

Availability and Consumption

Table 2.8 presents data on the availability of piped water supplied by the DJB to the citizens of Delhi. These figures suggest that the per capita availability of piped water supply has been growing steadily, and is at present well above the World Health Organization (WHO) recommendation of a minimum of 70 lpcd for urban areas. The per capita availability, in gross terms, has increased by nearly 135 per cent between 1951 and 2001 for households with piped water supply.

Table 2.8: Availability of Water in Delhi[48]

Year	*Average supply (million litres/day)*	*Per capita availability (litres/day)*
1951	190	108
1961	440	166
1977	785	190
1981	1,150	185
1991	2,160	231
1995	2,860	272
2001	3,250	254

The availability of water has been defined by water supply bodies as "total supply of water per person". This supply includes the transmission loss of water. The estimates take into account the approximate individual requirements of domestic consumers, industrial and commercial requirements, fire protection (1 per cent of the total demand), garden use (67,000 litres per hectare), free public hydrant supplies and special uses for hotels and other institutions. According to the Delhi Jal Board, the total loss is approximately 30 per cent. Of this, transmission and distribution losses account for 10 per cent, organisational losses such as the cleaning of water mains for 5 per cent, and thefts and pilferage for the remaining losses. The average per capita availability is arrived at by including the quantity actually consumed by industries and other public facilities along with domestic consumption. The average is therefore much above the actual per capita requirement of water. In fact, added to this is the total loss of 30 per cent, including theft and pilferage.

It is interesting to see how Delhi fares in comparison with other Indian cities. Table 2.9 presents the water supply situation across several major cities. Among the Indian cities for which figures are available in the study by Barah et al., Delhi's population coverage of water supply is high, and Hyderabad reportedly has 100 per cent of its population covered by piped water supply. However, in terms of per capita demand for water, Delhi's requirement is very high, and only about 65 per cent of the demand is met in aggregate terms. Hyderabad, with full coverage, is able to meet only 54 per cent of the demand. In terms of meeting per capita demand, Mumbai's performance remains the best at 76.1 per cent, while Chennai is able to fulfil only a meagre 23.5 per cent of its demand.

Table 2.9: Water Supply in Indian Cities[49]

City	*Population coverage of water supply (%)*	*Water demand*[50] *(lpcd)*	*Water availability (lpcd)*
Delhi	98.56	363	237
Mumbai	95.00	180	137
Hyderabad	100.00	120	65
Chennai	95.63	200	47

The total sewage outfall into the Yamuna is far more than can be accounted for against DJB supplies. Currently, about 1,470 million litres of raw water are being drawn daily from the Yamuna river. The standard norms demand that 80 per cent of this water should return as treated wastewater, i.e., 1,170 million litres. In the dry season, about 2,800 million litres of wastewater are being discharged into the Yamuna. This implies that a significant proportion of the daily requirement of water is being met by accessing groundwater.[51] Consumption of untreated groundwater has been repeatedly implicated as a causal factor in the incidence of cholera by a number of studies in Delhi.

It is interesting to take a look at the arbitrary standards for calculating requirements adopted by the Delhi Jal Board—270 lpcd for planned colonies, 153 lpcd for regularised colonies and 50 lpcd for unauthorised colonies and other areas.[52] Thus, a gross violation and undermining of WHO norms occurs right at the planning stage, with further inadequacies and inequities when it comes to actual distribution. It is evident that there is no scientific rationale behind this distribution, as the average for planned colonies is arrived at by adding the requirement of industries and wastage, whereas less privileged communities are provided with only half to one-fourth of the demand without actually explaining the reasons thereof. The DUEIIP report of 2001 does not identify the reasons for this inequity, though it criticises the state of affairs. The DCB and NDMC emerge as the most privileged areas with per capita supplies of 509 and 462 lpcd, respectively. At the other end of the spectrum, the Mehrauli Zone of the DJB has a per capita supply of 29 lpcd only.

Table 2.10: Water Connections and Consumption by Category of Consumer[53]

Year	*2001–02*	*2002–03*	*2003–04*	*2004–05*	*2005–06*	*2006–07*	*2007–08*
No. of metered connections (household/private) (in lakhs)	1,102,326	11,139,373	1,173,693	1,216,542	1,256,040	1,296,094	1,329,953
No. of unmetered connections	313,112	322,460	329,278	335,052	342,867	340,651	345,651
Domestic consumption in gallons (lakh kilo-litres)	9,296	9,624	9,770	9,842	9,770	10,976	11,102
Industrial/commercial consumption (lakh kilo-litres)	1,640	1,312	1,332	1,343	1,332	1,160	1,160
Per capita consumption (lpcd)	40	39.5	39	48.20	47.50	48	48

The production of treated water is 600 MGD. Total raw water available from surface water and groundwater sources is 630 MGD. Does the camouflaging of the industrial use of water affect the DJB statistics on water supply and consumption? To find an answer to this question, we may look at how the consumption of water by different categories in Delhi increased from1980–81 till 1999–2000 (Table 2.10).

In the last 20 years, the number of metered connections increased about 2.75 times, and unmetered connections about 2.25 times. In 1981, there were approximately 45,000 industrial units. Industries increased by 89 per cent for the period 1981–91; in 1991, there were 85,000 units. Industries increased by 47 per cent during 1991–96; there were 125,000 units in 1996. By 1999, there were 140,000 industrial units—a 12 per cent addition during 1996–99.[54] In 1990, 729,000 persons were employed in industries in Delhi, and 1,136,000 persons were employed in industries in 1996.[55] Between 1981 and 1999, industrial units increased by 211.11 per cent.

The DUEIIP report points out that in 2000, 37,000 industrial units were either located in conforming areas or had been proposed for regularisation.[56] Another 25,000 units were cottage industries or single-hand industries. The remaining 64,218 units were in non-conforming areas (about 50 per cent of the total units). Officially, industrial water consumption increased by only 166.80 per cent. Industrial consumption of water as a proportion of total water consumption decreased from 21.04 per cent in 1981 to 15.00 per cent in 1999. This is evidently an underestimation as a lot of water used by the industries is recorded as "domestic". The closure of industries has not made much difference.

Between 1981 and 1999, population increased by 115 per cent and domestic water consumption increased by 448 per cent. However, the increase in per capita consumption has been marginal during the period for which data is available (1990–91 to 1999–2000)—from 220.63 lpcd to 229.50 lpcd. The aggregate figures fail to capture the reality of the situation in terms of access to safe water sources and availability of adequate quantity across different socio-economic groups within Delhi.[57] Several studies have highlighted the lack of availability of an adequate quantity of water among poorer households.[58] There is variation in the exact quantity available to the households as reported by these studies.[59] However, they all highlight the fact that the urban poor of Delhi have very little access to an adequate quantity of safe piped water supply.[60] According to estimates made by the DJB, the population covered by piped water had grown from 48.6 per cent in 1967 to 90 per cent by 1992. The crucial question is, what proportion of this 90 per cent population's demand was met by piped sources of water?[61]

The DUEIIP report of 2001 explored the inequity in water supply. It observed that 10 per cent of the population had no piped water supply, and 30 per cent had grossly inadequate access. It estimated that, in 1995, nearly two-thirds of the population had substandard housing and infrastructure across different settlement types. Further, the DUEIIP reported that 40 per cent of the population in Delhi were below the poverty line. In essence, poverty coupled with settlements with poor infrastructure conditions implied that at least half the population of Delhi did not have access to more than 25 lpcd, and some had even less.

Barah et al. report that per capita consumption of water in Delhi ranged from 313 lpcd in affluent households to 140 lpcd in relatively less well-off households, and a meagre 16 lpcd for slum households in 1992–93.[62] Indirect evidence is provided for the question of distribution of water across socio-economic classes by a study conducted by the Asian Development Bank (ADB) in 1991–92 through the analysis of 1,000 water bills of households in Delhi sampled by social class (Table 2.11).

Table 2.11 : Analysis of 1,000 Water Bills[63]

Income class	*Monthly consumption (kl)*
Affluent class	47
Middle class	34
Lower-income group	25
Urban poor (with home connections)	21

The ADB study findings relate to consumers with legal metered connections who have relatively better availability of water. The households belonging to the lowest socio-economic group reported by Barah et al. are users of free public hydrant supply, and therefore receive lower quantities. It is again reiterated that the urban poor in Delhi receive water far below the WHO benchmark, and therefore remain highly vulnerable to waterborne diseases.

DRINKING WATER: MYRIAD PATHWAYS TO CONTAMINATION

Deep Tubewells

The deep tubewells are often not laid deep enough. Chlorinators need regular maintenance, and the use of chemicals needs to be carefully monitored. Safety of water supplies depends crucially on the human resources deployed. When chlorinators are out of order, it takes up to several weeks to set them right. Non-supply of bleaching powder may also be a source of potential breakdown of the safety chain. Outbreaks of cholera and other waterborne diseases (viral hepatitis A and E and enteric fever) have occurred in clusters supplied by deep tubewells lacking regular chlorination. Water extracted through deep tubewells (with chlorinators) is supplied in some resettlement and regularised colonies of the South and Central Zones and the rural areas. Deep tubewells are also the most important and often the only source of water supply in cooperative group housing societies (owned by the middle class), where they run without chlorinators almost as a rule.

Ranney Wells

Ranney wells have a minor contribution to make in the total water consumed in Delhi. The DJB operates Ranney wells in Narela, Civil Lines and Shahdara (South), zones that are located near the Yamuna. These are wells bored deep into the ground with lateral channels that facilitate the entry of subsoil water into the main bore. The water is drawn through pumps and supplied through a piped network after chlorination. The main risks of contamination lie in inadequate treatment of the water before consumption. Otherwise, like the municipal piped water supply, these wells are a relatively safe source of water.

"Sintex Tanks"

Now a generic term for large plastic storage tanks (the leading brand being "Sintex"), these tanks are placed in notified JJ clusters, and are regularly filled by tankers of the DJB. The tankers are filled from the different filling points of the DJB that receive piped supply. Contamination occurs due to people dipping their buckets and other containers into these tanks.

Tankers

Tankers of the DJB supply water by making trips to areas without piped water supply, where the community fills up its containers. It is quite common to see containers or rubber pipes being dipped into these tankers, leading to possible contamination. After the formation of the DJB, tanker services were greatly augmented; in the summer of 2002, there were about 1,000 tankers in operation in the field daily with each tanker making an average of about three to four trips. Unauthorised colonies have been included in the network of tanker supply in a major way. The Delhi Jal Board, through a notification in 2000, banned the sale of water through private tankers. Private water supply companies were directed to carry the message "not to be used for drinking purposes" on their tankers, and also not to sell it for that purpose. For bulk consumers such as hotels, food trades and congregations like marriage parties, private tankers continue to supply drinking water. The DJB also has facilities to provide drinking water through tankers for such occasions, on payment. The fact remains that private tankers, owned and operated by dominant groups from the peripheral villages of the South and Najafgarh Zones and adjacent districts of Haryana, continue to be a significant source of water supply for these bulk consumers.

Deep-Bore Handpumps/Pumps

Deep-bore handpumps are a suspect source, more likely to be unsafe than safe. In areas where sanitation is poor and open defecation is common, water tables up to depths of 60–80 feet maybe contaminated. In addition, technical flaws in not making such pumps deep enough also render them unsafe. Deep-bore pumps with attached filtration or treatment plants are safe. Contamination from deep-bore pumps with treatment facilities is rare, since these are better maintained as they belong either to institutions (hotels, commercial complexes) or to the more affluent.

Shallow Handpumps

Shallow handpumps are used mainly by the lower socio-economic groups, and usually draw contaminated groundwater from the superficial water table. The DJB, as a policy, paints these in red colour to signal the dangers involved in consuming this water. This practice started during the 1988 epidemic when large numbers of handpumps were painted red, but only a few were accompanied by written warnings—"not safe for drinking purposes". Despite such "warnings", handpumps remain the mainstay of water supply for the majority of the urban poor, as also for unauthorised colonies where piped supply is either not available, or is available in quantities that are insufficient due to the pressure being low or inadequate duration of supply. Even though mothers (and often fathers) in households may collect drinking water from safe sources that entail paying for the water or incurring travel costs, it is very often the case that children playing in the open drink water directly from the handpumps.

Problem of Booster Pumps

Booster pumps have become a common means of augmenting water supply in homes in middle- and upper-income groups. These pumps augment quantity at the cost of the quality of water. They are notorious for sucking in contaminants through minor cracks in the pipelines (if present). In 1994, booster pumps in conjunction with faults in the piped supply caused a major hepatitis E outbreak in Govind Puri and Kalkaji Janta Flats (Central Zone) along with sporadic cases of cholera between January and March. Manual boosters are installed by puncturing DJB pipelines in low-income colonies (typically in resettlement colonies and JJ clusters), with public hydrants to augment supply, particularly in low-pressure situations. They are as harmful as electrically operated booster pumps.

COMPROMISES, NOT CHOICES

Given the ground realities of water sources and water supply networks, it is important to examine the accessibility of safe water sources and the availability of adequate safe water in different colonies. In the absence of adequate safe water, communities take recourse to accessing unsafe sources to meet their requirements, and thus become vulnerable to waterborne diseases including diarrhoeal diseases (see Figures 2.2–2.5).

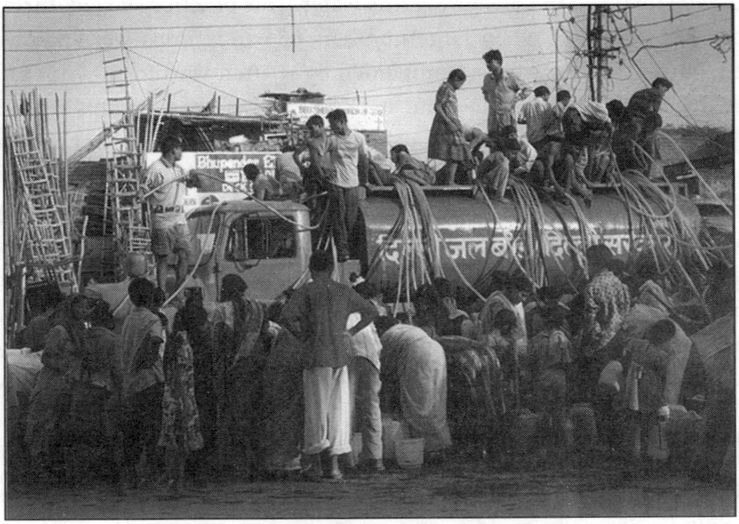

Figure 2.2: Water Scarcity in a South Delhi Slum. Photograph by author.

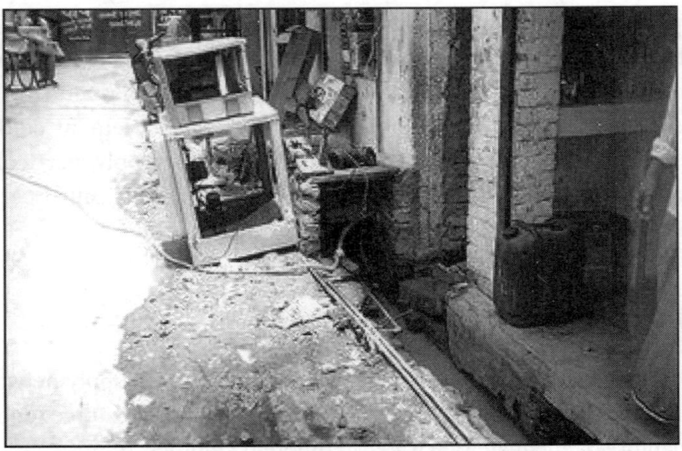

Figure 2.3: Water Pipelines Passing through Open Drains.
Photograph by author.

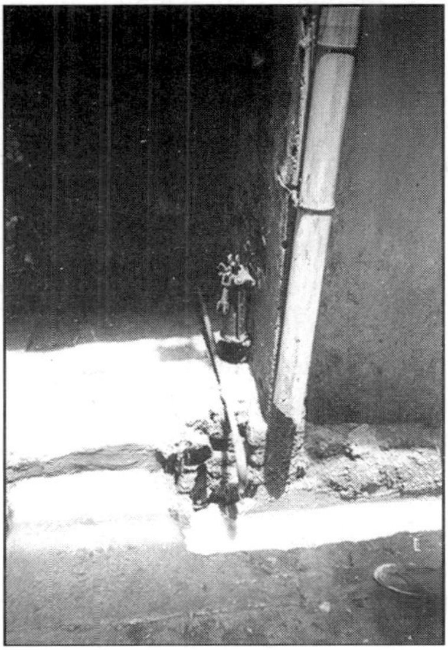

Figure 2.4: An On-line Booster in an Urbanised Village.
Photograph by author.

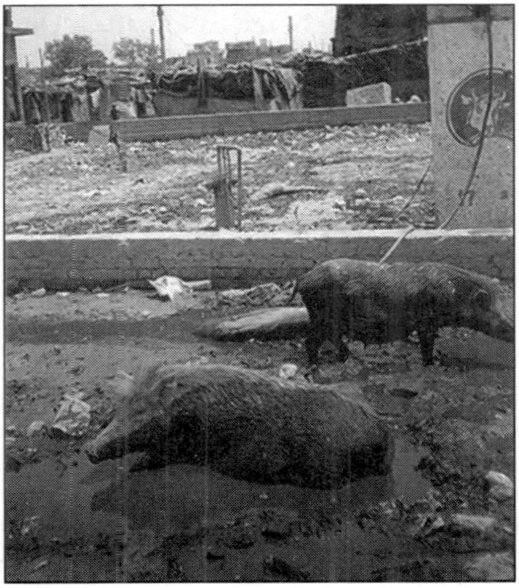

Figure 2.5: A Deep-Bore Pump amidst Unhygienic Conditions.
Photograph by author.

Inadequacy forces people to supplement the piped supply with alternative means, varying according to affordability for the household, and with consequences for the quality of the water procured. There are three main alternatives—handpumps, electric (motor) pumps and booster pumps. Handpumps are found across all income classes. The higher socio-economic classes (comprising better-informed residents) generally do not use handpumped water for drinking. Lower socio-economic groups who face both limited access to piped supply and limited resources to invest in alternatives (other than shallow handpumps) are exposed most to the risks of consuming contaminated water. The lowest-income groups reside in the slum clusters. To cater to these clusters, pipelines have been laid and public hydrants/public standposts have been installed. Water supply is generally intermittent, and the per capita availability is inadequate to meet even drinking and cooking requirements. Water from safe sources is also provided to these communities through storage tanks and tankers (plied by the DJB). These households cannot afford individual handpumps, and shallow handpumps have been built through community initiatives.

When a slum cluster is relocated to a new site, safe water supply is always one of the most critical vulnerability factors. The responsibility of providing safe water to a relocated cluster belongs to the Slum and JJ Department. In the 1990s phase of relocation, these clusters faced severe water supply problems. There were diarrhoeal disease outbreaks in some of these clusters, including the deaths of several children that took place on account of drinking contaminated water from a private tanker. Cholera began to be reported regularly from some of the newly relocated clusters. In a few clusters, where the Housing and Urban Development Corporation (HUDCO) was involved in the provision of basic amenities, the situation was better.

Households in unauthorised colonies are relatively better off socio-economically than communities residing in the resettlement colonies and slum clusters. They depend, however, entirely on individual initiatives for procuring water. While shallow handpumps remain a major source through which groundwater is accessed, electric pumps are also popular among the middle-income groups residing in unauthorised colonies. Deep-bore tubewells are found mainly among the upper-income categories, as these call for substantial investments. The middle-income groups install tubewells of relatively less depth, and the water drawn is not of satisfactory quality.

The summer and monsoon months create a set of circumstances that expose lower-income groups to much greater levels of contamination of their water supplies. During summer, the demand for water goes up while the supply of water is often reduced due to a fall in the raw water made available from the river (Yamuna) upstream. This shortage in water availability (primarily due to increased demand) is reflected in higher domestic storage of water. Storage practices therefore become crucial in determining the quality of the water being used by a particular household. The risks of contamination faced by the poorer households is greater, since they can least afford the better means of storage, and also because they are hit the hardest by shortfalls in piped supply. As a result, greater domestic contamination occurs in these families as they have less water available for maintaining domestic and personal hygiene.

During the rainy season, the problem is quite different. The soluble nature of faecal and other waste matters implies greater and faster dispersion of the wastes. As a result, groundwater gets contaminated more easily during this period than during the dry months. Contamination of groundwater in turn means that all income classes who are dependent on it get affected. The poor are least able to take steps to purify this water.

Two systems of purification are followed at the household level. Among the poorest sections (JJ clusters and unauthorised colonies), the municipal authorities distribute chlorine tablets on a regular basis for use in all containers where water is stored by the household. The higher socio-economic classes undertake individual initiatives like filtration devices and/or boiling the drinking water.

The quality of water available to a household is also determined by the method of waste disposal, which in turn is dependent on neighbourhood factors and the available infrastructure. The relationship between the quality of water and the manner of waste disposal is particularly important when water is drawn from individual sources. In planned areas, with proper sanitary latrines and sewerage systems, accumulated wastes pose less of a threat to the water available to the household. Resettlement colonies are serviced by community latrines, which are generally connected to septic tanks. Septic tanks need careful adherence to standards during construction and subsequent maintenance. Improper maintenance of these tanks is an important cause of groundwater contamination. With the water table getting contaminated, households that access handpumps are at greater risk. The depths from which water is drawn, as well as the extent to which the water table is contaminated, would determine the actual extent of exposure. The service provider is responsible for maintaining these community latrines as well as the septic tanks. In addition, open defecation (mostly by children) is a major contaminant of the superficial water table.

Unauthorised colonies do not have any sewer lines. Communities living in slum clusters cannot afford to construct individual sanitary latrines. As a result, open defecation becomes a major cause of groundwater contamination. In higher-income settlements, sanitary latrines are connected to individual septic tanks. Due to improper construction and maintenance, water table contamination is common. Thus, for all those who are forced to rely on individual initiatives for their water supply, ensuring proper waste disposal methods becomes critical to maintaining the quality of the water consumed. Solid waste collection and disposal is beyond the realm of the individual household. This is an obligatory function of local bodies under the acts governing them. While these services are deficient to varying extents in slum clusters, resettlement colonies and urbanised villages, unauthorised colonies are not entitled to such services owing to their legal status (or rather, the lack of it). As the area under occupation increases within an unauthorised colony, the groundwater gets increasingly contaminated, more so where open defecation is a common practice.

In households in unauthorised and regularised colonies, residents who can afford it construct sanitary latrines that are connected to septic tanks, as sewerage services are non-existent. Almost as a rule, the households also have handpumps. Due to improper construction of septic tanks, it is often the case that the septic tank contaminates the groundwater that the handpump draws. As a result, faecal contamination of drinking water occurs, giving rise to waterborne diseases and especially diarrhoeal diseases.

There is a greater felt need for water supply than for sewers. Water pipes are also technically much easier to install than sewer connections, which often require demolition of existing toilets. As a result, it is common in regularised colonies to find water connections without adequate sewer connections. Individuals in such cases discharge their wastes into street drains. These street drains end in open nullahs, which often do not have smooth flows and are not equipped to handle large volumes of liquid waste. As more and more vacant land is brought under construction for residential (and commercial) purposes, the drains become clogged owing to increasing amounts of liquid waste discharges (and also the dumping of solid waste). When water pipes are laid in these regularised colonies, they cut across these existing street drains. Water supplied through these pipes is susceptible to contamination from the stagnant or poorly flowing street drains. Later, when sewer lines are laid down, the water and sewer lines are in close proximity. In such situations, where intermittent water supply is a rule, contaminants often get sucked in from the sewer lines through minor cracks and other damages in the pipes whenever there is negative pressure in the water lines.

The primary responsibility for maintaining water quality surveillance lies with the Delhi Jal Board. Each water treatment plant has its own water quality surveillance team and laboratory that check water quality in the areas served by water from the plant. Quality checks in water treatment plants are rigorous; there are possibilities of contamination of piped water supplies during the transmission process, though. This was confirmed through informal interviews with members of the water quality surveillance teams. Cross-checking among different units or by central units can make the system transparent and effective.

The MCD and the National Institute of Communicable Diseases (NICD) also maintain water quality surveillance on a random basis through their field staff. Several NGOs and the mobile health services of the Directorate of Health Services have also joined in this endeavour. Discussions with these agencies revealed that:

- Shallow handpumps, almost as a rule, test unfit for human consumption.
- Deep-bore tubewells also often test unfit—particularly in areas that are endemic for waterborne diseases.
- Tankers and community-level storage tanks of the DJB generally tested fit.

- Public hydrants were also safe by and large, except for instances of focal contamination.
- Illegal piped connections sometimes failed the test because of tampering of pipelines and resultant contamination.
- Often, the service pipes of individual households were not properly maintained or passed through drains; in those cases, water from the consumer end of the household tested unfit though the main supply was fit for human consumption.
- Domestic contamination of a laboratory-proven safe supply was high, and was a matter of concern as this can be tackled by correcting factors associated with storage—intermittent supply, irregularity and inadequacy—as also by improvement of personal hygiene.
- Drawing of water by the use of on-line boosters also renders the piped supply unsafe, as has been established by laboratory tests.

P. Dhar tested water samples from 23 colonies/areas of Delhi vulnerable to waterborne diseases during the vulnerable season.[64] The study reported that:

- Overall, 72 per cent of non-piped sources and 34 per cent of piped sources tested unfit.
- Ninety-three per cent of shallow handpumps tested unfit.
- All deep-bore tubewells failed the test.
- Legal piped supply in individual households and public hydrants tested unfit for 37.5 per cent and 31.6 per cent of the samples, respectively.
- Sixty per cent of illegal piped supplies in individual households tested unfit.
- One hundred per cent of deep-bore handpumps tested unfit.

It can thus be concluded that the groundwater in Delhi is highly contaminated, irrespective of the depth from which it is accessed. Piped water supply is also liable to be contaminated for a complex set of reasons. In-migration coupled with a high intrinsic growth rate poses challenges to the provision of housing and infrastructure, to which the state has failed to respond adequately. Though resource constraints may exist in absolute terms, Delhi, being the capital city, has always had the privilege of higher resource inputs as compared to other metropolitan cities. The distribution and utilisation of resources for planning and maintenance of infrastructure has been disproportionate, resulting in large groups of population remaining deprived of civic amenities. The planning process has not accounted for the needs of the underprivileged; whatever facilities are available for these sections are for the most part a positive fallout of "votebank politics". The implications of this for public health is immense. Lack of adequate safe water supply and of safe disposal of solid and liquid wastes has had obvious impacts in terms of waterborne diseases. The following chapter describes the time trends of cholera in India, including the arrival of the El Tor strain in Delhi and the city's subsequent emergence as one of the hotspots of cholera in the country. *Vibrio cholerae* El Tor succeeded due to failures in providing the minimum basic amenities for the vulnerable population in Delhi.

NOTES

1. The decadal growth rate of the urban population was +106.58 per cent.
2. Francois Bernier, *Travels in the Mogul Empire*, trans. Archibald Constable, reprint (Delhi: Low Price Publication, 1989), 274.
3. Jagmohan, *Rebuilding Shahjahanabad* (New Delhi: Vikas, 1975).
4. Municipal Corporation of Delhi (MCD), *Civic Guide* (New Delhi: MCD, 1995).
5. Narayani Gupta, "Military Security and Urban Development: A Case Study of Delhi 1857–1912", *Modern Asian Studies* 5, no. 1, 1971, 61–77.
6. The lowest socio-economic category for whom Lutyens had planned for housing, were clerks in the government services.
7. Ritu Priya, "Town Planning, Public Health and Urban Poor: Some Exploration from Delhi", *Economic and Political Weekly* 28, no. 17, 1993, 824–34.
8. Stephen Legg, *Spaces of Colonialism: Delhi's Urban Governmentalities* (Oxford: Wiley Blackwell, 2007), 164.
9. Priya, "Town Planning, Public Health and Urban Poor".
10. Ibid.
11. V. K. R. V. Rao and P. B. Desai, "Greater Delhi—A Study in Urbanisation 1940–57", Planning Commission, Government of India, New Delhi, 1965.
12. The 1981 census reported a population of 6.2 million.
13. Priya, "Town Planning, Public Health and Urban Poor".

14. Ibid.
15. V. Nath, "Planning for Delhi and National Capital Region: Review of Plan Formulation and Implementation", *Economic and Political Weekly* 30, no. 35, 1995, 2194–202.
16. Nath, "Planning for Delhi and National Capital Region".
17. MCD, *Civic Guide.*
18. Delhi Development Authority (DDA), *Master Plan for Delhi, 1990* (New Delhi: DDA, 1990).
19. MCD, *Civic Guide.*
20. Ibid.
21. Ministry of Environment and Forests, Government of India, and Planning Department, Government of the National Capital Territory of Delhi. *Delhi 21: Delhi Urban Environment and Infrastructure Improvement Project (DUEIIP)* (Delhi: Government of India and Government of NCT of Delhi, 2001), http://delhiplanning.nic.in/Reports/Delhi21/Delhi-21.pdf (accessed 4 March 2012)(henceforth DUEIIP report).
22. DUEIIP report, 6. The Government of Delhi has consistently argued that its lack of proper control over key agencies like the Municipal Corporation of Delhi and the Delhi Development Authority is a major obstacles to planned development.
23. Nath, "Planning for Delhi and National Capital Region".
24. P. G. Dhar Chakravarti, "Delhi's Ongoing Debate on Informal Settlements and Work Places: Issues of Environmental Jurisprudence", Paper presented at the International Workshop on Coping with Informality and Illegality in Human Settlements in Developing Cities, Leuven and Brussels, Belgium, 23–26 May 2001.
25. MCD, *Civic Guide; Census of India*, Provisional Population Totals 2001: NCT of Delhi.
26. Directorate of Economics and Statistics, *Delhi Statistical Handbook, 2008* (New Delhi: Government of Delhi, 2008).
27. Department of Planning, *Economic Survey of Delhi, 2001–02* (New Delhi: Government of National Capital Territory of Delhi, 2002).
28. Directorate of Economics and Statistics, *Delhi Statistical Handbook, 2002* (New Delhi: Government of Delhi 2002); Directorate of Economics and Statistics, Delhi Statistical Handbook, 2008.
29. DUEIIP report.
30. Priya, "Town Planning, Public Health and Urban Poor".
31. Pay-and-use Jan Suvidha complexes with toilets and bathrooms are provided at the community level; mobile toilet vans are deployed wherever Jan Suvidha

complexes cannot be provided. More such pay-and-use complexes have been constructed recently under the Yamuna Action Plan.

32. DUEIIP report.
33. Ibid.
34. M. Munasinghe, "The Economist's Approach to Sustainable Development", in *Making Development Sustainable: From Concepts to Action*, eds. I. Serageldin and A. Steer, Environmentally Sustainable Development Occasional Paper Series No. 2 (Washington, D.C.: World Bank, 1994), 13–16.
35. Central Pollution Control Board (CPCB), *Status of Solid Waste Generation, Collection, Treatment and Disposal in Metrocities* (New Delhi: CPCB, 2000).
36. Tata Energy Research Institute (TERI), *Tata Energy Data Directory and Yearbook (TEDDY) 1999/2000* (New Delhi: TERI, 1999).
37. Mufeed Sharholy et al., "Municipal Solid Waste Management in Indian Cities—A Review", *Waste Management* 28, no. 2, 2008, 459–67.
38. DUEIIP report.
39. Ibid.
40. CPCB, *Management of Municipal Solid Waste in Delhi and Suggested Action Plan*, http://www.cpcb.nic.in/Highlights/2006/MUNICIPAL SOLID WASTE MANAGEMENT[1].pdf (accessed 12 December 2010).
41. Munasinghe, "The Economist's Approach to Sustainable Development".
42. Narayani Gupta, *Delhi between the Two Empires, 1803–1931: Society, Government and Urban Growth* (Delhi: Oxford University Press, 1981).
43. Personal communication, Office of the Chief Executive Officer, Delhi Jal Board, 2000.
44. Personal communication, Office of the Additional CEO, Delhi Jal Board, 2000.
45. P. Kumar and C. R. Babu, "Valuation of Ecological Functions and Benefits: A Case Study of Wetlands Ecosystem along the Yamuna River Corridors of Delhi Region", Mimeograph, Institute of Economic Growth, Delhi, 2001.
46. P. Kumar and Babu, "Valuation of Ecological Functions and Benefits".
47. Central Ground Water Authority, cgwb.gov.in/GroundWater/CGWA per cent20guidelines per cent20for per cent20NOC per cent201.pdf (accessed November 2010).
48. Personal communication, DWSSDU, 1997.
49. B. C. Barah, V. Sipahimalani and P. Dhar, "Urban Water Supply and Sanitation", in *Economic Instruments for Environment Sustainability*, ed. U. Sankar and O. P. Mathur (New Delhi: National Institute of Public Finance and Policy and Madras School of Economics, 1998), 53–65.

50. Water demand: assessment of requirements by the different water supply agencies.
51. DUEIIP report.
52. Ibid.
53. Directorate of Economics and Statistics, *Delhi Statistical Handbook 2008.*
54. DUEIIP report.
55. Directorate of Economics and Statistics, *Delhi Statistical Handbook 2000* (New Delhi: Government of Delhi, 2000).
56. DUEIIP report.
57. Barah et al., "Urban Water Supply and Sanitation".
58. R. Dasgupta, "Mapping Cholera Vulnerability in Delhi: An Ecosocial Perspective", *Asian Journal of Water, Environment and Pollution* 7, no. 1, 2010, 19–26.
59. A. Kundu, "Urban Development, Infrastructure Financing and Emerging System of Governance in India: A Perspective", *Social and Human Sciences* 4, no. 15, 2001, http://digital-library.unesco.org (accessed 7 January 2004).
60. Marie-Helene Zerah, "Household Strategies for Coping with Unreliable Water Supplies: The Case of Delhi", *Habitat International* 24, no. 3, 2000, 295–307.
61. P. Dasgupta, "Valuing Health Damages from Water Pollution in Urban Delhi, India: A Health Production Function Approach", *Environment and Development Economics* 9, no. 1, 2004, 83–106.
62. Barah et al., "Urban Water Supply and Sanitation".
63. Asian Development Bank, Water Utilities Data Book, 1993, http://www.adb.org/documents/books/second_water_utilities/second_water_utilities.pdf (accessed 4 March 2012).
64. P. Dhar, "Economic Issues Relating to Water Contamination and Waste Disposal: A Case Analysis of Urban Development in Delhi" (Unpublished diss., Jawaharlal Nehru University, 2000).

3

Time Trends of Cholera

The Rise and Fall of Vibrio Strains

The history of cholera epidemics, spanning over nearly two centuries, makes for an interesting study of disease dynamics over time, given the changing biological nature of the agent. The classical biotype caused cholera pandemics in India from 1817 to 1964, till the arrival of *Vibrio cholerae* El Tor. The early history of cholera in India has been closely linked with large religious fairs such as the Kumbhmela and the states response to them. The close association with the melas led to the spread of cholera to adjacent north Indian states. The expansion of the railway network and the consequent mobility of populations added a new force to the spread of the disease.

Ideas regarding the causality of cholera and preventive strategies emerged in India in the nineteenth century. Classical cholera declined in a major way after the 1920s, but was replaced by *Vibrio cholerae* El Tor. This marked the beginning of the seventh (and current) cholera pandemic, which first affected India in 1964. While Bengal was the home of classical cholera, the El Tor strain established itself in other states of India and acquired a new pattern of endemicity. The fast-expanding urban milieu and the emergence of the urban poor as a sizeable population group saw the emergence of cholera as an urban health problem. Yet another "novel" strain appeared in 1992–93, triggering a possible eighth pandemic. But the new strain (O139 Bengal) failed to prevail over El Tor, which soon regained its primacy.

PANDEMICS OF THE CLASSICAL BIOTYPE

In the colonial history of India, cholera occupied an important place as a public health problem and as a political issue. Hospital boards were established in Madras and Calcutta in 1786, as prior to that year "no regular reports on the incidence of cholera among the Europeans and the native soldiers were available".[1] The west was not much concerned about cholera till Europe was affected during the 1830s, when the disease was treated with the same concern as the import of yellow fever from West Africa and the West Indies.[2] Collection of data did not begin until the late 1860s; figures available for reported deaths during the nineteenth century are therefore not considered accurate.

Cholera was monitored during the nineteenth century and the first half of the twentieth century by deaths and/or annual mortality rates. This was on account of the high case fatality rate (CFR) of cholera. Better statistics were available from the 1870s. Mortality data began to be collected systematically with the epidemic of 1865 in Bengal. Between 1817 and 1865, an estimated 15 million deaths occurred in British India, and a further 23 million deaths are estimated to have occurred between 1865 and 1947.[3] During the last quarter of the nineteenth century, on an average, the annual cholera mortality rate of British India was 1.75 per thousand population. In 1874, this rate was at a low of 0.16 per thousand. British India was badly affected in 1900; cholera mortality peaked to 3.70 per 1,000 in 1900 and later stabilised to about three per thousand by 1906. Though it is customary to describe the history of cholera in terms of pandemics, scholars disagree on the dates of onset and the duration of successive pandemics.

First Pandemic

During the last quarter of the eighteenth century, cholera was prevalent both in the eastern and in the western coastal areas of India and also beyond the subcontinent. The first pandemic originated in 1817, first reported on 23 August by the civil surgeon of Jessore (now in Bangladesh). The basin between the Ganga and the Brahmaputra rivers experienced storms and very heavy rainfall in early August. Calcutta was affected at about the same time, and the disease spread beyond the borders of Bengal.

This was confirmed by the Calcutta Medical Board; the epidemic affected 195,935 square miles of Bengal Province.[4] Later during the year, cholera was reported outside Bengal. The army of the Marquis of Hastings then camping at Bundelkhand was severely affected. In 1818, cholera spread to northern India. Agra and Delhi were affected in 1818; Punjab reported its first case in 1820.

No overall estimates of mortality are available for the epidemic of 1817–21. On the basis of mortality figures for certain areas of Bengal and among troops of the East India Company, Moreau de Jonnes, a French physician, calculated that during 1817–31 cholera affected one-tenth of the population of British India and killed one-sixteenth. De Jonnes, whose methodology has been criticised, postulated an average annual mortality of 1.25 million and a total of 18 million deaths for the period. Other estimates put the total cholera deaths for India at 40 to 50 million.

Whatever the approximations may be, the 1817 epidemic came nearly three decades after the last recorded epidemic of the 1780s; the population was immunologically vulnerable, resulting in a high attack rate and mortality rate. It is important to recognise that 1815 and particularly 1817 were years marked by extremely heavy rainfall, severe floods and harvest failures. The year 1816 was extraordinarily hot and dry. Though the most severe epidemics have later been associated with famines, there was no famine in Bengal or other parts of India during that period. However, the poor and the undernourished were the worst affected in the 1817–21 epidemic. Though European residents were alarmed at the spread of cholera, they were not seriously affected. They were protected partly by relatively healthy living conditions and later (by the 1850s) by the emphasis on clean drinking water and personal hygiene. Mortality among slum dwellers in Calcutta was high, in comparison to the "higher classes of Native and Europeans".[5] This pattern was also confirmed from observations in Bombay and Madras.[6]

Second and Third Pandemics

The second pandemic also originated in Bengal in 1826 and spread to upstream regions of the rivers Ganga and Yamuna. It reached Punjab after affecting the United Provinces and Delhi in 1827. During a later, resurgent phase of the second pandemic, cholera again reached Delhi by an indirect yet interesting route. Cholera was raging in southern Bengal in 1840. Troops were being sent from Calcutta (and Madras) to China. These troops from Calcutta were considered to have "exported" cholera from Bengal to the Straits Settlements and then into China—affecting first Chushan Island outside Shanghai in July 1840, and then, over the next two years, various parts of the mainland. The spread of cholera followed the trade routes from China, affecting Kashgar, Yarkund, Kokand and Bukhara in succession, leaving a trail of death in these trading centres. Cholera reached Kabul in 1844 from Bukhara, which had earlier been affected in 1829 following a direct spread from India. In 1844, however, it returned to India, reaching Punjab, from where it extended south-west to Karachi and south-east to Delhi, affecting both these cities in 1845.

The third pandemic, following a recrudescence in India, was conspicuous for its spread to countries that had till then not been affected seriously by the disease. During the later phase of the pandemic in 1859, there was a spurt of cases in Bengal. The disease spread to Persia, Mesopotamia and Arabia, and thereafter to Russia.

Fourth Pandemic

The fourth pandemic began in 1863. There was a major epidemic in Mecca in 1865, considered by some scholars to have been imported from India by Haj pilgrims. Others disagreed and opined that the outbreak was a result of a recrudescence of infection already present in Mecca. However, all agreed that the infection had spread from Mecca to a large number of countries. The earliest instance of a cholera epidemic spreading widely from the Kumbhmela occurred in April 1867 at Hardwar, and the mela was recognised as a transmission route for the first time during this pandemic.[7]

The year 1877 was an epidemic year in India. In Madras Presidency in 1877, mortality due to cholera was 12.20 per 1,000. Four districts also experienced famine at this time; in those districts, mortality due to cholera rose to 20–25 per 1,000. Overall, at the height of the epidemic, cholera accounted for about 10 per cent of the annual mortality.[8] The poor were the worst affected when cholera epidemics coincided with famines.[9] This was evident in the second half of the nineteenth century, a period of frequent and widespread famines—in Madras Presidency in 1866 and 1877, and in Bombay Presidency in 1877 and 1900.

In Madras Presidency, the cholera epidemic of 1869–71 resulted in nearly 100,000 deaths. Cholera declined to low levels in 1873 (440 deaths) and 1874 (313 deaths). In 1875, there were 94,546 deaths, and the situation became worse in 1876 with 148,193 deaths. Drought and famine began in the Presidency at this stage of the epidemic, and annual mortality rose to 357,430 in 1877. Though the famine reached its peak in September 1877, cholera mortality was already showing a downward trend from February. Undoubtedly, however, cholera mortality tended to peak when the famine was at its most severe. In Madras Presidency during the 1877 famine and epidemic, cholera mortality was 18 per 1,000 in the 10 districts worst affected by famine, whereas in the six districts that were least affected, cholera mortality was 4.6 per 1,000.[10]

Hot and dry conditions, though not conducive to the survival of *Vibrio cholerae*, were responsible for the scarcity of drinking water. Villagers accessed fewer available sources of water, which were liable to contamination and acted as sources of infection. Consumption of roots, leaves and other surrogate foods in desperation during famine conditions was generally responsible for diarrhoeal diseases. The mobility of famine-affected communities in search of food and their concentration in relief camps facilitated the spread of the disease. The inadequate medical relief provided by the state failed to compensate for family and community care systems, which collapsed in such disaster situations. The association of famine and high cholera mortality underscored the fact that issues of poverty, food availability, hygiene and medical relief were not handled well by the colonial regime.

Fifth and Sixth Pandemics

The fifth cholera pandemic caused considerably less havoc than the previous four pandemics. It was during this pandemic (generally agreed to have occurred from 1881 to 1896) that Robert Koch, studying the outbreaks in Egypt and Calcutta, proved in 1883–84 that cholera was the result of a gastrointestinal infection. There were epidemics in India in 1881, with particularly severe outbreaks in Punjab, especially in Lahore. In 1891, there were 169,013 deaths in the Kumbhmela at Hardwar. Rogers considered that following the fair, cholera spread to the United Provinces and Punjab, and then spread by overland route to Afghanistan, Persia, southern Russia and other countries of Europe in the 1892–95 phase of this pandemic.[11] A similar situation occurred in 1894 following the Allahabad Kumbhmela.

The sixth pandemic lasted for nearly 25 years. Cholera cases in India had begun to increase since 1899, with major outbreaks in Calcutta and Bombay in 1900. Madras was also affected. Since 1900, cholera had begun spreading from India to other countries. There was a resurgence of cholera in some countries between 1908 and 1910; some authors have linked this to the increase in cholera cases in India during 1905–08. There were 189,955 cholera deaths in India in 1904. Between 1905 and 1908, there were an average of about 526,000 deaths each year. There were nearly 150,000 deaths in the 1906 Kumbhmela at Allahabad during this phase; the mela is also considered to have contributed to the epidemic. In 1909, deaths declined by about half to 227,842.[12] The high incidence of cholera in Punjab was linked to the spread of infection from melas at Hardwar.[13] Zurbrigg links malaria deaths in Punjab not only to climatic factors, as per the conventional epidemiological understanding.[14] She highlights the importance of the role of famines (hunger and malnutrition).[15] Epidemics of cholera in Punjab in 1901, 1906 and 1908 can clearly be correlated with famine conditions. In fact, in 1908 there were no fairs; yet there was an increased incidence of cholera.

The sixth pandemic ended in the early 1920s, following which there was a general decline in mortality due to cholera. Between 1900 and 1920, the annual mortality rate in India declined from about 112 per 100,000 to about 50 per 100,000. The decline continued; in 1947 there were about 30 cholera deaths per 100,000 population, and by 1963 this had decreased to 4.3 cholera deaths per 100,000 population.[16] The 1920–63 phase of cholera in India is characterised by an endemic situation in different states with some fluctuations. There were two peaks in this phase—1927–31 and 1941–45. El Tor cholera began to be detected in India in 1964. Epidemic increase of cholera cases in 1924 occurred simultaneously in Bengal, Bihar, Orissa, Assam and the United Provinces as early as March–April. With the onset of the monsoon, cases peaked in Bihar and Orissa. Punjab was affected in July, but the epidemic did not proceed to the North-Western Frontier Provinces (NWFP).

The years 1925 and 1926 were not epidemic years in India, and cholera remained generally confined to Bengal. Meanwhile, from Punjab, cholera spread to Kashmir in April 1925, where the epidemic continued till October, with the north Kashmir province being the worst affected. In south India, the months of January in both years (1925 and 1926) reported the maximum cases; the infection spread to Ceylon as well. Cases of cholera began to rise again from April 1927 in the Bengal and Madras Presidencies, followed by the United Provinces, Bihar and Orissa. Soon it spread to Punjab, the Central Provinces, Hyderabad and Bombay Presidency. Peaks were recorded in Bengal in November 1927 and March 1928, and cholera affected Bihar, the United Provinces and Punjab earlier than the usual months in 1928. Madras Presidency was affected in June 1928, with the south-eastern districts being the worst affected. Nearly 90 per cent of the deaths in 1928 were reported from the United Provinces, Bihar, Orissa, Bengal and the Madras Presidency. During 1930, cholera remained at high levels in Bihar, Orissa and the United Provinces, but Bengal registered a decline. This epidemic began in Bengal and, by April, had affected the United Provinces (and Bihar and Orissa). It also spread westward into Punjab. The epidemic of 1927 lasted in western India (Bombay and Central Provinces) till 1931, though registering a lower level of deaths.

Cholera declined sharply in 1932; a further decline in 1933 was of particular interest considering the fact that the Kumbhmela was held at Hardwar after a period of 12 years.[17] An epidemic in Bengal, Bihar, Orissa, United Provinces and Central Provinces was responsible for the peak in 1934–35. The 1938 Kumbhmela at Hardwar is considered to have played a major role in the epidemic situation in Punjab and other parts of northern India. Though the mela started in February, cholera cases began to rise only after summer set in, during April. The first case was reported from Punjab on 9 April. In the next week, 11 districts up to Lahore were affected, and 16 other districts in the week after that. From there it took just one more week for cholera to reach NWFP. In Punjab, there were 70,622 deaths, as against 6,341 deaths in the previous year. Bengal also reported a large number of deaths in 1938: 71,133 in contrast to 32,700 in 1937. Central Provinces reported 45,332 deaths, whereas there were only 1,107 deaths in the previous year. The public health commissioner of the Government of India chose not to blame the Hardwar mela, perhaps because the administration was already cautious of taking anti-religion positions.[18] The epidemic was attributed to floods; others reasoned that floods had occurred in Bengal in October 1938.[19]

Cholera cases were reported from the Ganges valley during 1941, from where the disease spread further to Punjab, Sind and NWFP. A similar pattern was observed in 1942. Forty-seven per cent of the deaths occurred in Bengal. Madras (25 per cent), Bihar (11 per cent) and Assam (3 per cent) were the other affected provinces. In contrast to the general trend, cases in Bengal did not decline during the monsoon (July–August); instead, they continued to rise and reached a peak in October. The tail of the epidemic continued into 1945.

The 1941–45 epidemics coincided with the Second World War, and have been attributed to serious shortages of food on account of the war—food meant for civilian consumption was stockpiled for the army. Another factor of serious concern was that civilian medical officers had joined the army in large numbers, thus leaving gaps in the health services infrastructure. Further, medical and sanitary stores were diverted to the army.

From 1948, cholera in Punjab showed a consistent downward trend. There were epidemics in Bihar in 1950 and 1952–53, in Madras in 1948 and 1950, and in Uttar Pradesh in 1948 and 1952–53. There were also epidemics in Bengal in 1948–50.Thereafter there was a general decline. The mean annual death rate declined steadily from 1891–1915 (ranging between two and three) to about one in 1935, and thereafter to 0.29 in 1955; the reduction was slowest in the endemic districts. The incidence rate and death rate were at lows of 3.68 and 1.99 per 100,000 persons, respectively, in 1955. The incidence rate registered an increase in 1963 to about 12.66 per 100,000.[20] The first El Tor case was reported from India in 1964.[21] The seventh pandemic caused by *Vibrio cholerae* El Tor began in 1961 in South-East Asia, and by 1963 had begun to affect countries of mainland Asia.

REGIONAL PATTERNS

Between 1910 and 1954, five states—Bengal (29 per cent), Bihar and Orissa (25 per cent), United Provinces (17 per cent) and Madras (14 per cent)—accounted for 85 per cent of the deaths.[22] In his presentation at the Conference of the Far Eastern Association of Tropical Medicine in Calcutta in 1927, A. J. H. Russell divided the Indian provinces on the basis of cholera mortality as follows:[23]

1. Assam, Bengal, Bihar, Orissa and the United Provinces: average incidence was high and variation was less from year to year.
2. Bombay Presidency, Central Provinces, Punjab and NWFP: sudden peaks of cholera occurring at infrequent intervals; infection was not endemic in these areas and was imported from other areas from time to time.
3. Madras Presidency: the northern and central groups of districts were epidemic areas while the southern group was an endemic area.

Pollitzer, however, classifies the Indian states into two groups on the basis of the prevalence of cholera:[24]

1. Regions where epidemics occurred occasionally and which remained free from infection for considerable periods. These included Punjab, Delhi, United Provinces (Uttar Pradesh), Central Provinces (Madhya Pradesh), Hyderabad, Mysore and Bombay.
2. Areas where the disease was maintained at a high level (endemic) and at times assumed epidemic proportions. These consisted of Bengal, coastal Orissa and some districts of Assam and Bihar.

Swaroop computes the average mortality rate from cholera for 10 years with the lowest mortality (1901–45), and uses the magnitude of this average as a rough measure of endemicity.[25] According to his observations, the principal regions in which cholera was highly endemic in India were:

- located generally around rivers
- areas of high population density
- low-lying land tracts, not more than 500 feet above sea level
- areas of high absolute humidity and rainfall

In other words, these areas were:

1. The delta region in Lower Bengal, formed by three rivers—Hooghly, Damodar and Rupnarayan

2. At or around the confluence of the rivers Ganga and Brahmaputra and Meghna in East Bengal (now Bangladesh)
3. In the deltaic zone of the four rivers of Orissa—Mahanadi, Brahmani, Baitarini and Subarnarekha
4. Northern Assam and the Brahmaputra valley
5. Patna and Gaya districts of Bihar where the Gandak, Sone and Gogra rivers join the Ganga
6. The low-lying river basins of United Provinces (Uttar Pradesh), beginning from the junction of the Ganga and Jamuna at Allahabad and extending through Varanasi to the points where the Gomti and the Sone join them
7. Madras Presidency, in the Cauvery delta
8. Madras Presidency, in the delta formed by the Krishna and Godavari rivers around the Colair lake

Cholera generally spread from Bengal through the United Provinces (Uttar Pradesh) and Punjab, north-west to Afghanistan. This route of spread was described by Brydenin 1874 as the "northern epidemic highway".[26] Similarly a "southern epidemic highway" was also described, along which the disease spread from the United Provinces through central India southwards to Madras and Bombay.

SEASONAL TRENDS

Pollitzer notes shifts in the seasonal trends in cholera as one proceeds westward from Bengal, the endemic home of cholera, on the basis of mortality figures between 1900 and 1920.[27] He demonstrates that cholera peaked in Bengal between September and January, followed by a second peak during March–April; incidence fell to a minimum during the months of June, July and August. Cholera appeared in a mild epidemic form in Bengal in the dry seasons. But storms and tidal waves that brought saline water inland were associated with cholera epidemics, as in 1876 and 1897. There was, however, considerable variation within different regions of Bengal. Winter was found to be unfavourable for the spread of cholera in Bihar and the United Provinces. The seasonal peak was reached in these two states in the spring. In Punjab, peak incidence was during the monsoon

(July and August). In Madras Presidency, there were two cholera peaks that were correlated to the south-west monsoon in June, July and August and the north-east monsoon during November and December.

A. B. Fry, on the basis of district-level data, demonstrated in 1925 that change in seasonal incidence patterns took place in the Bhagalpur division of Bihar between Rajshahi and Patna.[28] Purnea District was shown to have peak incidence during spring; for Bhagalpur, which lay further west, summer and the rainy season were the peak period. Fry concluded that not only did the seasonal pattern change in the Bhagalpur division, but the endemic pattern of cholera in East Bengal gave way to an epidemic pattern. Based on the mean monthly cholera deaths for five Indian provinces, and represents the seasonal trends.

Seasonal variation is of importance, as epidemics originating in Bengal generally spread westward upto Bihar or the United Provinces during the same year, subsiding during winter. The westward progress resumed only during the following year. This time table was generally followed unless the occurrence of epidemics in fairs or festivals accelerated the progress of the disease. Following the recrudescence in the United Provinces each year, the disease followed the land route to Punjab. There were arguments against the notion of early researchers that prevailing winds exerted a direct influence in propagating cholera infection.[29]

It was also argued that in the north-western parts of India, including Punjab and the United Provinces, the moisture-laden south-west monsoon promoted the spread of cholera that was imported through the boats sailing up the Ganges. Drought years were also equally prone to cholera. The survival of *V. cholerae* showed a decrease rather than an increase *pari passu* with an increase of ambient temperature. Other factors were therefore obviously responsible for the increased prevalence of cholera during the summer months. Flugge postulated in 1893 that hot weather led to an increased consumption of raw water, other cold drinks and cold foods like fruits, salads and jellies, all of which were liable to be contaminated with *V. cholerae*.[30] The lowering of the level of rivers, other surface water sources and groundwater in wells that occurred in late summer was also critical since, if those waters became contaminated with *V. cholerae*, they were liable to maintain a high level of vibrios, which thrived better in concentrated water containing organic matter.

Rogers studied the relationship between cholera and seasonal trends, and concluded that rainfall and relative humidity could not explain the epidemiological pattern of the disease.[31] He observed that cholera incidence was minimum during the south-west monsoon in Assam and Lower Bengal, but maximum in Punjab during the same season. He argued that mean temperature showed a closer relationship to cholera incidence, as cholera was at its minimum during winter in Punjab, United Provinces, Central Provinces and the Deccan area, but not so in Lower Bengal. Russell was of the opinion that relative instead of absolute humidity was of epidemiological importance.[32] At the same time, he also stressed that the "clue to the cholera problem was not to be found in any individual climatic factor". Koch laid emphasis on the issue of rainfall being a crucial determinant of cholera.[33] The rains washed the cholera-infected faeces into tanks or ponds, thereby contaminating the drinking water source.

THE VIBRIO TRAVELLED . . .

In addition to geographical and climatic issues, travel (including caravans, railways, ships and the travellers themselves) has also been considered as a determinant in the transmission of cholera. Punjab, among the Indian provinces, remained relatively unaffected by cholera. The first reliably authenticated infection occurred in Punjab in 1820. In the next 35 years, there were only five epidemics—in 1827, 1845, 1852 and 1855. Railway traffic was opened in Punjab in 1860. Large epidemics followed in 1861, 1862, 1865, 1867, 1869, 1872, 1875, 1879 and 1881. The population remained the same, and the meteorological conditions did not change; only the traffic accelerated, with the cholera focus in Bengal.

Whenever water and sanitation were taken care of, cholera decreased among travellers accessing various modes of transport. Koch observed in 1885 that "the introduction of sanitary improvements, particularly the provision of pure waterworks water in place of *Hooghly* water in 1874 led to a marked decrease of the cholera incidence on ships leaving Calcutta with *coolies* [seasonal labourers] for Assam and other ports".[34] It is interesting to quote Napier in this context:

> that normal railway travel on business or pleasure does not tend to spread the disease to any great extent on account of the control that can be exercised over passengers, and that, though the sanitary arrangements are far from perfect, especially at the small stations, there are latrines and a safe water supply. Such travellers of course come from all grades of society, but even the poorest are seldom destitute, and the fact that they are travelling usually indicates that they can afford the ordinary necessities of life.[35]

CHOLERA AND THE MILITARY

In British India, cholera was one of the most important causes of sickness and mortality among the troops. The main causes of death among British soldiers in India between 1830 and 1846, as reported by the Royal Commission on the Sanitary State of the Army in India in 1863, were dysentery and diarrhoea (32 per cent), fevers (23 per cent), diseases of the liver (10 per cent) and cholera (10 per cent). In contrast, only 6 per cent of European soldiers died in combat or of wounds. Simultaneously, troop movements were held responsible for the spread across rural India. Large-scale troop movements from Bengal to northern India were considered to have facilitated the spread of the epidemic of 1917. During 1857–58, there was a repetition of this pattern on account of the Sepoy Mutiny. In the aftermath of the Mutiny, cholera posed a serious threat to the well-being of European soldiers on whom the colonial rulers were heavily dependent. Cholera became the preoccupying concern of the new sanitary commissioners in the 1860s. Investigations into cholera (and venereal diseases) established that the sanitary and medical security of the military could not end at the barrack gates. Such measures had to be extended into adjacent urban and rural areas and to the indigenous general population. After 1861, cholera in cantonment areas and military camps was generally prevented, a fact that has been considered a significant (if underlying) factor in the increased security of British power in India.

CHOLERA AND PILGRIMAGES: UNHOLY NEXUS?

The widespread dissemination of the cholera pandemic that had its origins in the Indian subcontinent became a symbol of fear in the west.

In 1831, Moreau de Jonnes identified religious pilgrimages and troop movements as two of the critical determinants in the spread of cholera in India. Faeco-oral transmission of *Vibrio cholerae* through reservoirs and watercourses that provided water for drinking, washing and bathing was the main source of infection in India. Mass bathing at the Kumbh and ArdhKumbhmela sat Hardwar and Allahabad and the ritual sipping of water provided efficient routes of transmission. The practice of pilgrims bringing back Ganga water for their relatives and friends to sip ensured the propagation of the infection. The congregation of people has consistently been considered a warning signal in the literature on cholera. The fact that safe water and sanitary measures could ward off such risks has been overlooked.

The Kumbhmela at Hardwar in April 1867 was attended by nearly three million people. Only 19 people were treated for cholera during the mela. The disease was considered to have actually spread during the mass bathing on 12April, and disseminated across northern India by the dispersing pilgrims. Similarity with famine conditions have been drawn in view of the poverty of the pilgrims, the conditions under which they travelled and their crowding together in insanitary conditions—perhaps an overplayed claim. Contamination of the water of tanks and wells along the routes of the pilgrims also infected towns and villages. Nearly a quarter of a million people are estimated to have suffered from the disease in this epidemic, and about half of them died.[36]

Banerjea demonstrated in 1951 that, overall, the average death rate from cholera in the years during which no Kumbh or ArdhKumbh fairs were held was 1.6 times lower than during festival years.[37] During March and April each year, 116 fairs with a total gathering of about 250,000–300,000 were held in the United Provinces (most of them in the eastern districts), when meteorological conditions were favourable for the spread of cholera. Kumbh and ArdhKumbh fairs were estimated to attract nearly three million and two million people, respectively, at Allahabad and about one million and half a million, respectively, at Hardwar. Banerjea reported cholera deaths in the Kumbh and ArdhKumbh fairs at Allahabad and Hardwar from 1879 to 1948 (Table 3.1).[38]

Table 3.1: Cholera Deaths in Kumbh and ArdhKumbh Fairs, 1879–1948[39]

Hardwar			*Allahabad*		
Year	*Fair*	*Deaths*	*Year*	*Fair*	*Deaths*
1879	Kumbh	35,892	1882	Kumbh	89,372
1885	ArdhKumbh	63,457	1888	ArdhKumbh	18,704
1891	Kumbh	169,013	1894	Kumbh	178,079
1897	ArdhKumbh	44,208	1900	ArdhKumbh	84,960
1903	Kumbh	47,159	1906	Kumbh	149,549
1909	ArdhKumbh	21,823	1912	ArdhKumbh	18,894
1915	Kumbh	90,508	1918	Kumbh	119,746
1921	ArdhKumbh	149,667	1924	ArdhKumbh	67,000
1927	Kumbh	28,285	1930	Kumbh	61,334
1933	ArdhKumbh	1,915	1936	ArdhKumbh	6,793
1938	Kumbh	70,622	1942	Kumbh	7,662
1945	ArdhKumbh	77,345	1948	ArdhKumbh	52,604

Cholera in the United Provinces (based on cholera death rates) generally increased during the years in which the Kumbh and ArdhKumbh fairs were held. In some instances, the rise in cases occurred during the year following the fair; for instance, in 1880, 1892, 1910, 1913 and 1938. There were, however, exceptional years when fairs were held but the incidence of cholera was low, as during 1933 and 1942. A similar exception occurred during 1888, at a time when cholera prevention measures were not well developed at the fairs. It is significant that in 1887 and 1908, cholera mortality in the United Provinces was particularly high despite the absence of religious congregations. While these figures establish the association between the religious fairs and an increase in cholera mortality rates, not each of these peaks is attributable to the fairs. In fact, some of these increases have been attributed to the increased incidence during those periods in Bengal, from where the infection was likely to have been imported. Punjab was generally also affected along with the United Provinces. However, the epidemic rise of cholera mortality in Punjab in certain periods does not correlate with fairs. Food scarcity was associated with the increase in deaths during epidemics of cholera in Punjab in 1901, 1906 and 1908.[40]

To a lesser extent than the Kumbh and ArdhKumbhmelas, the temple of

Jagannath at Puri, pilgrimage sites at Nasik and Pandharpur (Maharashtra), Tirupati (Andhra Pradesh) and Kanchipuram (Tamil Nadu) have all been implicated at different times as being sources of epidemic cholera. The location of Hindu religious places along rivers and the periodicity of the major festivals perhaps contributed to the epidemicity of cholera. Initially, colonial reports on cholera did not look for associations between the disease and pilgrimages. The International Sanitary Conference at Constantinople in 1866 made particular efforts to protect Europe from cholera originating from Asia. Taking a strong contagionist line, reference was made to Hindu pilgrimages (with particular mention of Puri) and Haj congregations of Muslims at Mecca (as a second stage of relay). Sanitary commissioners, appointed in the aftermath of the conference, were asked to investigate the causes of cholera epidemics. The Government of India (by then directly under the Crown) instituted inquiries into the sanitary state of major pilgrimage and festival sites. Drawing on the case of the Hardwar outbreak of 1867, the reports pointed to a close association between cholera and pilgrimage. Epidemiological association between cholera and Hindu pilgrimage gave rise to the expected antipathy among the ruling classes.

Sanitary Commissioner of Bengal Dr David B. Smith made scathing observations on the public health scenario of Puri. Similar reports emanated from other parts of India as well. The medical and sanitary assault on cholera took an anti-Hindu stance. It not only condemned the pilgrims but also accused Hindu priests of compromising on public health standards for pecuniary interest. In 1916, the sanitary commissioner to the Government of India recommended that preventive actions should be taken at fairs and also along the routes that the pilgrims took to the fair, including major railway stations. The pilgrims were categorised as a "dangerous class" who required special surveillance and regulatory measures. This high-risk approach made it appear possible to control cholera by controlling those most obviously implicated in its transmission. Asia's poor pilgrims were held on par with the slum dwellers of industrial Europe. Strict control over pilgrims and pilgrimages, including quarantines, were instituted to protect cantonments and municipalities. Pilgrim tax was recommended to pay for additional sanitary measures. This was not implemented due to the obvious political fallouts, particularly after the promise of religious toleration offered in Queen Victoria's proclamation in the aftermath of the 1857 Mutiny. Pilgrimages thus came to be tolerated as a "necessary evil", with the hope that with the spread of western education and ideas, pilgrimages would lose their traditional appeal and Indians would value sanitation and hygiene. In practice, sanitary surveillance at the pilgrimage centres was tightened. J. M. Cunningham, Sanitary Commissioner of the Government of India, with his anti-contagionist views, opposed quarantines and sanitary cordons as he considered these measures ineffective. In 1892, the Government of NWFP ordered the breaking up of the Mahavarunimela in Hardwar following an outbreak of cholera among those already assembled. Two hundred thousand pilgrims en route to Hardwar were turned back. This caused a public outcry. The proposed legislation for conferring powers on the government to disperse fairs and religious assemblies on sanitary grounds was quietly dropped by the viceroy. Till the beginning of the twentieth century, it was considered inevitable that cholera would occur at fairs and pilgrimages.[11] The responsibility of the state was not given due consideration. Funds, expertise and institutions for this job were lacking.

Waldemar Haffkine tested the anti-cholera vaccine in India during 1893–96. The ruling medical establishment remained cautious. As with the banning of fairs and festivals, there was a fear of public reaction if compulsory anti-cholera vaccination was introduced. Before 1914, only soldiers, prisoners and tea estate workers were inoculated. Even as late as 1930, the suggestion of compulsory inoculation of pilgrims at the Allahabad Kumbhmela was rejected by the government. At a time when the Congress civil disobedience movement was at its peak, this was absolutely a political decision. In 1936, compulsory inoculation of pilgrims was introduced at Pandharpur. In 1940, the Central Advisory Board of Health recommended that provincial and state governments introduce vaccination in more festival centres. In 1945, vaccination was employed as a compulsory prophylactic measure at the Hardwar Kumbhmela.

CHOLERA THEORY AND SANITARY POLICY

The spread of the first pandemic beyond the confines of the Indian subcontinent stimulated interest in theories of causation and evolving strategies of control. European theories of aetiology ranged from the electrical state of the atmosphere, the operation of the climate on the soil providing the right condition for the germination of the cholera seed and contagion, to transmission of the cholera germ in water (Snow's theory).[42] The debate acquired fresh importance after British troops were affected severely by cholera in the 1860s. The dominant view then was that cholera was basically a "disease of locality", like malaria. At the same time, Snow's theory was gaining ground in England. While in England the approach was to devise sanitary policies, the policy pursued in India was to impose internal and maritime quarantines.

One of the first investigators was Dr James L. Bryden, the first statistical officer of the newly formed Sanitary Department. His main tasks were to establish the limits of the geographical distribution of the disease, the duration of the epidemics, the influence of meteorological conditions, the routes of transmission, and control of the disease. Bryden's natural history approach needs to be considered against the background of Enlightenment science. He adopted William Farr's Liebigian nosology and statistical methods. By 1866, Farr was in agreement that cholera spread through contaminated water. Bryden, on the other hand, believed that there were two processes operating in the causation of cholera. He likened the pathogenic organism to a seed that underwent cycles of reproduction and decay. For epidemic spreads, Bryden hypothesised that cholera seeds were transported beyond the endemic area by monsoonal air currents. This theory was carried forward by James McNabb Cunningham, the sanitary commissioner from 1866 to 1884. The localist/atmospheric cholera theory became a powerful tool against advocates of quarantine and those who sought more direct interventions in public health by the government.

Annesley Charles DeRenzy, the then sanitary commissioner of Punjab, was a critic of Bryden's hypothesis and the consequent inaction of the government. He himself was a believer in Snow's hypothesis. In fact, Bryden never thought that the improvement of water supply was important. DeRenzy opposed the huge expenditure that was incurred in the implementation of the Contagious Diseases Act. He advocated that resources would be better utilised through grants to municipal commissions and improvement of water supplies in the cantonments. During the 1850s, Francis MacNamara, Professor of Chemistry at Calcutta

Medical School, initiated and later improved a large water supply scheme in Calcutta. These scientists did not receive any credit; DeRenzy was transferred from the civil medical services to a remote station in Assam.

The 1867 epidemic originating from the Hardwar Kumbhmela led to an inquiry. Along with Bryden, the other investigator was John Murray, Inspector-General of Hospitals for the North-West Provinces. Murray concluded that the "germ of epidemic cholera appears to reside in the evacuations of a person suffering from the disease".[43] Murray also recommended strict regulation of water supply and provision of camps for the pilgrims. His recommendations were reiterated by the MacKenzie Committee commissioned by the Madras government, but was rejected by the Indian government on grounds of cost. By 1870, the Indian government decided to discontinue *cordons sanitaire*. In 1873, the Government of India's Sanitary Commissioner J. M. Cunningham, realising that the success of sanitary measures lay in the cooperation of the local communities, advised that municipalities must form centres from which education in "sanitary matters should spread among the people".[44]

At about the same time, the subsoil water theory of the German hygienist Max von Pettenkofer achieved international recognition. The critical factor was considered to be the presence of a porous soil and abnormally high levels of groundwater. In 1870, a scheme for registration of subsoil water levels was instituted in Madras and later extended to other provinces. No direct linkages could be established to the incidence of cholera, and the measure encountered opposition. It was finally discontinued by the Army Sanitary Commission in 1879. The hypothesis became obsolete with Koch's discovery of *V. cholerae* and the proof that the faeces of patients served as the immediate vehicle of transmission. Koch opposed Pettenkofer at the 1885 cholera conference. Virchow (1885) and Liebermeister (1896) also opposed Pettenkofer independently.[45]

The notion of "contagion" dominated the scenario till the 1870s. The analogy with smallpox continued to prevail. The outbreak of the disease in certain localities and the absence of cases among those who tended the sick were construed as evidence against its communicability. In fact, till the first half of the 1880s, official medical doctrine in India continued to diverge from prevailing opinion in Britain. The German Cholera Commission with Robert Koch arrived in Calcutta in December 1883, after working for several months on cholera in Egypt. The "Egyptian" bacillus was isolated from a water tank; several people who regularly drank water from that source were diagnosed with cholera. While Koch demonstrated the existence of the comma bacillus, he failed to establish causality. What he demonstrated was a mere association between the presence of large numbers of the bacterium in the intestines of cases and its absence in persons free from the infection. Further, there was no conclusive evidence based on animal models. The thrust of research had, however, shifted from the locality to the laboratory.

Sir Joseph Fayrer, Surgeon-General at India Office Council in London, argued that proof of cholera's contagious character would imply strict international regulations, including quarantine, over India's overseas trade. A two-member British commission dispatched to Calcutta in 1884 ruled that Koch's bacillus was innocuous and could not be the cause of cholera. The Government of India stressed the control of local factors. Cholera inoculation developed by Haffkine also met with limited success.[46] Following Gaffky's analysis of the cholera epidemic of Hamburg, the critical role of water was firmly established. In 1894, Metchnikoff established causality by drinking water containing the comma bacilli and inducing cholera in himself, and also producing the disease in rabbits.

Meanwhile, British India, as the "factory of cholera", was subjected to international censure. The plague epidemic of 1896–97 (the Bombay Plague) put further pressure on the British administration to improve public health measures. The International Sanitary Conference in Venice called for a more interventionist role of the government. At about the same time, the bacillus theory gained more credence. Medical researchers and advisors argued the importance of climate, physical environment and social behaviour as contingent factors. The environmentalist school converged with their contagionist opponents in condemning the climate, the soil and the people of India for being responsible for cholera. By the 1890s, the contagionist theory had finally gained official acceptance; the state and its health officers opted for more active policies towards the control of cholera. By the early twentieth century, there was general agreement among public health authorities in India regarding the relevance of specific measures against cholera (particularly water supply), but merely as part of a general sanitary programme.

Table 3.2: Epidemic Years and Average Inter-epidemic Interval of Cholera, 1900–63[47]

Years	*Epidemic years*	*Average inter-epidemic interval*
1900–24	1900, 1903, 1905–06, 1908, 1910, 1915, 1918–19, 1921 and 1924	1.75 years
1925–47	1927–30, 1935–36 and 1941–45	2.25 years
1948–63	1948, 1953, 1957–58 and 1963	3.25 years

The time trends of cholera in India correspond well with the global pandemic till the 1920s, when the sixth pandemic came to a close. There was a sharp decline following the 1877 epidemic (fourth pandemic). The fifth pandemic began in 1881; the rising trend of 1879–80 was explained by the increase in cases in the United Provinces following the Kumbhmela at Hardwar in 1879. Following the decline of this phase, there was a rise in cases during 1885, possibly due to the ArdhKumbh fair at Hardwar. The rising phase from 1889 and the peak in 1900 mark the beginning of the sixth pandemic; its resurgent phase is evident in the sharp, rising trend of 1905–08.[48] Cases increased in the United Provinces and Punjab in 1913 following the Allahabad ArdhKumbh in 1912; there were relatively fewer cholera deaths (18,894) during the mela itself. There was a steady decline from that point till 1918 when, following the Kumbhmela at Allahabad, north Indian states saw a rise in the number of cases. The 1921 ArdhKumbhmela at Hardwar witnessed 149,667 deaths at the mela itself; the disease spread to adjacent areas of Punjab and the United Provinces, resulting in a sharp rise in cases (460,000) and deaths (446,817), with a case fatality rate of more than 97 per cent for the country as a whole. The sixth pandemic ended in 1923 (Figure 3.1); cases and deaths were the lowest recorded, at 80,000 and 71,504, respectively.

Barua and Greenough, commenting on the global situation of cholera during 1926–60, observe that:[49]

- Cholera disappeared from Europe after 1925.
- Cholera, however, did not remain confined to the Indian subcontinent.

- Cholera kept occurring regularly in Asian countries.
- The origin of the 1947 epidemic of Egypt remained undetermined, but was not caused by pilgrims from Mecca nor by British troops returning from India.

There was a general decline in the all-India trend; each successive epidemic up to 1938 appeared to decrease in magnitude, except in the case of the epidemic (1941–45) during World War II and the food scarcity occasioned by the war. After 1919, cholera incidence during the inter-epidemic periods also became lower. Individual provinces, however, showed considerable heterogeneity in the length and severity of epidemics.

In Europe and North America, cholera was endemic in industrial cities and urban slums. In India, cholera remained by and large a disease of the rural poor. During the 1860s and 1870s, the model of sanitary reform in Britain was implemented to some extent in the major Indian cities, particularly with respect to improved water supplies. These made an impact on urban mortality, but slum dwellers derived only very marginal benefits from these initiatives. Between 1841 and 1865, the annual reported deaths due to cholera in Calcutta ranged from 2,500 to 7,500. The sewage system was started in Calcutta in 1865, followed by filtered water supply in 1869. Following these measures, cholera deaths dropped sharply. Despite the rapid expansion of the city, in the second half of the nineteenth century, annual cholera mortality reached the figure of 3,000 only once during 1895; otherwise it remained well below that level. Similar benefits were observed in Bombay and Madras following the provisioning of water and sewerage. Despite these advances, when the cholera epidemic and famine coincided in Madras Presidency in 1877, and the rural poor migrated to Madras city in large numbers, urban mortality reached the highest levels. Piped water supply and sanitation did not improve in small towns and less so in villages; cholera therefore continued to affect these settlements.

The absence of major famines has been considered crucial to the decline of cholera. There were no major famines after 1908. Cholera also gradually declined thereafter, only to peak again with the Bengal famine during the Second World War. Cholera mortality began to decline in the early decades of the twentieth century. Population was growing, and there was no evidence to suggest any remarkable socio-economic improvement for the majority of the people. It has been hypothesised that sanitary precautions and medical interventions, rather than a better standard of living or improved socio-economic standards, are the most plausible explanation for the decline. It must also be remembered that, globally, the sixth pandemic was on the decline at the same time, and the declining trend in India should be considered in the context of that trend. After 1923, public health services were expanded or established in various parts of India, with efforts to control primarily epidemic diseases. Cholera disappeared from Europe at about this time, following the development of sanitary engineering services.[50] Cholera declined in most countries of the world, including Asian nations, in the mid-1920s, thereby marking the decline of the sixth pandemic.

W. S. Harris reported in 1913 that the provision of piped water supplies in the towns of the United Provinces had led to a great reduction in cholera.[51] However, he added that the fact that cholera had not been eliminated completely was because infections continued to be disseminated through unsafe sources of water supply and the movement of pilgrims. The provision of piped water supplies to towns in Bombay state resulted in a sharp decline in the incidence of cholera.[52] Cholera prevailed in areas where the provision of water supplies was not adequate or where communities were dependent on unsafe sources of water.[53] The incidence of cholera declined sharply in district towns of Bengal where water supply was provided, as compared to the rural areas of the corresponding districts.[54]

The decline of cholera through the first half of the twentieth century was also the story of declining deaths, attributed to several extrinsic factors:

- Improvement of the case reporting system
- Detection of clinically mild cases
- Prompt hospitalisation of those with severe dehydration and shock (cholera gravis)
- Development of "herd immunity"[55]

Case fatality rate has been calculated on the basis of reported cases and deaths.[56] Data constraints have been pointed out earlier. The cholera statistics (and reporting) in India focused primarily on deaths and mortality rates.[57] Available data on cholera in Europe suggests that CFR did not exceed 50 per cent. On the contrary, CFR calculated on the basis of available data in India (1920 onwards) suggests a very high rate till the 1950s. Importantly, examining the trends, it may be observed that the declining trend began during the mid-1950s. The decline was sharp; CFR decreased from nearly 89 per cent in 1955 to 34 per cent in 1963.

THE SEVENTH PANDEMIC

The outstanding feature of the current, seventh pandemic of cholera is that its causative agent is *Vibrio cholerae*, biotype El Tor. El Tor was first isolated by Gottslich in 1905, and the claim of its identification with classical *V. cholerae* was overruled for two reasons:

- Its haemolytic activity
- The failure to establish an association between these strains and clinical cholera or even diarrhoea; all such strains were recovered from wells, surface waters or the stools of "healthy" pilgrims returning from Mecca.

The decision to absolve *V. cholerae* El Tor from choleragenic activity was accepted internationally, and continued to prevail in spite of repeated outbreaks (with El Tor as the pathogen) that were clinically indistinguishable from cholera. The most conspicuous of these outbreaks, and the ones that have a direct relationship to the present pandemic, were the four recorded outbreaks in Sulawesi (Celebes), Indonesia, during 1937–38, 1939–40, 1944 and 1955–57. The recurrence of these outbreaks and the repeated recovery of this vibrio from the stools of persons with mild diarrhoea marked the island as an endemic focus for *V. cholerae* El Tor infection. El Tor disease began its upsurge in an epidemic form in Macassar, its usual focus. Soon it spread to the central and northern areas of the island. It spread to Java in May, flagging off the first trip of the current pandemic. Pandemic, by definition, is a continuous show or record of sequential dissemination of a disease globally. The seventh pandemic of cholera is described in terms of three distinct geo-chronological phases:[58]

- First period (1961–62): affecting all the countries of South-East Asia
- Second period (1963–69): affecting the countries of mainland Asia
- Third period (1970 to date): Middle East–Afro–European phase

Phase I

It is generally accepted that the January 1961 outbreak in Sulawesi was the precursor of the seventh pandemic of cholera. From there it spread to Java in May and to Sarawak in July. By August, the disease had been reported in Kalimantan (Borneo), Macao and Hong Kong. The Philippines experienced its first batch of cases in September, and Sumatra and Timor were infected in November. In 1961, there were 12,197 cases with 1,969 deaths in these territories; the causative agent in all these cases was *V. cholerae* El Tor. The WHO convened a Scientific Group on Cholera Research to study the problem. Noting that the disease caused by El Tor was clinically indistinguishable from that caused by *V. cholerae* classical, the group recommended that cholera should be defined in the International Sanitary Regulations as including cholera El Tor. The 15th World Health Assembly in April 1962 ratified this decision.

The pandemic continued to spread further and, by end-1962, all the states of South-East Asia were affected—Sabah in January, Taiwan in July and Irian Barat (formerly West New Guinea) in October; during 1962 there were 13,393 cases with 1,977 deaths. Considering the geo-placement of the affected territories, seaborne spread of the infection was hypothesised. Initial cases in the concerned countries were reported in coastal areas or among fishermen/boatmen, who also showed a higher carrier rate than among the contacts of cases living permanently on land.[59] The most critical question is why the disease began to spread outside Sulawesi (which was already an endemic area) in 1961 and not earlier. For cholera, a disease with man as its only "source vector", the factors necessary for pandemic flare-ups are:

- Volume of infection (the degree of prevalence of the disease) in the endemic area
- Number of persons leaving the endemic area
- Susceptibility of populations with whom these persons come in contact during the journey and at the destination

The 1961 outbreak in Sulawesi spread to different sections of the island. There were large-scale troop and civilian movements within Indonesia; emigration was also on a higher scale than before. Adjacent South-East Asian countries had been free of cholera for at least a decade and a half.

When the infection was introduced, it easily established a foothold in the susceptible population. At the same time, economic restructuralisation was going on in these countries with the large-scale introduction of mechanised high-sea transportation and travel. The countries affected in 1961 reported an additional 11,611 cases and 1,457 deaths in 1962.The pandemic was on its way to the Asian mainland in 1963.[60]

There were several microbiological characteristics that facilitated the spread of the El Tor strain. The proportion of mild and subclinical cases was high. The ratio of severe cases to mild or subclinical cases was reported to be 1:5 for classical cholera and 1:25 to 1:100 for El Tor cholera.[61] The carrier state also lasted longer, resulting in the spread of unapparent infections. Further, the viability of El Tor outside the human body is high, resulting in greater spread from infective material than the classical variant.

Phase II

While mainland Asia was affected in 1963, all territories of the Western Pacific region that had experienced the pandemic during 1961–62 were again infected. Malaysia was the first country to be affected in May, while all other countries of the Indo-Chinese peninsula (Singapore, Thailand, Cambodia and Burma) except Vietnam reported cholera by December 1963. Vietnam joined the pandemic in January 1964. Two more El Tor invasions were recorded that year—in the Republic of Korea in September and in East Pakistan (Bangladesh) in December. It is interesting to note that the infection spread to all countries through ship passengers, except Cambodia where the infection was imported from Thailand by railways.

On 1 April 1964, Barua et al. diagnosed the first El Tor cholera case in India from a patient in Calcutta.[62] During 1964–66, Mukherjee and Basu isolated (on the basis of phage typing) 2,970 vibrio strains in different outbreaks in India; in their opinion, El Tor cholera had entered India in March 1964 through the port of Madras.[63] They opined that in both cities (Calcutta and Madras), the infections were likely to have been carried by the sea route by Indian repatriates from Burma. They observed that although cholera El Tor appeared in East Pakistan in December 1963, for several months it was confined to the eastern districts. The movement of refugees to India occurred mostly from the western districts, and was unlikely to have been responsible for importing the infection.

West Pakistan was affected during the first week of June 1965, having been free of the disease since January 1961. Though Bangladesh (East Pakistan), India and Pakistan were the home of classical cholera, they responded quite differently to the El Tor pandemic. In Bangladesh, the classical variety continued to dominate. In Pakistan, both biotypes continued to coexist and the classical type caused a major epidemic in 1968. In India, the classical biotype had been almost completely replaced by 1966. However, classical vibriore surfaced in Calcutta, Assam and Orissa in 1968–69. The reason for this differential behaviour is incompletely understood.[64]

El Tor cholera began to spread westward from Pakistan. Afghanistan was affected in the first half of July 1965. In the next two weeks, all four eastern provinces of Iran were suffering heavily from El Tor cholera. Iranian health authorities claimed that the infection had been introduced by opium smugglers. Though the July epidemic in Afghanistan was a mixed one, only El Tor travelled to Iran. On 21 August 1965, the USSR notified its first case, and a year later Iraq became a part of the pandemic.

Notifications of cholera as per the norms of the International Health Regulations ceased with the threat of a further westward spread. Unwarranted panic prevailed, and some countries adopted measures that were reminiscent of past centuries. The range of measures was incredible and included disinfection of mail and printed matter; prohibition of importation of tinned fruit, iron beams, carpets, teak and mineral ore; prevention of the entry of the westbound Orient Express with 70 passengers for more than a week; prevention of passengers from disembarkation from a plane, including a minister of health, for many hours in the heat of a summer's day; and detention of cholera vaccine at an airport for three days because the plane sent to collect it could not get permission to land. The result of these restrictions was the announcement of freedom from infection without adequate proof of surveillance and/or because of international refusal to notify the presence of the disease. Officially, a lull was reported in the spread of the pandemic from 1967 to 1969 as no new territories were affected, except Laos in 1969. Some epidemiologists apprehended that such halt was unusual and not sustainable. In the history of cholera pandemics, a pandemic never retreated once it had crossed the Caspian Sea or Mecca, from where dissemination was rapid. During

1967–69, El Tor cholera continued to be reported from the previously affected areas, in many of which the disease had established endemicity. It reappeared in Malaysia and Singapore (1968) and in Hong Kong, Macao and the Republic of Korea (1969) after being quiescent in those territories for five years or more. During 1969, vigilant health authorities detected eight imported cases in Japan and one in Australia.

Phase III

Africa was affected during the 1970s, and the death rate was one of the highest in the world. The worst affected communities were the displaced and refugee populations in Somalia and Zaire.[65] From 1973, sporadic endemic infections related to the seventh pandemic strain were reported in the United States along the Gulf Coast of Louisiana and Texas. These infections were traced to the consumption of locally harvested contaminated shellfish. Cases in other US locations were traced to the consumption of shipped-in Gulf Coast seafood.[66] The seventh pandemic reached Latin America in 1991. Beginning from the Peruvian coast in January 1991, the infection was carried by fishermen to Ecuador and Columbia. It then spread to all nations of South and Central America and also to Mexico. In the earliest affected communities, the case fatality rate was to the tune of about 30 per cent, later dropping to an overall cumulative rate of about 1 per cent.[67]

Exploring the patterns of cholera in Mexico during 1991–96, Boroto and Martinez-Piedra note that cholera recurred each year during summer.[68] Cholera incidence was 2.5 times higher in coastal areas than in interior areas. Cases typically occurred in less urbanised areas where access to safe water and sanitation was lacking. In low-lying plains, hydrological conditions made it difficult to achieve and maintain high sanitation standards. The authors argue that hydromorphic soils hindered the construction of appropriate sewage disposal systems. Low infiltration rates favoured the overflow of the soakage pits of septic tanks, especially if the pits were not emptied and cleaned regularly. Underground water was close to the surface (within 1 metre) in affected communities, thereby resulting in a high probability of groundwater contamination with faecal matter. Downstream residents were recognised as a particularly vulnerable group in this study, wherever upstream pollution was high.

In a study of epidemic cholera in Ecuador, the route of transmission was identified as principally through contaminated drinking water and, to a lesser extent, through contaminated seafood.[69] In a study of 63 cases and 126 controls, the most important vulnerability factor identified was the lack of potable water supply at the household level; in its absence, communities accessed water by illegal tapping of municipal pipes, or purchased water from tankers. Storage containers with wide, uncovered mouths were identified as risk factors, as not only were they liable to contamination by hands, but residual chlorine also evaporated rapidly. Consumption of beverages from street vendors was another critical risk factor.[70] *Helados* sold by street vendors were identified as responsible for the transmission of epidemic cholera in Guatemala in 1993.[71] *V. cholerae* is not killed by freezing. Sixty per cent of helado samples had a pH of ≤4.5, the pH level above which *V. cholerae* survives. Forty per cent of the helado samples tested suggested the use of unsafe water.

During the 1990s, cholera continued to affect refugee camps in African nations that were ravaged by war and famine. Rwandan refugee camps around Goma, Zaire, were badly affected. Cholera was also reported in Europe, from Romania and the Black Sea states of the former Soviet Union where public health systems had broken down.[72] During the same period, cholera outbreaks were reported from Karachi, Pakistan; the outbreaks were observed to be independent of rainfall, while civil unrest and crumbling infrastructure emerged as critical determinants.[73]

EL TOR SPREADS IN INDIA, FAR AND WIDE

Several factors contributed to the rapid spread of El Tor infection inside India:[74]

- Land travel as the main route of spread
- Propensity of *V. cholerae* El Tor to eliminate cases of the classical biotype
- Invasion of El Tor cholera in areas in India which either had never been cholera-affected and/or had been free of the disease for years
- The higher proportion of mild cases and carriers in El Tor outbreaks compared to outbreaks of classical cholera

- Longer persistence of the carrier state for the El Tor strain than for the classical biotype
- Longer viability of El Tor outside the human body

Following its introduction in 1964, cholera spread rapidly across India. In 1965, cholera was reported from Delhi, Gurgaon, Surat and Madras. El Tor cholera was reported from Gurgaon during July–September and spread upto Rewari.[75] The CFR was 12.1 per cent during the initial phase and later declined to 3.7 per cent. Contaminated wells were identified as sources of infection.[76] More than 1,800 cases of El Tor cholera were reported from Uttar Pradesh.[77] Cholera was reported from Ahmedabad, Gujarat, in 1966.[78] During the same year, it was also reported from the Andaman and Nicobar Islands.[79] In 1968, cholera was reported from the arid districts of Rajasthan—Sikar, Churu and Pali were the affected areas.[80] Pal and Misra reported in 1969 that strains isolated from Rajasthan in 1968 were similar to those isolated earlier from Delhi, indicating the spread from Delhi to adjacent states.[81]

In an epidemiological study of *Vibrio cholerae* El Tor outbreaks in Indore city in 1968, Mittal et al. observed that cases were reported from among communities without household water supply (who accessed water from public taps) and sanitary latrines (defecation in open fields and to a lesser extent in public latrines).[82] A high fly index was also reported.[83] Cholera was detected in Lucknow in 1969.[84] The areas affected were densely populated, partially sewered, and environmental sanitation was poor. The poorest sections of the community were affected. A significant association was established between "bazaar-purchased food" (street food) and cholera. El Tor cholera was reported sporadically from all the municipal wards of Baroda in April–May 1970.[85] Cholera was reported during June–August 1972 from Aurangabad town.[86] Residents of bastis (slums) were the worst affected; the risk factors identified were inadequate water supply and improper drainage and sewage disposal.

Kashmir was affected in 1971. Simultaneously, in 1970–71, there were reports of classical cholera outbreaks from West Bengal, Madhya Pradesh and Orissa following the Bangladesh Liberation War, with the arrival of hundreds of thousands of refugees from East Pakistan (Bangladesh) and their rehabilitation in different parts of these states.

In February–March 1977, cholera outbreak was reported from Manipur, a state that till then had not been affected by the El Tor invasion. The outbreak occurred among a group of about 2,500 labourers working on a river project. They were living in shanties and accessing well and river water for drinking. Defecation was carried out in the open and was considered to have contaminated the drinking water sources. Contaminated municipal piped water supply was incriminated in different outbreaks in Indore in 1980, Bhavnagar in 1987 and Ahmedabad in 1988. In 1988, there was a major epidemic in Delhi, which will be taken up for detailed discussion in the next chapter.

NEW ENDEMIC STATES

Bengal was traditionally the "home" of classical cholera. Post-1964, the distribution of cholera within India underwent a change. States with low or zero incidence gradually became endemic for cholera. Severe epidemics (particularly following fairs and festivals) with high mortality had been replaced by endemic foci and low mortality.[87] Sen Gupta and Kapoor observed in 1969 that large numbers of cases had been reported from Assam, Gujarat, Tamil Nadu, Mysore, Rajasthan and Delhi between 1964 and 1968.[88] While the attack rate declined during this period in Bihar, Madhya Pradesh, Orissa, West Bengal and Tripura, it increased in Andhra Pradesh, Assam, Gujarat, Kerala, Tamil Nadu, Maharashtra, Mysore, Rajasthan and Delhi.

During 1965–75, 16 or more states were reporting cholera, compared to 6–10 states that used to report cholera earlier. Cholera was reported from states that had been free of cholera for a long time—Kerala, Gujarat, Haryana, Punjab and Rajasthan—or from areas that had never known the disease—the Andaman and Nicobar Islands.[89] In the 25 years after the introduction of the El Tor strain, Maharashtra, Tamil Nadu, Karnataka, Kerala and Delhi accounted for about 80 per cent of the reported cases. In 1994, 1995 and 1996, Delhi accounted for 45.10 per cent, 57.81 per cent and 20.47 per cent, respectively, of all cases reported from the country.

A LESS FATAL FACE

Cholera had declined in India by the mid-1950s.In 1955, 14,167 cases and 5,250 deaths were reported. Even before the introduction of El Tor cholera in 1964, there had been a steady decline in the incidence and CFR in India. The annual death rate from cholera (per thousand population) dropped from 1.58 in 1900–24 to 0.17 in 1948–63 and further to 0.0017 in 1964–68.[90] Epidemics also became less frequent. The CFR from cholera declined from 49.34 per cent in 1950 to 35.64 per cent in 1963. The arrival of the El Tor strain was marked by a sharp and steady reduction in CFR.[91]

The incidence of cholera cases doubled from 1962 to 1963, and remained at that level during 1964. *Vibrio cholera* El Tor was identified in India for the first time in 1964. The incidence rate declined progressively during the 1960s. There was a rise in the incidence rate during 1971–73. This coincided with the arrival of larger numbers of Bangladeshi migrants (following the Liberation War of Bangladesh), when cholera spread to several Indian states. Thereafter, the incidence rate declined to about one per 100,000 cases, with minor fluctuations across years. The death rate declined sharply, with El Tor replacing the classical biotype across the country. Though the incidence rate increased during 1971–73, the death rate continued to decline even during those years. There has thus been a steady, systematic decline in the death rate. In 1964, 20,000 cholera deaths were reported in the country, while only 10 cholera deaths were reported in 1994[92]—the death rate declined from 3.620275 per 100,000 to 0.001036 per 100,000 during this period.

The CFR declined because of the intrinsically milder nature of the El Tor strain when compared to the classical strain. Before the arrival of the El Tor strain, there had already been a sharp decline in the CFR of classical cholera between 1956 (43.06 per cent) and 1963 (35.15 per cent) (Figure 3.3). Despite the introduction of the new strain (El Tor), the CFR continued to decline to 19.49 per cent in 1969. Though cases declined in 1970–71, there were relatively more deaths and the CFR increased marginally. This was followed by a phase of steady decline. The reduction in CFR started from the mid-1950s. From 1920, for three-and-a-half decades, CFR remained in the range of 80–90 per cent. In the next decade-and-a-half, CFR decreased by 70 per cent, when the WHO introduced oral rehydration therapy (ORT). In another decade-and-a-half, following the introduction of ORT, there was a slower decline by nearly 20 per cent. As with many other diseases, the peak reduction had been attained before the discovery/ application of the specific therapeutic agent.

Figure 3.1: Incidence Rate, Death Rate and CFR of Cholera, 1964–98[93]

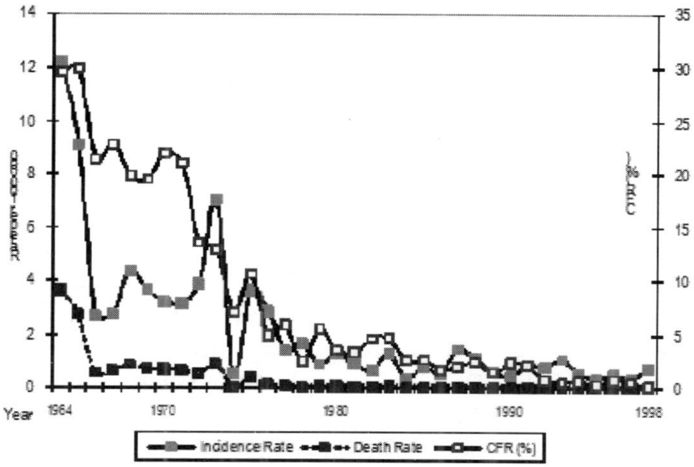

In the endemic states, cholera does not show a stable endemicity. It demonstrates seasonal fluctuations and is also prone to focal epidemics. The seasonal incidence varies between different regions of the country and is subject to change in the same endemic pocket. In some states, the peak incidence is in August. In West Bengal (and Bangladesh), there has been a shift in peak incidence from summer and early winter to autumn. Compared to the classical biotype, El Tor cholera has a higher infection-to-caseratio (i.e., in apparent infections and mild cases), and is therefore prone to endemicity.

The seventh pandemic spread to all continents; trade, commerce and faster modes of travel facilitated that spread. Countries experiencing war, civilian strife and famine were pictures of familiar vulnerability. Spreading across the Indian states, *Vibrio cholerae* El Tor established itself in new areas. Notwithstanding the introduction of a new strain, the incidence and death rates fell consistently. The new endemic foci were predominantly urban areas—a repetition of the endemic pattern in industrial towns of North America and Europe a hundred years earlier. The vulnerability of poorer communities living without basic services was exposed. Even where piped water supplies had been established, there were problems of maintenance and contamination leading to focal outbreaks. Water storage, food safety and personal hygiene issues gained in importance.

O139 BENGAL: THE NEWEST KID ON THE BLOCK

Two letters were published in the 13 March 1993 issue of *Lancet* reporting cholera outbreaks in India and Bangladesh; the microbiological features suggested the involvement of a hitherto unknown strain. The first letter was by Ramamurthy et al., of the National Institute of Cholera and Enteric Diseases (NICED), Kolkata.[94] They referred to a cholera-like outbreak in Chennai, Tamil Nadu, that began in October 1992 and continued till the end of November 1992. Forty-nine representative strains of that outbreak were examined by NICED. In January 1993, 28 and 48 more strains of *V. cholerae* were received from Madurai and Vellore, respectively, for microbiological characterisation. By November 1992, more than 95 per cent of the isolates were of non-O1 type, and, like the strains from south India, were "untypable". Serological tests on 124 strains revealed that they were not agglutinable with the O1 antiserum or with any of the monoclonal antibodies against factors A, B and C of *V. cholerae* O1. The strains were categorised as *V. cholerae* non-O1. Except for one, all other strains from Chennai were not agglutinable against the 138 antisera available at the National Institute of Health, Japan, indicating the possibility of a new serotype. These non-O1 strains had the unusual trait of producing cholera toxin (CT). Most of the strains were resistant to cotrimoxazole (98 per cent), streptomycin (92 per cent) and furazolidone (86 per cent), but were sensitive to other commonly used antibiotics including tetracycline. The similarity in the biochemical, serological and toxigenic status of the strains of *V.cholerae* non-O1, the association with an outbreak in Chennai, and the isolation of similar strains from widely separated regions of India were interpreted as being of epidemiological significance, indicating the clonal spread of a "novel" non-O1 serotype.

In the other letter, John M. Albert et al. from the International Centre for Diarrhoeal Diseases Research, Bangladesh (ICDDR,B) in Dhaka reported an outbreak in mid-January 1993 of acute watery diarrhoea that resembled cholera.[95] The outbreak occurred in southern Bangladesh, and adults were the most-affected group. By the middle of February, about 10,000 people had been affected and the estimated deaths were to the tune of 500. Sixty-seven per cent of the rectal swabs cultured from the field outbreak had yielded non-O1 *V. cholerae*. Seventy per cent of the swabs cultured from the admitted patients at the ICDDR,B also yielded *V. cholerae* non-O1. The non-O1 strains could not be identified with any of the known types, and the pandemic potential of this "novel strain" was recognised. The strain was isolated in Pakistan and Nepal as well.[96] There was another resurgence of O139 in Pakistan in 2000–01, coinciding with a similar trend in India.[97]

It was the unusual feature of the outbreaks of cholera that alerted investigators in Vellore, Chennai, Madurai and Kolkata. Non-O1 vibrios had never been associated with any clinical disease, or, more importantly, with epidemic spread. Microbiological investigations of these outbreaks indicated that these isolates produced copious amounts of the cholera toxin (CT), though they were non-O1. Investigators at Kyoto University, Japan, had previously developed grouping sera for all recognised non-O1 *V. cholerae*, and they had been enumerated from 02 to 138. The new CT-producing non-O1 *V. cholerae* did not group with any of these 137 serogroups; hence it was designated O139.

The O139 serogroup organisms were indistinguishable from other serogroups of *V. cholerae* in terms of morphology, cultural characteristics and biochemical reactions. It was resistant to Mukherjee's IV and V phages that were specific to *V.cholerae*. It did not agglutinate with O1 antiserum. But all strains of O139 that had been tested produced CT. The amount of toxin produced by the Madras strain was 10.4–80 ng/ml, which corresponded to the level produced by the wild strains of *V. cholerae*. In the south Indian studies, *V. cholerae* had been found to be sensitive to tetracycline but resistant to cotrimoxazole and furazolidone. Using the O139 antiserum, 518 strains received from different parts of India during November 1992 were examined (Table 3.3).

Table 3.3: Reported Serogroups of *V. cholerae* in Some Indian States[98]

State	*No. of Strains*	*O139*	*O1*	*Per Cent of Non-O139 Isolation*
Andhra Pradesh	3	3	0	100
Karnataka	4	4	0	100
Maharashtra	16	16	0	100
Tamil Nadu	298	271	13	91
West Bengal	197	186	0	94
Total	518	480	13	93

Of the 518 samples tested, 93 per cent were of the O139 type. Serogroup O139 dominated in all the states from which samples were received. There were early indications that the disease was spreading across different states of India. The non-O139/non-O1 strains did not produce any cholera toxin. At that stage, Sachdeva et al. were of the opinion that "the O139 serogroup was spreading rapidly and was in the process of replacing El Tor *V. cholerae*".[99] The rapidity of the spread of the O139 strain was reminiscent of the spread of El Tor in 1964. By 1965, about 89 per cent of the *V. cholerae* isolates from different parts of the country were of the El Tor type. In Kolkata, the O139 variety had completely displaced the El Tor serogroup by May 1993.

MAPPING THE SPREAD

Jesudasan and Jacob John trace the time sequence of the appearance and spread of the O139 serogroup.[100] The earliest detection of the strain was in September 1992 from an outbreak in Vellore, Tamil Nadu. In the following month, the strain was isolated from an outbreak in Chennai. In Kolkata, the strain was identified in November 1992. In December 1992, there were reports of the new strain from southern Bangladesh and by February–March 1993, cases were being reported from central and northern Bangladesh. Outbreaks were reported from Bangkok, Thailand, in April 1993.

Investigators in Tamil Nadu (Vellore, Madurai and Chennai), Karnataka (Mysore and Amaravati), Andhra Pradesh (Visakhapatnam) and Maharashtra (Nagpur) had sent strains of non-O1 *V. cholerae* isolated from patients with cholera during October 1992 to the NICED in Kolkata for characterisation. In all these batches of samples, *V. cholerae* O139 was identified. The authors hypothesised that this clone had first appeared in the southern Indian peninsula (Vellore, Chennai, Madurai or Mysore) and then spread both inland to Nagpur, Wardha, Rohtak and Ludhiana, and along the coast of the Bay of Bengal to Visakhapatnam, Kolkata and Bangladesh. The infection also spread to Bengaluru, Pune, Jodhpur, Jabalpur and Delhi. Within six months, *V. cholerae* O139 had spread from south India to Bangkok, providing evidence of the epidemiological propensity of the strain to survive and spread in a context of ever-increasing human movement across countries for trade and other purposes. This prompted some experts to forecast the spread of the O139 strain as the beginning of a possible "eighth pandemic".

Jalgaonkar and Fulehave studied the *Vibrio cholerae* O139 outbreak in Yavatmal (Maharashtra) in 1993 that marked the first reported incidence of the new infection from western India.[101] This outbreak occurred between March and July 1993. Thirty-four strains of *V. cholerae* were isolated from 154 patients admitted with cholera at Shri Vasantrao Naik Government Medical College and Hospital, Yavatmal. Of these 34 strains, 26 were non-O1 and eight were O1 El Tor vibrios. In July 1992, seven strains of El Tor vibrio Ogawa, belonging to T2 phage, were also isolated from that region. The O139 isolates were found to be sensitive to gentamicin (95.65 per cent), tetracycline (75 per cent), ampicillin (54.16 per cent), cotrimoxazole (50 per cent), chloramphenicol (40.74 per cent) and streptomycin (11.23 per cent). Naranget al., at the M. G. Institute of Medical Sciences at Sevagram in Wardha (Maharashtra), isolated 44 strains of *V.cholerae* O139 between April and August 1993 [102] All the strains were sensitive to tetracycline, erythromycin, gentamicin, ciprofloxacin and norfloxacin, but were resistant to cotrimoxazole and polymyxin B (50 IU). Narang et al. reported an increase in the incidence of *V. cholerae* since 1990, when 15 strains were isolated as against four in 1989. The number of isolations was 36 in 1991 and 39 in 1992. In 1993, 54 strains were isolated, of which 44 were O139 and 10 were El Tor Ogawa; no further strains of O139 were isolated after August 1993. It was concluded that it would be difficult to predict whether the new strain would acquire epidemic proportions, while other researchers were predicting the advent of the eighth pandemic.

At the same time as the Maharashtra outbreaks, O139 was reported from Haryana. Sabherwal and Sikka cultured 116 stool samples at Rohtak Medical College in 1994.[103] These samples were collected from patients belonging to Rohtak and the neighbouring areas. Of these strains, 27.27 per cent belonged to the O139 serogroup. At about the same time, Prabhakar et al. studied stool samples at the Christian Medical College, Ludhiana, in Punjab.[104] These samples were collected from patients admitted to the hospital between May and August 1993. Of the 41 strains of *V. cholerae* isolated, 35 were of the O139 type. Clinically, all the O139 cases suffered from diarrhoea and vomiting, but without any cellular exudates in stools. Twenty-four were adults and 11 were children. Tetracycline emerged as a drug of choice in Ludhiana, as sensitivity was 100 per cent.

Though the initial indications of the epidemic spread of a new strain were obtained from different parts of Tamil Nadu (and investigated by the NICED, Kolkata), the worst-affected region was the contiguous districts of southern Bangladesh and 24 Parganas (South) District of West Bengal. Between November 1992 and May 1993, 52,000 persons were affected in 24 Parganas (South) District. Over 11,000 were admitted at various health centres and hospitals of the district; 688 died. During this period there were an estimated 100,000 cases and 10,000 deaths in southern Bangladesh. Most of the cases in both countries were adults, pointing to the introduction of a new organism in a population without pre-existing immunity. Watery diarrhoea and severe dehydration were recorded in most cases. *V. cholerae*non-O1 was known to be ubiquitous in tropical aquatic environs; 24 Parganas (South) District in India shares the same estuarine ecosystem with Bangladesh. In addition, there are regular population movements and trading (particularly fishing and forest-based activities) between the two countries.[105] The Infectious Diseases Hospital (IDH), Kolkata, admitted large numbers of cases from the Kolkata suburbs and 24 Parganas (South) District. Table 3.4 reports the details of the acute diarrhoeal cases admitted to the hospital in 1993, including the O139 cases.[106]

Table 3.4: Acute Diarrhoea Cases at the IDH, Kolkata, 1993[107]

Month	*Acute diarrhoea cases, <10 years age*			*Acute diarrhoea cases, >10 years age*			*Total diarrhoea cases*		
	M	*F*	*CFR*	*M*	*F*	*CFR*	*Acute diarrhoea*	*O139*	*Age>10 years*
	No.	*No.*	*Per cent*	*No.*	*No.*	*Per cent*	*No.*	*Per cent*	*Per cent*
January	392	251	15.55	399	306	65.24	1,348	35.0	52.3
February	369	244	16.31	506	480	36.51	1,599	28.0	61.7
March	526	386	20.83	2,613	1,854	36.48	5,379	44.9	83.0
April	517	406	43.33	5,311	3,161	26.91	9,395	54.1	90.2
May	513	366	45.51	2,718	1,891	22.99	5,488	54.2	84.0
June	425	337	18.37	998	914	17.78	2,674	55.1	71.5
July	393	245	23.51	1,288	1,082	20.67	3,008	53.4	78.8
August	363	302	24.06	1,323	1,421	20.40	3,409	60.8	80.5
September	529	412	20.19	1,897	1,605	21.41	4,443	57.3	78.8
October	549	367	22.92	2,112	1,331	20.33	4,359	51.0	79.0
November	287	224	11.74	917	762	13.69	2,190	41.2	76.6
December	260	159	7.15	501	310	32.06	1,230	11.1	66.0
Total	5,123	3,699	24.14	20,583	15,117	25.54	44,522	50.43	80.2

Note: M: male; F: female; CFR: case fatality rate per 1,000 cases.

During 1993, *Vibrio cholerae* O139 accounted for 50 per cent of admissions of acute diarrhoea cases at the IDH, Kolkata. Cases were reported throughout the year, with peaks during August, September and October. Of the acute diarrhoea cases, 80.2 per cent were aged over 10 years, suggestive of a new strain; the CFR among this group was as high as 65.24 per cent in January, but later declined. In an in-depth study of 113 patients of O139 cholera at the IDH, a distinct clinical entity was described that was characterised by painless, watery diarrhoea, vomiting, dehydration and absence of fever.[108] The illness was generally a severe, life-threatening infection with dehydration (85 per cent). None of the patients had blood in the stool, but abdominal cramps were recorded in 44.3 per cent of cases. Thus, the disease was clinically indistinguishable from a typical, severe O1 cholera, with the exception of the cramps.

The NICD, Delhi, reported a large series of both O1 and O139 cholera outbreaks (Table 3.5).[109]

Table 3.5: *V. cholerae* O139 Isolated at NICD from Different States, 1993[110]

State	Samples	Isolation (Per Cent) of	
	No.	V. cholerae	O139
Andhra Pradesh	9	0.0	66.7
Assam	4	0.0	0.0
Bihar	17	0.0	5.9
Delhi	2,850	24.4	29.2
Gujarat	5	0.0	0.0
Haryana	122	10.7	27.9
Karnataka	89	1.1	52.8
Madhya Pradesh	37	0.0	35.1
Maharashtra	44	0.0	15.9
Rajasthan	28	3.6	39.3
Tamil Nadu	2	0.0	50.0
Uttar Pradesh	66	0.0	62.1
Total	3,273	21.7	30.3

Out of 423 samples received from different states in the country, except Delhi, 38.1 per cent were confirmed as *V. cholerae* O139. The isolation rate in Delhi was 29.2 per cent. Isolation rates from south Indian states and Uttar Pradesh were higher, in the range of 50–60 per cent. The number of total samples tested in Delhi is high, as it included the routine testing of all diarrhoea cases admitted at the IDH, Delhi, whereas the samples from other states included only suspected clinical cases of O139 cholera.

Till 1993, non-O1 vibrios had been associated with sporadic cases or relatively confined outbreaks of diarrhoea.[111] The incidence of non-O1 *V. cholerae* was reported to be 5–10 per cent of the hospitalised cases in Kolkata,[112] and 1–3 per cent in Bangladesh.[113] The isolation rate of *V. cholerae* O1 was 12.2–40.9 per cent between 1983 and 1992. Although during 1993 there was a sudden spurt in the isolation rate of *V. cholerae* non-O1 (O139), the isolation rate of *V. cholerae* O1 remained similar to the previous years. The isolation rate of *V. cholerae* O139 was twice as high as that of *V. cholerae* O1 from April to June in 1993.Thereafter, the isolation rate of *V. cholerae* O139 declined and the isolation rate of *V. cholerae* O1 increased.

Resistance to cotrimoxazole was as high as 94.5 per cent in northern

India. Strains in Maharashtra were also resistant to cotrimoxazole, but not to that extent. Resistance to cotrimoxazole and furazolidone was also reported from Bangladesh and southern and eastern states of India.[114] While some strains of non-O1 vibrios cause diarrhoea mediated by NAG-ST, only rare strains have been known to produce CT. Although it was clear that the O serogroup specificity and CT production are unrelated properties, for all practical purposes agglutination with O1 or O139 antisera is sufficient to label a given strain of *V. cholerae* as choleragenic. The O1 variety does not have invasive properties and it does not cause bacteraemic illness. In contrast, non-O1 organisms occasionally cause invasive illness. In cholera-endemic areas, many adults are immune, at least partially, to the O1 serogroup; thus, children are more affected than adults. In the outbreaks due to O139 vibrios, a higher-than-expected proportion of adults were affected, indicating that all communities were epidemiologically naive to this clone.

Outbreaks of O139, despite spreading rapidly, did not culminate in the "eighth pandemic" of cholera. It did not eliminate the El Tor strain as hypothesised by some experts. Even at the stage when it was spreading rapidly, El Tor and O139 coexisted in a cholera outbreak in Garhi village, Delhi.[115] By the beginning of 1994, El Tor had resumed its dominance in Bangladesh, and this trend continued in 1995. Mahalanabis et al. have studied 502 cases of O139 cholera patients and 63 cases of O1 cholera in Dhaka (by systematic sampling of 1,854 cases). They report that there were differences in vulnerability factors between the two variants of cholera.[116] They observe that only 1.6 per cent of O1 cases had in-house potable drinking water, compared to 7.2 per cent of O139 cases. Further, 30.7 per cent of O139 cases had access to sanitary latrines while only 9.1 per cent of O1 patients had access to this facility.In India, O139 continued to flare up later at different points of time, but no specific risk factors could be identified. *Vibrio cholerae* El Tor soon regained its position as the dominant strain.

Cholera never lost its status of being a political disease; *haija* (Hindi for 'cholera') still retains a certain political connotation in Delhi. This chapter has traced the response of the colonial regime to different facets of the disease in order to gain a holistic understanding of the various forces at work, beyond the paradigm set by traditional biomedical epidemiological models. The history of cholera in India corresponds closely to the history of pandemics. Poverty, lack of social security, the failure of the state to provide equitable basic services (and protect socio-economically and politically weaker communities) and poor public health engineering standards stand out as vulnerability factors. Though the decline of cases and deaths may seem impressive, the emergence of endemic urban pockets of cholera is a matter of both shame and concern.

Among the endemic states, Delhi stands out prominently. While civil society grapples with the social, economic and political priorities of provision of basic, essential infrastructure, the pathogen throws up new challenges, exposing the gaps. *Vibrio cholerae* O139 Bengal was able to raise the spectre of an eighth pandemic because of these intrinsic weaknesses. The following chapter will examine the time trends of cholera in Delhi against the backdrop of the 1988 epidemic that was remarkable not so much for its magnitude as because it highlighted the plight of poor communities and the faulty provisioning of services in the capital city of India.

NOTES

1. R. Pollitzer, *Cholera* (Geneva: World Health Organization, 1959), 13.
2. R. Pollitzer, "Cholera Studies", *Bulletin of the World Health Organization* 10, no. 3, 1954, 421–61.
3. Pollitzer, "Cholera Studies".
4. David Arnold, "Social Crisis and Epidemic Disease in the Famines of Nineteenth-Century India", *Social History of Medicine* 6, no. 3, 1993, 385–404.
5. David Arnold, *Colonizing the Body: State Medicine and Epidemic Disease in Nineteenth-Century India* (Delhi: Oxford University Press, 1993), 166.
6. Pollitzer, "Cholera Studies".
7. Ibid.
8. E. Whitcombe, "Famine Mortality", *Economic and Political Weekly* 28, no. 23, 1993, 1169–79.
9. Plague accounted for an estimated 10 million deaths between 1896 and 1921, and malaria for nearly twice that number.
10. Arnold, "Social Crisis and Epidemic Disease".
11. L. Rogers, "The Incidence and Spread of Cholera in India: Forecasting and Control of Epidemics", *Indian Medical Research Memoirs*, no. 9, 1928.

12. M. Yacob, "Epidemiology of Cholera in the Punjab", *Indian Medical Gazette* 79, 1944, 383.
13. Pollitzer, "Cholera Studies".
14. S. Zurbrigg, "Hunger and Epidemic Malaria in Punjab, 1868–1940", *Economic and Political Weekly* 25, no. 1, 1992, 2–26.
15. Zurbrigg links famine conditions to prices, but at the same time acknowledges the limitations of this approach.
16. K. C. Patnaik and P. N. Kapoor, *Statistical Review of Cholera Problem in India, with Particular Reference to Endemicity* (New Delhi: Central Bureau of Health Intelligence, 1967).
17. There were only 1,915 deaths—the lowest ever figure in the series of Kumbh and ArdhKumbhfairs from 1897 to 1948. A. C. Banerjea, "Note on Cholera in the United Provinces", *Indian Journal of Medical Research* 39, 1951, 17–40.
18. Arnold, "Social Crisis and Epidemic Disease".
19. Pollitzer, "Cholera Studies".
20. Patnaik and Kapoor, *Statistical Review of Cholera Problem in India.*
21. Dhiman Barua, "History of Cholera", in *Cholera*, ed. Dhiman Barua and William B. Greenough III (New York: Plenum Publishing Corporation, 1992), 16.
22. Patnaik and Kapoor, *Statistical Review of Cholera Problem in India.*
23. A. J. H. Russell, "Statistical Studies in the Epidemiology of Cholera", *Transactions of the Seventh Congress of the Far Eastern Association of Tropical Medicine, 1927* (Calcutta, 1929), 2: 131.
24. Pollitzer, "Cholera Studies".
25. S. Swaroop, "Endemicity of Cholera in India", *Indian Journal of Medical Research* 39, no. 2, 1951, 141–83.
26. J. L. Bryden, *Vital Statistics of the Bengal Presidency. Cholera Epidemics of Recent Years Viewed in Relation to Former Epidemics: A Record of Cholera in the Bengal Presidency from 1817 to 1872* (Calcutta, 1874).
27. Pollitzer, "Cholera Studies".
28. A. B. Fry, "Cholera in Bengal: Past and Present", *Indian Medical Gazette* 60, 1925, 301.
29. Pollitzer, "Cholera Studies".
30. R. Münch, "Review: On the Shoulders of Giants, Robert Koch", *Microbes and Infections* 5, no. 1, 2003, 69–74.
31. Rogers, "The Incidence and Spread of Cholera in India".
32. A. J. H. Russell and E. R Sundararajan, "The Epidemiology of Cholera in India", *Indian Medical Research Memoirs*, no. 12, 1928.
33. Pollitzer, "Cholera Studies".
34. Ibid.

35. L. E. Napier, "Cholera", in *The Principles and Practice of Tropical Medicine* (New York: Macmillan, 1946), 370.
36. Arnold, *Colonizing the Body*, 192.
37. Banerjea, "Note on Cholera in the United Provinces".
38. Ibid.
39. Ibid.
40. Zurbrigg, "Hunger and Epidemic Malaria in Punjab".
41. R.B. Lal, "Fairs and Festivals in India", *Indian Medical Gazette* 72, 1937, 96.
42. Mark Harrison, *Public Health in British India: Anglo-Indian Preventive Medicine 1859–1914* (London: Cambridge University Press, 1994), 99–116.
43. Harrison, *Public Health in British India*, 106.
44. Ibid.
45. Ibid.
46. Pollitzer, "Cholera Studies".
47. Patnaik and Kapoor, *Statistical Review of Cholera Problem in India.*
48. In 1891, 169,013 persons died at the Kumbhmela at Hardwar and the epidemic spread to the United Provinces.
49. Barua, "History of Cholera", 15.
50. Ibid.
51. W. S. Harris, "The Effect of Pipe Water Supplies in the Reduction of Cholera in Urban Areas", *Tropical Disease Bulletin* 3, 1913, 486.
52. E. Benjamin, "Cholera in Bombay Province" (Bombay, 1949).
53. Free provision of water to the entire population through public standpipes was able to eliminate cholera from every state of the Malay Peninsula
54. K. Subrahmanyan, "Note on the Importance of Environmental Sanitation in the Campaign against Cholera", Unpublished working document, WHO/Cholera/12, World Health Organization, Geneva, 1951.
55. The notion of herd immunity is a controversial one. It was generally agreed by different authors of the period that herd immunity acquired through an epidemic protected for three to four years. It was argued by others that while an individual outbreak may fail to produce good herd immunity, immunity may eventually be acquired through repeated cholera infections.
56. Patnaik and Kapoor, *Statistical Review of Cholera Problem in India.*
57. Bhatty, "Cholera in South Asia".
58. Barua, "History of Cholera", 16–23.
59. Ibid.
60. Ibid.
61. W. H. Masley, "Principles and Practice of Cholera Control", Public Health Papers No. 40, World Health Organization, Geneva, 1970.

62. Barua, "History of Cholera", 16.
63. Ibid.
64. Ibid.
65. R. Lan and P. R. Reeves, "Pandemic Spread of Cholera: Genetic Diversity and Relationships within the Seventh Pandemic Clone of *Vibrio cholerae* Determined by Amplified Fragment Length Polymorphism", *Journal of Clinical Microbiology* 40, no. 1, 2002, 172–81.
66. *Morbidity and Mortality Weekly Report* 40, no. 13, 1991, 225–27.
67. *Morbidity and Mortality Weekly Report.*
68. R.J. Borroto and R. Martinez-Piedra, "Geographical Patterns of Cholera in Mexico, 1991–96", *International Journal of Epidemiology* 29, no. 4,2000, 764–72.
69. J. T. Weber et al., "Epidemic Cholera in Ecuador: Multidrug Resistance and Transmission by Water and Seafood", *Epidemiology and Infection* 112, no. 1, 1994, 1–11.
70. D. Koo et al., "Epidemic Cholera in Guatemala, 1993: Transmission of a Newly Introduced Epidemic Strain by Street Vendors", *Epidemiology and Infection* 116, no. 2, 1996, 121–26.
71. Helados are a food item prepared from crushed ice, similar to the *chuskis* (ice candy) sold in the streets of Delhi and north India.
72. *Independent*, "Cholera Kills 12 in South Russia", 11 August 1994.
73. A. Sheikh et al., "Cholera in a Developing Megacity: Karachi, Pakistan", *Epidemiology and Infection* 119, no. 3, 1997, 287–92.
74. D. M. Mackay,"Cholera: The Present World Situation", *Transactions of the Royal Society of Tropical Medicine and Hygiene* 73, no. 1, 1979, 1–2.
75. Classical cholera outbreaks were earlier reported during 1958 and 1960; routine testing for cholera of the stool samples of patients admitted with acute diarrhoea at the Infectious Diseases Hospital, Delhi, started from 1965.
76. R. R. Arora and B. S. Misra, "Epidemiological Features of Outbreaks of Cholera in India: A Review", *Journal of Communicable Diseases* 7, no. 2, 1975, 84–89.
77. Patnaik and Kapoor, *Statistical Review of Cholera Problem in India.*
78. Arora and Misra, "Epidemiological Features of Outbreaks of Cholera in India".
79. Subarna Roy et al., "Molecular Tracking of the Lineage of Strains of Vibrio cholerae O1 Biotype El Tor Associated with a Cholera Outbreak in Andaman and Nicobar Islands, India", *Tropical Medicine and International Health* 10, no. 6, 2005, 604–11.
80. Arora and Misra, "Epidemiological Features of Outbreaks of Cholera in India".

81. S. C. Pal and B. S. Misra, "Laboratory Investigation of Cholera Epidemics in Delhi and Rajasthan during 1968", *Journal of Communicable Diseases* 1, no. 1, 1969, 14–17.
82. M. C. Mittal, E. M. Beckett and M.S. Pathak, "An Epidemiological Study of Gastroenteritis (Cholera El tor) Outbreak in Indore City, 1968", *Journal of Communicable Diseases* 1, no. 1, 1969, 54–59.
83. Though flies may carry *Vibrio cholerae*, and are an indicator of poor sanitation, they are currently not considered vectors of importance as far as cholera is concerned.
84. P. K. Saxena, B. G. Prasad and J. K. Bhatnagar, "A Study of Cholera Cases (El tor) among the Cases of Gastroenteritis Admitted to Infectious Diseases Hospital, Lucknow during 1969", *Journal of Communicable Diseases* 2, nos 1–4, 1970, 162–80.
85. S. C. Pal et al., "Cholera El Tor in Baroda", *Journal of Communicable Diseases* 4, nos 2–3, 1972, 140–49.
86. S. R. Sen Gupta et al., "Epidemiological and Clinical Profile of Cholera in Aurangabad Town during 1972", *Journal of Communicable Diseases* 6, no. 1, 1972, 4–10.
87. Roy et al., "Molecular Tracking".
88. S. K. Sen Gupta and P. N. Kapoor, "Trends in Incidence of Cholera in India", *Journal of Communicable Diseases* 1,1969, 3–4.
89. M. I. D. Sharma, "Problem of Cholera in India", *Journal of Communicable Diseases* 7, no. 2, 1975, 79–83.
90. Sen Gupta and Kapoor, "Trends in Incidence of Cholera in India".
91. Ibid.
92. Ministry of Urban Affairs. *Report of the National Commission on Urbanisation*.
93. Computed by the author.
94. T. Ramamurthy et al., "Emergence of Novel Strain of *Vibrio cholerae* with Epidemic Potential in Southern and Eastern India", *Lancet* 341, no. 8846, 1993, 703–4.
95. John M. Albert et al., "Large Outbreak of Clinical Cholera Due to *Vibrio cholerae* Non-O1 in Bangladesh", *Lancet* 13, no. 341, 1993, 704.
96. Vibha Sachdeva et al., "Widespread Emergence of *Vibrio cholerae*O139 in India", *Southeast Asian Journal of Tropical Medicine and Public Health* 26, no, 2, 1995, 342–46.
97. K. Jabeen and R. Hasan, "Re-emergence of *Vibrio cholerae* O139 in Pakistan: Report from a Tertiary Care Hospital", *Journal of Pakistan Medical Association* 53, no. 8, 2003, 335–38.

98. Adapted from Sachdeva et al. "Widespread Emergence of *Vibrio cholerae* O139 in India".
99. Sachdeva et al., "Widespread Emergence of *Vibrio cholerae* O139 in India".
100. M. V. Jesudasan and T. Jacob John, "The Appearance and Spread of *Vibrio cholerae* O139 in India", *Indian Journal of Medical Research* 99, 1994, 97–100.
101. S. V. Jalgaonkar and R. P. Fule, "Cholera Outbreak Due to *Vibrio cholerae* Serogroup O139 in Yavatmal (Maharashtra) in March–July, 1993", *Indian Journal of Medical Research* 99, 1994, 101–2.
102. P. Narang et al., "Changing Patterns of Vibrio cholerae in Sevagram between 1990 and 2005", *Indian Journal of Medical Microbiology* 26, no. 1, 2008, 40–44.
103. U. Sabherwal and Rama Sikka, "Emergence of *Vibrio cholerae* Serogroup O139 in Haryana in May–June 1993", *Indian Journal of Medical Research* 99, 1994, 105–6.
104. H. Prabhakar, M. Lal and H. Kaur, "Outbreak of Gastroenteritis Due to a New Strain of Non O Group 1 Vibrio cholerae, in Ludhiana in May–August 1993", *Indian Journal of Medical Research* 99, 1994, 107–8.
105. R. Dasgupta, "District Health Profile Series-I, 24-Parganas (South), West Bengal 1992–93", Working Paper Series No. 1, Jawaharlal Nehru University, New Delhi, 1995.
106. S. K. Bhattacharya et al., "Clinical Profile of Acute Diarrhoea Cases Infected with the New Epidemic Strain of *Vibrio cholerae* O139: Designation of the Disease as Cholera", *Indian Journal of Medical Research* 27, no. 1, 1994, 11–15.
107. S. K. Bhattacharya et al., "Clinical Profile of Acute Diarrhoea Cases".
108. Ibid.
109. Sachdeva et al., "Widespread Emergence of *Vibrio cholerae* O139 in India."
110. Personal communication from the National Institute of Communicable Diseases.
111. Ramamurthy et al., "Emergence of Novel Strain of *Vibrio cholerae*".
112. Ibid.
113. Albert et al., "Large Outbreak of Clinical Cholera".
114. Sachdeva et al., "Widespread Emergence of *Vibrio cholerae* O139 in India'
115. R. Dasgupta, "Cholera Outbreak in Garhi", Proceedings of the Conference of the Indian Association of Epidemiologists, New Delhi, 19–21 November 1995.
116. D. Mahalanabis et al., "An Epidemic of Cholera Due to *Vibrio cholerae* O139 in Dhaka, Bangladesh: Clinical and Epidemiological Features", *Epidemiology and Infection* 112, no. 3,1994, 463–71.

4 Cholera in Delhi, 1965–2000

EL TOR ARRIVES IN DELHI, TO STAY

After 1947, there was a general decline of classical cholera in the country. Following its introduction in India in 1964, El Tor cholera began spreading to other Indian states.[1] This was to be expected with the introduction of a new strain of which the population did not have immunological experience. In 1965, El Tor cholera was reported from several states, including Delhi.[2] There were two major watersheds in the period between 1965 and 2000. A major epidemic in 1988 raised several administrative, infrastructural and managerial issues. In the aftermath of the epidemic, a series of steps was taken for the prevention and control of diarrhoeal diseases. Despite these measures, there was another spurt of cases in 1994–95 owing to the introduction of a new strain, the O139 Bengal (Figure 4.1; Appendix Table A.1).

Figure 4.1: Cholera Cases and Deaths in Delhi, 1965–2000[3]

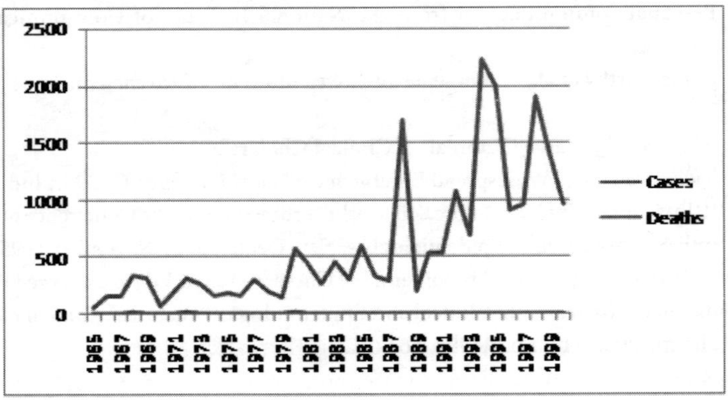

In 1965, the first El Tor cholera case was reported during the week ending 8 May, and the last case in the week ending 2 October. The initial phase of spread of the El Tor infection was not as explosive as might ordinarily be expected when a new strain is introduced. Only 55 cases were detected in Delhi in 1965. Infection spread to Delhi from adjacent Uttar Pradesh, where more than 1,800 cases were reported in 1965.[4] Epidemiological studies investigating El Tor cholera in Delhi demonstrated that most of the patients belonged to lower socio-economic groups and were living in unauthorised colonies without proper water and sanitation services.[5] The exact mode of transmission could not be established in most cases, and no relationship could be established between one case and another.

During 1966 and 1967, there was an upward trend; the onset of the first case, however, was delayed to the second half of June and the last case was reported in the second half of October. In 1968, there was a new high of 333 cases, and the "season" lasted till November. The year 1969 saw cholera being reported as early as April, continuing up to November. The year 1970 was a particularly low-incidence year with only 63 cases. The onset was unusually delayed to July, and the last case was reported in December. The April–November pattern was restored in 1971, and the number of cases also rose appreciably. The National Institute of Communicable Diseases (NICD) reported that the incidence of cholera in 1968 and 1969 was as high as 27 per cent and 30 per cent, respectively, of all diarrhoeal cases admitted in the IDH.[6] This declined to 6 per cent from 16 per cent between 1970 and 1975, with the exception of 1972, when the incidence rose to 24 per cent.

Despite fluctuations in this period, the five-year moving average trend-line shows an upward trajectory. Cholera cases reached a plateau during the 1970s. The first half of the 1980s saw a considerable increase in the case load, culminating in the 1988 epidemic. There was a temporary lull following the epidemic. With the emergence of the new O139 strain, there was another sharp rise that continued till the late 1990s. Overall, the rising trend continued. Following the introduction of the El Tor strain, there was an increase in the number of deaths, which peaked at a maximum of 22 in 1980. There was a steady decline of deaths thereafter and zero mortality was achieved in 1990. No deaths were reported from the O139 strain.

The trend-line for the incidence rates (per 100,000 population) of cholera cases in Delhi demonstrates an increasing trend over the years. Significantly, this is in contrast to an overall declining trend over the corresponding period in India (Figure 4.2). The CFR was as high as 9 per cent in 1965. But this dropped sharply during the following years, settling in this phase of the epidemic at a 2–4 per cent level that continued through the 1970s. Though the incidence rate continued to rise steadily over the 1980s and 1990s in Delhi, the CFR dropped further to zero, in keeping with the national trend. The CFR was relatively higher in the earlier high-incidence years of 1980 and 1985. It registered a sharp decline after 1980, only to rise to a 3 per cent + level in 1985. In 1986 it dropped sharply to 0.3 per cent, and even the 1988 epidemic recorded a CFR of only 0.47 per cent. The 1988 epidemic recorded the second-highest incidence rate in this 25-year series, 20.02 per 100,000; the rate was highest in 1994 at 21.02 per 100,000. In 1989, the number of cases decreased by as much as 90 per cent, but the CFR rose marginally to 0.5 per cent. Since 1990, no cholera deaths have been reported and the CFR dropped to zero.

Figure 4.2: Incidence Rate and CFR of Cholera in Delhi, 1965–2000[7]

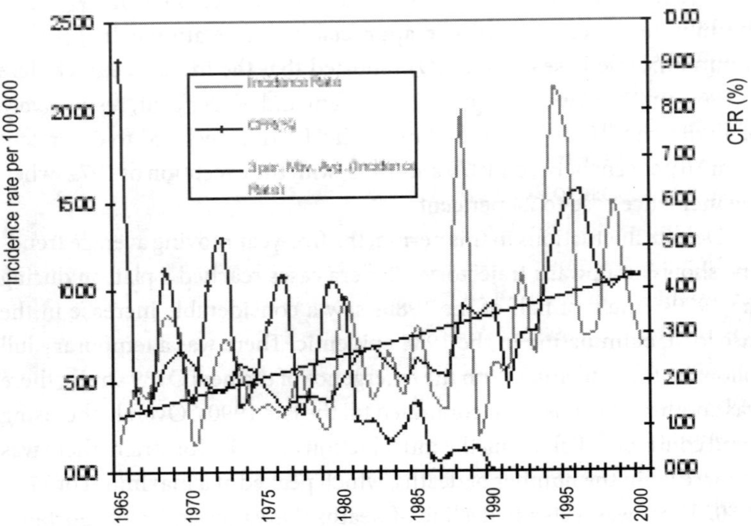

Cholera has been reported among very young children in Delhi. Neonates have also been diagnosed with *V. cholerae*. In a sentinel surveillance centre that treated 8,714 cases of acute watery diarrhoea among under-5 children, 0.7 per cent were clinically suspected of cholera. Half of the suspected cases were confirmed by the laboratory, and in each case the serotype was Ogawa. A quarter of these cases were infants, the youngest being three months old.[8] Most of the families reported using groundwater in addition to municipal supply. A later case series from another sentinel centre reported Inaba as the dominant serotype among paediatric cases (under 12 years).[9] Through the 1990s, several case series have reported increasing antimicrobial resistance, up to 90–100 per cent in hospitalised cases, particularly to common antibiotics such as nalidixic acid and cotrimoxazole.[10]

While El Tor cholera is generally marked by low mortality, other factors that have possibly played a role in bringing down mortality include the sensitisation of both the community and the health administration. The system of referral to the IDH on clinical suspicion of cholera is as prevalent among the large formal medical institutions as among informal practitioners. The possible role of host–agent adaptation also merits consideration.

TRENDS IN GASTROENTERITIS INCIDENCE

Sentinel surveillance of gastroenteritis (GE) cases was instituted in 13 index hospitals of Delhi following the 1988 epidemic. The number of index hospitals was later increased to 22 in 1993. These 22 index hospitals are fairly representative of the geographical areas of Delhi, but by no means do they represent a complete picture of the case/disease load. Figure 4.3 shows the incidence rate per 100,000 population and the CFR of reported gastroenteritis cases from 1988 to 2000.

The trends in GE and cholera during 1988–2000 make for an interesting comparison. Following the 1988 epidemic, both declined sharply. The declining trend continued up to 1991in the case of gastroenteritis. Cholera cases, meanwhile, increased about two and a half times in 1991 from the 1990 level, and this continued into 1992 as well. Gastroenteritis figures have been on the rise since 1992. There was an acute rise in 1993, which is

Figure 4.3: Gastroenteritis in Delhi: Incidence Rate and CFR, 1988–2000[11]

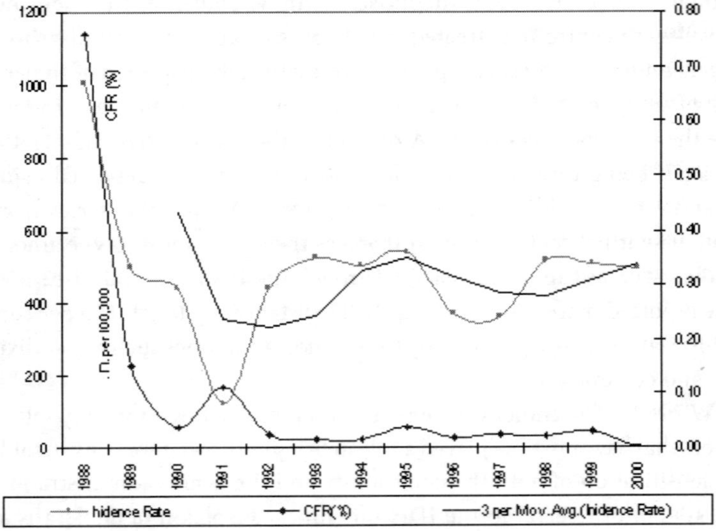

attributable partly to the import of *Vibrio cholerae* O139 and partly to the fact that the number of index hospitals went up. Though the O139 epidemic lasted throughout 1994 and 1995, the GE incidence rate showed a marginal decline in 1994, rising again in 1995. Since 1996, however, gastroenteritis and cholera trends have moved in an identical fashion.

The 1988 epidemic recorded 84,792 GE cases and 643 deaths. During the epidemic, only eight cholera deaths were recorded, and most of the deaths were notified as GE deaths. The Voluntary Health Association of India (VHAI) report elaborated that the concerned authorities went to great lengths to deny that a cholera epidemic was at hand, and also that there was a "clamp down" on information.[12] In such a situation, it is possible that cholera deaths were denied and the cause simply recorded as gastroenteritis. Also, cholera notification demands laboratory confirmation; not all GE cases were tested for cholera in the epidemic situation. Thereafter, GE deaths and CFR registered a sharp drop. In contrast to the cholera situation, reported GE deaths decreased to zero at the end ofa decade, in 2000.

ZERO MORTALITY: TECHNICAL SMOKESCREEN

The Maharishi Valmiki Infectious Diseases Hospital is the referral centre in Delhi for diagnosing and reporting cholera cases. Gastroenteritis cases are admitted at all hospitals; on clinical suspicion, these are referred to the IDH. Some institutions perform the hanging drop test for clinically suspected cases, and refer only those found positive by this test. These referred cases are by and large clinically stabilised in their primary care institution. But this is not to imply that deaths do not occur at the IDH, where the primary causes of deaths are certified as some other factor, including aspiration of vomitus and other respiratory or cardiac complications. It is often the case that laboratory confirmation of cholera is received after the death. In none of these situations is the case certified as a cholera death. Such deaths average about three to six per year. The "corrected" CFR would thus be similar to the national picture rather than suggesting a zero-mortality scenario.

The WHO recommends that Part I of the death certificate should deal with the *immediate* cause and the *underlying* cause that triggered the events leading to death. The notion of underlying cause is the "essence of the international death certificate". It is defined as:

1. The disease or injury which initiated the train of morbid events leading directly to death, or
2. The circumstances of accident or violence which produced the fatal injury

Part II of the certificate records any significant associated diseases that contributed to the death but did not directly lead to it. Cholera should, therefore, feature at least as the underlying condition if not the immediate cause.

Kumar et al. have explored the epidemiological features of 75 GE deaths in 22 index hospitals in Delhi during 1990–92.[13] Seventy-five per cent of the deaths occurred in the under-5 age groups, and more than half of the total deaths were of infants. The majority of deaths were of people from slum areas. Over half the households from which these deaths were reported did not have access to piped water supply, and about a similar proportion lacked access to sanitary latrines. The majority of deaths in the series were reported during May–September, and the vulnerability factors for incidence of cases identified by the researchers included scarcity of drinking water, increased consumption of unsafe water and contamination of subsoil water. In a case series of 264 paediatric admissions, it was found that only 22 per cent of the patients were prescribed oral rehydration solution (ORS) (there was no difference in this regard between public and private sector physicians), though 40 per cent were administered intravenous fluids and 64 per cent received antibiotics.[14]

SEASONAL TRENDS

The monthly incidence data for cholera in Delhi, as reported by the NICD, is analysed for the period 1977–2000. These comprise only reported cases of patients admitted at the IDH whose stool samples were tested for cholera, and therefore do not reflect the actual case load in the community. The data has been grouped into four quarters, namely, January–March, April–June, July–September and October–December.

January to March has traditionally been a cholera-free period in Delhi. There was an increased incidence of winter cholera cases in Bangladesh that was followed by the O139 epidemic. Cholera during the winter was reported for the first time in the 1990s when the O139 epidemic was unfolding. Two cases were reported from Govindpuri, Central Zone.[15] The same area later witnessed a major hepatitis E outbreak, which lasted from the end of January to March 1994. The cholera cases and hepatitis outbreak were attributed to the supply of unchlorinated water from a deep tubewell. A cholera case also occurred in January 1999 in Narela. Cholera had never been reported during March till 1996, when cases were reported from the Central, Civil Lines and South Zones and became a common feature in these zones. Thus, there has been a rising trend in winter cases of cholera since 1994, with most of these cases being diagnosed as O139 cases. Cholera was reported for only eight months in 1977, while it was reported for 11 months in 1999 and 2000, a pointer to the increasing levels of endemicity of the disease in Delhi.

Summers in Delhi (April to June) are marked by high temperatures and water scarcity. Diarrhoeal diseases, including cholera, follow naturally. A definite increasing trend in the incidence is observed during the summer months. The 1990s saw water scarcity in the summer and a sharp rise in the incidence rate of cholera cases. The incidence rate for the summer months doubled from the 1980s level (1981–90), with an average of 1.53 per 100,000 population, to 3.42 per 100,000 population in the 1990s (1991–2000). With the onset of the O139 phase in 1993, the average incidence rate in 1991–95 rose to4.04 per 100,000; during 1996–2000 this rate declined to 2.81 per 100,000, still nearly double the rate of the 1980s.

July to September is the rainy season in Delhi, accounting for 75 per cent of the annual rainfall. These months account for a significant proportion of the annual cases of cholera with a correlation coefficient of 0.95. The average incidence rate during 1981–2000 was about 4.80 per 100,000, except for 1991–95 when it increased to 7.14 per 100,000 population.

Thus, over two decades, the incidence rate in the rainy season (July–September) remained at nearly constant levels, barring fluctuations due to the O139 strain. This is in contrast to average incidence rates during the summer season (April–June), which doubled over the 1990s as compared to the 1980s, with a sharper rise if the peak O139 phase is taken into consideration.

October–December represents the "tail" of the cholera season. Since 1991, cholera cases have been reported every December. Simultaneously, there has also been a rise in the number of cases of cholera being reported during November. While the average annual incidence rate during 1981–90 was 0.28 per 100,000, the corresponding rate during 1991–2000 was 0.74 per 100,000, a nearly three-fold increase. Interestingly, the rise in the average annual incidence rates in winter cases was greater for the period 1996–2000 (0.84 per 100,000 population) as compared to 1991–95 (0.64 per million), indicating rising endemicity.

Table 4.1 presents the ratio of the number of cases occurring during the summer months (April–June) to the cases occurring during the monsoon months (July–September) during 1994–2000 for the zones in which the annual incidence of cholera is observed to be high, i.e., Central, South, Shahdara (N), Shahdara (S), Civil Lines, Rohini and Narela.

Table 4.1: Ratio of Summer to Monsoon Cases for the Major Municipal Zones[16]

	1994	*1995*	*1996*	*1997*	*1998*	*1999*	*2000*
Central	1.00	1.14	1.47	0.53	0.42	2.15	4.61
South	0.94	1.10	0.97	0.58	0.52	2.32	2.24
Shahdara (N)	0.13	0.25	0.31	0.35	0.21	1.02	0.66
Shahdara (S)	0.21	0.31	0.62	0.41	0.50	2.56	0.60
Civil Lines	0.26	0.30	0.35	0.26	0.51	0.82	0.44
Rohini	0.18	0.19	0.07	0.16	0.18	0.48	0.34
Narela	0.29	0.37	0.15	0.35	0.26	1.24	1.00
All Zones	0.36	0.47	0.45	0.34	0.35	1.25	0.96

The picture *within* each zone remains fairly consistent till 1998, with a low standard deviation across years, except for the Central and South Zones. The proportion of cases reported in the monsoon is higher (more than double) than that reported in the summer for most of these zones. During 1999 and 2000, a marked rise is observed in the ratio in the Central and South Zones, the proportion of cases in summer being much higher than in the monsoon season. Cholera incidence by seasons is widening as the disease becomes endemic at higher levels, indicating indigenous transmission increase in early summer and in winter (Figures 4.4 and 4.5).

Figure 4.4: Seasonal Trends in Central, South and Shahdara (South) Zones[17]

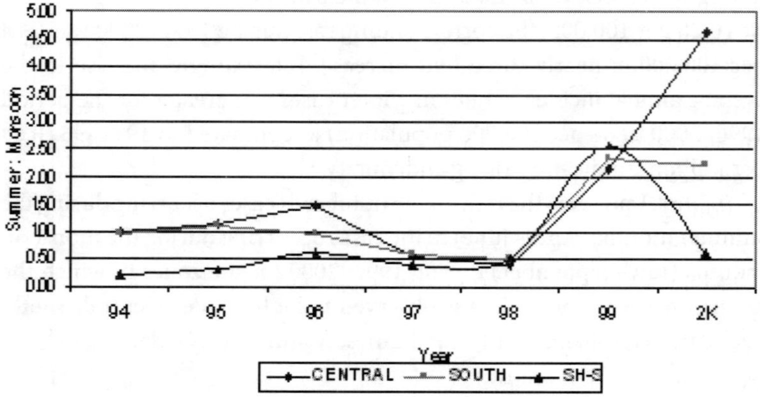

Figure 4.5: Seasonal Trends in Shahdara (North), Civil Lines, Rohini and Narela Zones[18]

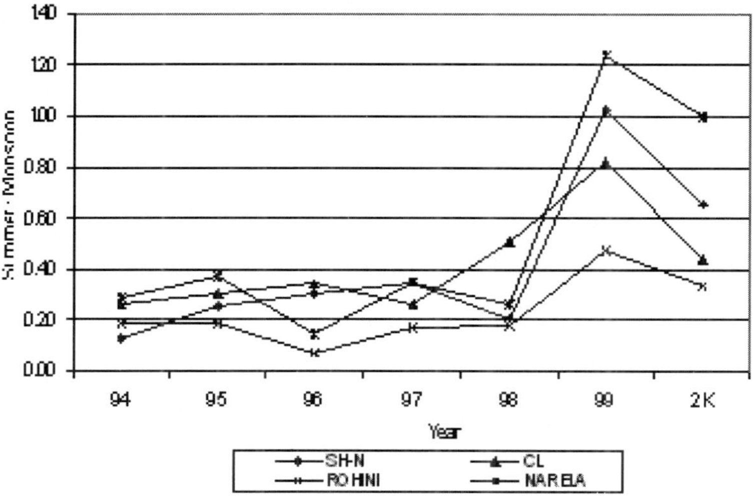

O139: NEW STRAIN, OLD CRISIS

The year 1994 marked another watershed with the introduction of the *Vibrio cholerae* O139 strain. This was an epidemic year, with 2,226 cases, and the trend continued in 1995 with 1,989 cases. Detection of O139 cases had, however, begun in 1993, though the peak isolation was in 1994. Cases declined following the subsidence of the O139 strain.

Non-O1 vibrios were being isolated regularly from stool samples in Delhi, much before the O139 epidemic (Table 4.2). Non-O1 isolation rates were similar to those reported from Bangladesh, but lower than those from Kolkata. The isolation rate ranged between 0.5 and 3.0 per cent. Remarkably, following the introduction of the O139 strain, isolation of non-O1 vibrios rose to 29.2 per cent. The month-wise break-up of the 1993 situation (Table 4.3) reveals that the peak isolation rate was in May. This tapered off in later months, though no month was free of it.

The NICD investigated several cholera outbreaks in Delhi and other states.[19] In 1993, 2,850 stool samples from Delhi were tested, of which 29.2 per cent yielded *V. cholerae* O139 and 24.4 per cent *V. cholerae* O1. Of

Table 4.2: Cholera Cases (O1 and Non-O1) in Delhi, 1983–93[20]

Year	*Samples no.*	*O1 no.*	*O1 rate per cent*	*Non-O1 no.*	*Non-O1 rate per cent*
1983	1,969	455	23.1	60	3.0
1984	2,051	305	14.9	10	0.5
1985	2,543	587	23.1	69	2.7
1986	1,770	330	18.6	41	2.3
1987	1,579	285	18.1	60	3.8
1988	4,164	1,702	40.9	26	0.6
1989	1,620	197	12.2	32	2.0
1990	2,006	533	26.6	14	0.7
1991	1,917	537	28.0	12	0.6
1992	2,783	1,075	38.6	52	1.9
1993	2,850	697	24.4	831 (O139)	29.2

Table 4.3: Isolation of *V. cholerae* in Delhi, 1993[21]

Month	*Samples no.*	*O1 no.*	*O1 rate per cent*	*Non-O1 no.*	*Non-O1 rate per cent*
January–March	60	0	0	0	0
April	219	8	3.7	73	33.3
May	710	155	21.8	290	40.8
June	564	117	20.7	201	35.6
August	505	133	26.3	141	27.9
September	432	109	25.2	81	18.8
October	206	107	51.9	37	18.0
November	32	10	31.3	1	3.1
December	5	0	0.0	0	0.0
Total	2,850	697	24.4	831	29.2

423 samples collected from other states of the country, 38.1 per cent were confirmed to be *V. cholerae* O139. Sixty-four strains of non-O1 isolated from Delhi during 1991 and 1992 were tested serologically with O139 antisera. None of them was found to agglutinate with *V. cholerae* antisera, confirming that O139 had arrived in Delhi during 1993.

Till 1993, non-O1 vibrios had been associated with sporadic cases or relatively confined outbreaks of diarrhoea.[22] The incidence of non-O1 vibrios was reported to be 5–10 per cent of the hospitalised cases in

Kolkata.[23] The corresponding figure for Bangladesh ranged from 1 to 3per cent.[24] The NICD reported that, in Delhi, 54per cent of laboratory-confirmed cases were O139 infections.[25] Importantly, both *V. cholerae* O1 and O139 were isolated from 12 children at the IDH.[26] In Delhi, *V. cholerae* O139 was demonstrated to coexist with El Tor, discounting the then prevailing notion that O139 could replace El Tor in the manner in which El Tor had earlier replaced classical vibrios.[27]

During 1995, 1,988 cases of *V. cholerae* O1 and only one case of the O139 serogroup were isolated from Delhi. In 1997, O139 cases in the months of May, June and July accounted for approximately 3per cent of the cases, while in 1998 this proportion rose to about 20per cent. Incidentally, the cholera cases reported from Delhi showed a steep rise from 956 in 1997 to 1,908 in 1998.This increase is attributable to the re-emergence of the O139 strain, a signal for increasing O139 surveillance. By 2005, the majority of infections were O1, and a shift was observed from Ogawa to Inaba; new phage types 4, 16 and 25 were isolated. Significantly, 96 per cent of the O1 isolates were multi-drug-resistant.[28] The NICD had reported the re-emergence of *V. cholerae* O139 in a different locality in Delhi; similarities were reported with strains from Ahmedabad in contrast to earlier similarities with strains from Kolkata.[29]

THE 1988 EPIDEMIC: THE BEGINNING

Delhi experienced a cholera epidemic in 1988. That the capital city could suffer from such an epidemic not only shook the country, but also led to major changes in the approach to control strategies in Delhi. The plight of the urban poor and the lack of urban basic services were brought into focus. The knee-jerk responses and the obsession with vaccination during this epidemic offer a textbook case of how not to manage a cholera epidemic. Over the years, cholera has emerged as a political issue and has been used by community leaders to scare a complacent administration into action on various civic problems—primarily relating to water and sanitation.

In 1988, the first cholera case was detected during April, as in earlier years. This was followed by an increase in reported cases during May and

June.[30] From late June, a spurt in the number of cases was noted, which reached its peak in July and August.[31] While some investigators attributed the source of the epidemic to a focal outbreak in Rajokri village, others opined that the epidemic had started in Brahmpuri and Gokulpuri areas of Shahdara (North) Zone.

Between 14 and 17 May 1988, 14 children from Rajokri, aged between 3 and 14, were admitted at the IDH with gastroenteritis. A preliminary survey of 248 households in the area on 17May detected 36 cases of GE and two deaths. Three wells considered to be the cause of the epidemic were disinfected, and 1,498 people were inoculated with the anti-cholera vaccine. The NICD conducted its investigation on 20 May and put the number of deaths at five.[32] By 19 May, 5,690 persons had been inoculated against cholera.

Rajokri is a village in Najafgarh Zone with a population of about 8,000. The village itself was not affected by the outbreak. The area that was affected was Rajokri Pahari on the outskirts of the main village. Rajokri Pahari had stone quarries and was inhabited by migrant labourers living in slums, without access to any basic services. "The entire environment appears to be highly polluted with thick dust particles all around coming out of the stone crushing operation in the area", recorded the NICD report.[33] There was no tap water, and the residents were defecating in the open in fields. Contractors had filled up two dry, shallow wells in the area with tanker water, and the labourers used this water for drinking. This contaminated water source was considered by the NICD to be the cause of the outbreak.

Stool samples of patients admitted at the IDH tested negative for cholera. The NICD had collected three stool samples from the community. These also tested negative for *Vibrio cholerae*, and were positive for *E. coli*. The MCD tested 11 water samples on 17 May, and all these samples were found to be unfit for human consumption. The NICD tested two samples from wells; one of these was fit and the other unfit for consumption.

The Director General of Health Services, in a communication issued earlier on 29 January 1988, had categorically ruled out the role of vaccination during an epidemic/outbreak. Interestingly, the then director-in-charge, NICD, recommended in her report on the Rajokri episode, dated 27 May 1988, that all the inhabitants of the village should be inoculated against cholera with anti-cholera vaccine. The subsequent thrust on inoculations (June onwards), though largely blamed on the prime minister, would have been guided by some technocrats.

Increase in Cholera Cases in Hospitals

In the last week of May, Safdarjung Hospital in New Delhi had also tested several GE patients from different areas of South, Central and Najafgarh Zones and found them to be positive for cholera. The affected areas were Govindpuri, Dakshinpuri, Mehrauli, Sadiq Nagar, Palam and Sagarpur. The information was communicated to the public health authorities and field action was taken for preventing further spread.

Two hundred and fifty-five cases of cholera were reported from Shahdara (N) Zone by 26 July. This accounted for nearly a third of the cases in Delhi until then. The worst-affected areas were Seemapuri, Gokulpuri, Ghonda–Maujpur and New Seelampur.[34] On 15 July, after repeated denials, the government admitted that there had been at least 30 cholera deaths since 1 July, most of them of children.

On 22 July, the prime minister visited some of the affected areas of Shahdara (North) Zone and an "action plan" was formulated. It was an eight-point (11, according to some reports) plan. The emphasis remained on vaccination (900,000 vaccinations within a week), cleaning up of the area within a week (later extended to two weeks) and the installation of permanent drinking water sources within 15 days.[35]

THE EPIDEMIC SPREADS

In 1988, 1,708 bacteriologically confirmed El Tor cholera cases were reported along with eight deaths. This was the highest number of cases recorded in a single year in Delhi since 1965; the corresponding figures for GE were 84,972 cases and 643 deaths. As many as 1,324 cases of cholera were reported during July–August 1988, with nearly 600 cases in the second half of July. Table 4.4 compares the figures for July and August for the preceding 10 years.

Table 4.4: Cholera in Delhi, July–August 1979–88[36]

	1979	*1980*	*1981*	*1982*	*1983*	*1984*	*1985*	*1986*	*1987*	*1988*
July	32	242	98	46	76	70	148	116	45	684
August	52	152	122	112	203	88	154	45	84	650
Total	84	394	226	258	279	158	302	161	129	1,324

Out of 2,873 diarrhoea stool specimens from the IDH, 1,324 (46 per cent) tested positive for cholera.[37] The peak of the 1988 epidemic was during the last week of July and the first week of August. The highest incidence rate of 77 per 100,000 was in the age group of 1–4 years, with decreasing attack rates in higher age groups, the lowest being in the age group of 25 years and above (10 per 100,000). Khanna et al. found that 6.6 per cent of the cases occurred in infants.[38] Dutta et al. reported an incidence rate of 55/100,000 among infants.[39] Overall, 73 per cent of the cases occurred in children below the age of 15. The ratio of males to females was 3:2 (780:544), indicating, to some extent, differential rates of accessing care.

Three hundred and seven deaths were reported from hospitals. While the exact cause cannot be ascertained (GE or cholera), micro studies revealed that most of the children who had died were malnourished and were already suffering from chronic diarrhoea.[40] Gastroenteritis in these children was accompanied by other complications including bronchitis, pneumonia or septicaemia. The National Institute of Health and Family Welfare was quoted by the VHAI as having reported that the incidence of diarrhoea among children in the slums and resettlement colonies of Delhi was more than four times the national average.[41] According to the VHAI, 6.6 per cent of cases occurred among infants.[42] Significantly, more than half the deaths during the epidemic were of infants.[43]

The Shahdara (43 per cent) and Civil Lines (29 per cent) Zones were the worst affected, accounting for 72 per cent of the total cases (Table 4.5). In terms of incidence, Civil Lines reported 85.7 cases per 100,000 population, while Shahdara reported 55.7 per 100,000. Both these zones are part of the riverine belt on the banks of the Yamuna, which is vulnerable to waterborne diseases. The highest proportion of cholera cases has consistently been observed every year from these two zones.

Table 4.5: Incidence of Cholera in the 1988 Epidemic[44]

Affected areas	*Mid-year estimated population (in '00,000s)*	*Cases*	*Incidence rate per 100,000 population*
MCD Zones			
City	5.19	10	1.9
SadarPahargunj	5.14	45	8.8
Karol Bagh	7.64	43	5.6
West	9.68	50	5.2
Civil Lines	5.93	508	85.7
Narela	2.83	48	17.0
Najafgarh	5.62	79	14.1
South	6.34	69	10.9
Central	6.77	26	3.8
Shahdara	10.47	583	55.7
NDMC	9.88	15	1.5
DCB	1.20	11	9.2

The affected colonies can be classified by their municipal zone and type of settlement, as shown in Table 4.6.

Table 4.6: Colonies Affected During the 1988 Epidemic[45]

Zone	*Colony*	*Settlement Type*
Shahdara	New Seemapuri, NandNagri, Sunder Nagri, Kalyanpuri, Trilokpuri	Resettlement
	Gokulpuri, Maujpur, Brijpuri, Bhajanpura, Khajuri, Karawal Nagar	Unauthorised
	Tahirpur, Johripur	Urbanised village
Civil Lines	Jahangirpuri	Resettlement
Rohini	Haiderpur	Urbanised village
Najafgarh	Mangolpuri, Sultanpuri	Resettlement

The areas earliest and worst affected were the resettlement colonies, particularly in Shahdara Zone. The epidemic later affected adjacent urbanised villages and unauthorised colonies. The 1988 epidemic is thus closely identified with the plight of the resettlement colonies. It is significant that the epidemic followed the collapse of services in these resettlement colonies subsequent to their being handed over by the DDA to the MCD, a key factor that will be explored in detail later in this chapter.

CAUSES OF THE EPIDEMIC

It is important to understand the background against which the epidemic occurred and the causes that explain an outbreak of this magnitude. The major factors include the settlement patterns of the affected colonies, the state of infrastructure and the administrative factors that went with it. Other issues include microbiological and behavioural factors.

Settlement Factors

In 1972–73, the Town and Country Planning Organisation (TCPO) reviewed and evaluated the master plan of Delhi. Among its major findings was a housing deficit of 380,000 in 1971, with little progress in housing facilities for low-income groups. The slum population (excluding squatters) was estimated to be nearly one million, and a total of about 1.5 million were living in substandard housing. Concern was also expressed about congestion in the urbanised villages and about environmental pollution.[46]

Slum clearance work received a major thrust following the TCPO review. This responsibility was transferred from the MCD to the DDA by the Government of India in 1974. Twenty-seven resettlement colonies were constructed in the peripheries of the city during this period, to relocate 120,000 squatter households. The resettlement colonies were site-cum-services schemes. Each family was provided a plot of 25 square yards. These colonies were provided with roads, parks, public toilets, shops, schools, dispensaries and community centres. Industrial areas were also provided for in nearby areas to provide employment. Further, these were planned areas, and appropriate and adequate infrastructure was expected.

Despite these guiding principles, there were several major deficiencies in the resettlement colonies.[47] The colonies were located at the periphery of the city on low-lying wasteland, often along drains and ditches in areas that were basically unsuitable for human habitation. In contravention of the caution urged by the master plan, the colonies were set up in the trans-

Yamuna area without developing an adequate drainage system. The area of individual plots was lowered from an initial allotment of 89 square yards (recommended by the DIT) to 25 square yards (allotted by the DDA).[48] Thus, little was done for the improvement of the "substandard" housing situation. Adequate water supply and proper waste disposal systems were not given due attention at the city level. The implementation of local-level systems also remained weak. The minimum standard of public latrines was fixed at one seat for 20–50 persons; in actual practice, one seat served 150 persons. Parks almost invariably deteriorated into dumping areas for solid wastes and wastewater due to the inadequacy of drainage and of solid waste collection and disposal systems.

The state of civic amenities and basic services that existed in the resettlement and other colonies was explored by the three-member committee appointed by the Supreme Court in response to Writ Petitions (Criminal) Nos 330 and 400 of 1988.[49] Detailed discussion of the deficiencies of basic services that were considered to have contributed to the epidemic is available from the report of this committee. Two other microstudies also provide valuable insights into the ground situation, and take into consideration the community's accounts and perceptions.[50] The expert committee went into considerable detail regarding the infrastructure situation; it quoted figures provided by the civic agencies themselves. Even by their own admission, the deficiencies were gross enough.[51] While the VHAI study took the various components of causality and control into account, it is incomplete to the extent that the report went to the press even while the epidemic was on.[52] Ritu Priya's findings from a case study of Sunder Nagri, the worst-affected colony, detail the vulnerability of such colonies in general.[53]

Water Supply

The availability of piped supply was inadequate in all the affected colonies in June 1988. In the resettlement colonies of Shahdara, less than a third had piped supply. The official standard was one water tap for every 30 families and one handpump for every 32 families. Each lane had one or two taps supplying water from the local deep tubewells. The supply was erratic, and residents reported that it was available for only three to four hours a week.

Lack of a reliable and adequate supply of piped water forced residents to draw their daily requirement from shallow handpumps that were installed both by the administration and also by residents at their own cost. The disposal of solid and liquid wastes in these colonies was grossly inadequate, leading to the contamination of groundwater and the subsequent consumption of unsafe water by the residents.

Quantitative inadequacies apart, there was a question-mark around the quality of water that was being made available to the residents through the piped supplies. The expert committee recorded that defects were detected in pipelines in several resettlement colonies, which led to contamination. The condition of pipelines in Sunder Nagri and Seelampur was worse, and they could not be commissioned in time.

Different agencies conducted laboratory tests for water quality during the epidemic period. The largest number of samples, 548, was tested by the Public Health Laboratory of the MCD. Other central agencies that conducted tests included the National Environmental Engineering and Research Institute (NEERI) and the Industrial Toxicology Research Centre (ITRC).[54] Baveja et al. also reported on a series of 60 samples.[55] Table 4.7 summarises the findings of these agencies and researchers.

Table 4.7: Bacteriological Fitness of Water During the 1988 Epidemic[56]

Source	*MCD*		*ITRC*		*NEERI*		*Baveja et al.*
	Sample no.	*Fit per cent*	*Sample no.*	*Fit per cent*	*Sample no.*	*Fit per cent*	*Fit per cent*
MCD	89	85.39	–	–	–	–	78.2
DDA	2	100.00	–	–	–	–	–
Piped supply	–	–	23	78.26	–	–	–
Tubewell	22	0.00	15	60.00	8	25.00	50.00
Handpump	391	1.02	30	46.67	73	21.92	33.3
Public Hydrant	–	–	–	–	19	57.90	–
Tanker	6	100.00	3	100.00	4	57.90	–
Trolley	15	0.00	–	–	–	–	–
Ice	23	0.00	–	–	–	–	–
Total	548	16.06	71	61.97	104	69.23	–

There are overlaps across categories of sources as reported by different agencies. None of these agencies specified whether the water sources reported were collected at the source or at the consumer end. For some sources, the sample size is small and interpretations need to be made with caution. All agencies tested for total coliforms to determine fitness for human consumption.

Considerable variation can be observed in the fitness of piped supplies. The critical issue is that for large piped supplies (including public hydrants), coliforms must not be present in 95 per cent of the samples taken throughout any 12-month period as per WHO guidelines.[57] The reported values fall far below the required standard. Most of the unfit MCD samples were from Civil Lines, Shahdara and South Zones, which reported the majority of cholera cases.

Tubewells emerged as the key source of unsafe water in the reports. These were generally the only source of piped water supply for the resettlement colonies. The failure to maintain the quality of tubewell water implied that the chlorination system was not functioning properly. This was entirely owing to the failure of the concerned agencies to chlorinate water drawn by deep tubewells; the problem was man-made and avoidable. Groundwater samples obtained from handpumps were also unfit for drinking. In the unauthorised and JJ colonies, where people were acutely dependent on groundwater because of lack of piped supply, contaminated groundwater led to the spread of infection.

A few samples were taken from tankers; the "100 per cent fit" results should be interpreted with caution. Most of the contamination of tanker water occurs while accessing it, often through the dipping of containers into the tanker or drawing water though rubber pipes. The VHAI study reported foreign bodies in tanker water, though the lack of laboratory testing of such samples means that evidence on whether such samples were bacteriologically fit or not is absent.

What is also of concern is that 100 per cent of the ice and water trolley samples were unsafe. These trades are subject to regulation and licensing. The failure of public health administration thus stood exposed. The consumption of these items being higher during the summer months, transmission of diarrhoeal diseases (and cholera) must have been greatly facilitated by consumption from such sources.

Dutta et al. collected water samples from known cholera foci of the city from May to October 1990.[58] They found that, overall, 43.3 per cent of the water samples were unfit for human consumption; 75.3 per cent of the handpump water samples and 9.7 per cent of tap water samples were unsatisfactory. When available, a sample from stored water and a sample of the primary source were also taken. The sample size of paired samples was small: 29 piped water samples and 14 handpump water samples. Of the 26 fit piped water samples, 18 (69.23 per cent) stored samples were reported to have tested unfit. Out of six handpump water samples, two (33.3 per cent) stored samples tested unfit. On the basis of such small samples, the authors argued that personal hygiene was one of the critical determinants in the spread of diarrhoeal diseases.

This study also made a retrospective analysis of behavioural factors through a case control study. Forty-four households reporting cholera cases in Shahdara during the 1988 epidemic were selected. From the same area, 300 unaffected households were also selected as controls. The study did not specify the factors for which the controls were matched. Moreover, the investigation was conducted two years after the epidemic. Still, the households reporting cholera cases in 1988 were taken as "cases". The relationship of certain household practices with the risk of being affected by cholera were studied among cases and controls. Statistically significant differences were reported for three variables. The storage of water in narrow-mouthed containers, the use of soap and water for washing hands before meals, storage of leftover food for more than six hours without refrigeration and consuming it later were identified as the risk factors.

Sanitation and Wastewater Disposal

According to the report submitted to the Supreme Court, 35 out of 44 resettlement colonies did not have proper sewerage systems. Out of a total of 543 regularised and unauthorised colonies, only 135 colonies had sewer connections. In 25 of these colonies, internal sewers were not operational for lack of pumps. As many as 221 colonies in this category in Shahdara lacked sewers. At many places, sewage was pumped into open drains, resulting in the collection of wastewater near houses.

Out of 1,583 septic tanks, 1,446 (more than 90 per cent) were choked with sludge; 1,234 km of open drains were silted up. Latrines and urinals were poorly maintained and there was indiscriminate defecation around the latrines, including the newly constructed ones. Though one lavatory seat was supposed to be provided for every seven families, in reality, as many as one hundred or more persons were actually using it.

Sullage drains were constructed by the DDA without proper slopes and outlets, making the disposal of wastewater difficult. On account of inadequate provision of garbage bins in the colonies, solid waste was often thrown into open drains, causing further stagnation. A number of sullage pumps were not working. Sullage was being pumped into bigger drains, which ultimately drained into major drains maintained by the Flood and Irrigation Department of the Delhi Administration. Low-lying land within the colonies facilitated the stagnation of water mixed with night soil and garbage. Groundwater was thus liable to be polluted easily because of the sandy loam soil and the high water table. Only about a tenth of the 59 sullage pumps were functioning when the outbreak started. The DDA was responsible for the removal of solid waste until the transfer of the colonies to the MCD on 1 June 1988. About 5,000 truckloads of garbage were piled up by the end of May 1988. Garbage bins were inadequately provided, and people tended to dump refuse at the roadsides or into drains near houses.

Administrative Lapses

The Committee on Reorganisation of Delhi Setup (Sarkaria Committee) published its report in December 1989. The report examined the administrative issues contributing to the epidemic, and pointed out the difficulties arising out of overlapping functions between the MCD and the DDA.

The overlap of functions between the MCD and other authorities concerned with the provision of infrastructure and basic civic services in areas being developed was of critical importance. Under the DDA Act of 1957, the central government, after consultation with the corporation, may declare any area in Delhi to be a "development area". After an area is declared a development area, the DDA performs all the functions and exercises the authority normally vested in a local body. After the development is complete, the DDA hands over the area along with the basic infrastructure and services, such as sewerage, drains, roads, water supply systems, parks and green spaces, to the MCD, which then assumes the responsibility for their maintenance. While the provisions of the law are clear, the process of handing over (as pointed out in the report) involved consultations and negotiations that often lasted up to several years. During the interim period, both the MCD and the DDA were inclined to neglect the maintenance of civic and other services in these areas, resulting in serious inconvenience, and indeed health hazards, to the residents of the area.

Squatters on land acquired for public purposes, known as JJ dwellers, were to be provided developed, serviced plots, and in some cases even tenements, as per certain decisions of the government. The implementation of this scheme, known as the Jhuggi-Jhonpri Relocation (JJR) Scheme, was originally entrusted to the MCD in 1960, but was transferred to the DDA in January 1968. Relocation was not one of the original objectives of the DDA; the responsibility for this work has been alternating between the DDA and the MCD. At the time of the epidemic, the policy emphasis was on *in situ* improvement of squatter settlements.

Under the Slum Areas (Clearance and Improvement) Act of 1956, areas lacking basic facilities were declared slum areas. Wherever development of such areas was not possible, they were cleared and occupants were provided "slum rehousing tenements". Twenty thousand such tenements had been allotted to slum dwellers under this scheme in different parts of the city. Dangerous katras (slum tenements) located within the slum areas were demolished and occupants provided with alternative accommodation. Under the Slum Clearance and Improvement Scheme, environmental improvement was carried out to improve the living conditions of slum dwellers. In 1988, this work was being done by the slum wing of the DDA, while maintenance services for slums were the responsibility of the MCD. The Sarkaria Report noted that the practice of shifting development and maintenance work relating to slums between the MCD and the DDA had also been criticised earlier by the Estimates Committee of Parliament.

Another function entrusted to the DDA was the provision of basic civic facilities in regularised (previously unauthorised) colonies and urbanised villages under the various schemes of the Delhi administration. The resources made available to the DDA were not sufficient to meet the actual expenditure incurred by it on the development of basic infrastructure facilities in these colonies and villages. These colonies, along with development work relating to urban villages, were transferred to the MCD on 1 April 1987.

Under the DMC Act of 1957, the MCD is responsible for providing basic services, including public health, drinking water, sanitation and solid and liquid waste disposal. Within the MCD, the Health Department provides medical services through dispensaries (belonging to different systems of medicine), hospitals, maternity and child welfare centres and maternity homes. The department is also concerned with the control of communicable diseases, management of outbreaks and health education. The Conservancy and Sanitation Engineering (CSE) Department maintains environmental sanitation, including open drains, and is responsible for the disposal of solid waste. Till the late 1970s, conservancy and sanitation responsibilities lay with the Public Health Division of the Health Department. Water supply, sewers and liquid waste disposal were managed by the Water Department. During 1988, the responsibility for cleaning septic tanks in the resettlement colonies was vested in the Engineering Department of the MCD.

The decision to transfer resettlement colonies from the DDA to the MCD had been under consideration for about four years. Without assessing available facilities, funds, equipment and manpower, the Delhi administration decided in May 1988 to transfer all 44 resettlement colonies to the MCD with effect from 1 June 1988. The Sarkaria Report pointed out that the necessary prerequisites were not paid adequate attention by the MCD before taking charge of these colonies. These included infrastructure for distributing water, sewage and drainage facilities, arrangements for transportation and disposal of garbage, adequate manpower to supervise the workers transferred from the DDA to the MCD, and funds for carrying out its responsibilities in these colonies.

The Lieutenant Governor of Delhi presided over a meeting on 12 May 1988 that decided upon the financial assistance that would be made available to the MCD by the Delhi administration. Rupees 200 million were allotted for setting up and maintaining machinery and purchasing all material and equipment for maintenance of water and sanitation services. Funds for this purpose were released nearly six months after the outbreak. The first instalment of Rs 50 million was released in January

1989. A sum of Rs 100 million was allotted for immediate repairs and for making the services operational. Funds were released about two weeks *after* the outbreak. A sum of Rs 1.06 billion was earmarked for additional facilities. The Lieutenant Governor directed on 12 May 1988 that the Delhi Administration should process this fund immediately. The actual release of the fund started from 10 November 1988, after the epidemic was already over. Till 31 March 1989, only Rs 263.6 million had actually been released.

A New Strain

The predominant serotype of the 1988 epidemic was *Vibrio cholerae* El Tor Ogawa (99.4 per cent). The isolation rate of 46 per cent of all diarrhoea cases admitted in the IDH was exceptional, compared to 10–27 per cent isolation rates observed in earlier years. The antibiogram observed in the 1988 epidemic differed from the previous years' isolates, when resistance to furazolidone was much lower and that to tetracycline greater. Khanna et al. suggested the possibility of the introduction of new strains into the environment.[59] The source and mechanism of spread of such a strain has remained unknown. *In vitro* susceptibility testing of the isolated vibrios showed 99per cent sensitivity each to tetracycline and chloramphenicol, 98per cent to streptomycin, 97 per cent to furazolidone and 94 per cent to ampicillin (Table 4.8).

Table 4.8: Resistance of *V. cholerae* to Furazolidone and Tetracycline[60]

	1980	*1981*	*1982*	*1983*	*1984*	*1985*	*1986*	*1987*	*1988*
Furazolidone	2.0	0.9	0	0.2	0.3	1.0	0	0	3.8
Tetracycline	2.8	5.5	4.5	8.5	0.3	5.5	2.0	3.5	0.8

The reasons for the sudden increase in cholera cases are unknown. This outbreak followed one of the worst drought periods in many areas. Similar experiences had also been noted in the past. It has been hypothesised that such drought conditions, apart from affecting the availability of safe drinking water and leading to the consumption of water from unsafe sources and the subsequent spread of diarrhoeal infections, may also increase the susceptibility of humans. It has also been hypothesised that, like *Vibrio parahaemolyticus*, *V. cholerae* O1 may have a natural reservoir in the aqueous environment. A sudden proliferation of the bacteria in the aqueous environment and its spread into drinking water sources like tubewells and handpumps could have contributed to the outbreak.

The residents of resettlement colonies were the most-affected group, owing to the near-total collapse of services following the transfer of these colonies from the DDA to the MCD. The existing level of provision of infrastructure and delivery of services was already far below reasonable standards. The affected communities were acutely dependent on groundwater drawn through shallow handpumps. Lack of sanitary latrines (and consequently open defecation) and improper waste disposal led to massive contamination of groundwater. Drought conditions also contributed to the problem. The shift in antibiogram suggested biological variation of the causative agent.

CONTAINMENT MEASURES

Rational principles of management of a cholera epidemic include provision of safe water, proper disposal of solid and liquid wastes of the community and the identification, isolation and treatment of the cases at the earliest. Though a cholera epidemic is usually associated with panic, yet cholera need not pose a major public health problem in a community that has a properly managed programme for the control of diarrhoeal diseases.

Sharing Information

The essence of a control programme is to inform the community of the appropriate control measures. The report submitted to the Supreme Court criticised the administration for failing to advise the community to administer oral rehydration to a patient of diarrhoea at the earliest, and to continue rehydration if needed after discharge from the hospital. The community was not advised to stop using handpump water for drinking purposes, to store water properly and use chlorine tablets or boil the water, or to maintain sanitation and personal hygiene. Further, the affected people should have been told not to have a false sense of security about the vaccine. The VHAI report[61] observed that mass media like All India Radio and Doordarshan (the state television) were not utilised.

The emphasis was on handbills and posters that were of little relevance to illiterate/semi-literate communities. Moreover, they were not distributed or displayed adequately. Interpersonal communication, a most powerful tool in a situation like this, was conspicuous by its absence.

The State of Medical Care

Initial care was provided largely by private practitioners; but it was costly and often irrational, comprising intravenous infusion, antibiotics and antidiarrhoeals in wrong and hazardous doses. Drugs like tonics, Liv 52 and Isaphgol were also prescribed. While a significant number of practitioners failed to provide information about oral rehydration, others prescribed expensive commercial ORS brands. Reasonably priced ORS formulations meeting WHO specifications were not available with chemists. The VHAI report of 1988 pointed out that, often, one ORS packet was given per family, which was inadequate for complete correction of dehydration in an individual patient, let alone of multiple cases in the same family. Further, correct information on dosage for different age groups was not properly disseminated; as a result, incomplete rehydration and complications were common. The staff of the school health services, who were making house-to-house visits for disseminating health education and promoting the use of ORS, was withdrawn for vaccination work, resulting in these components being "abandoned" for sometime.[62]

Clear guidelines regarding initial treatment—when to refer, where to refer, how to handle GE and suspected cholera cases and their contacts—were not provided to medical practitioners by the concerned health authorities. There was confusion regarding the admission and referral criteria for cholera cases, causing hardship to patients. Many of them reached the IDH directly without the remediation of dehydration. Facilities for stool examination and emergency care were available at the Guru Teg Bahadur and Hindu Rao Hospitals, but were inadequate to meet the patient load. Due to the overload of work, many children were discharged too early, and some of them died on their way home with the recurrence of diarrhoea and vomiting. This was attributed to the lack of clear guidelines whereby milder cases could have been tackled at peripheral levels/institutions, leaving the critical cases to hospital care.

Vaccination During the Epidemic

Despite a previous directive to the contrary by the Director General of Health Services, cholera vaccination was undertaken *after* the onset of the epidemic, in accordance with the action plan that was announced following the visit of the prime minister on 22 June. A target was set of achieving 900,000 inoculations against cholera in the trans-Yamuna area in one week (23 to 29 August 1988).

Jet injector machines were imported, as these were considered the "ideal answer to contingencies . . . where quality and the factor of time both are of essence".[63] These machines could deliver as many as 8,000 inoculations per hour. In another context, it was claimed that "the acceptability of jet injector machines among the people is high . . . people flocked by themselves and cent per cent people were inoculated in the villages" in the flood-affected areas of Orissa. The jetgun was thus projected as the surest and quickest way to contain the epidemic.

In Delhi, though the target was 900,000 inoculations, the administration procured 2,400,000 doses, of which as many as 2,361,000 doses were indeed administered. These included vaccines made available on demand to NGOs, political parties, security agencies, corporate organisations, religious bodies and the Super Bazar (a cooperative marketing organisation) for sale to the general public. In the first week of July, typhoid immunisation had also started. A total of 1,157,200 paediatric doses and 730,120 adult doses were administered. This was undertaken in the context of the perception of an increased risk of waterborne diseases. The whole exercise of vaccination was condemned by the report submitted to the Supreme Court as "an exercise in futility and mismanagement from the medical point of view". The estimated cost of this exercise was put at Rs 10 million or more. More importantly, the emphasis on vaccination detracted from attention to rational oral rehydration therapy.

Evaluation of Control Measures

On 7 August 1988 (the epidemic had just begun to show a downward trend at this point, and the control measures were fully operational), teams from the Union Ministry of Health and Family Welfare inspected different areas affected by the epidemic and other areas from which cholera cases had been reported, for the evaluation of control measures. Their findings are a commentary on the control measures that were instituted.

No cholera immunisation was undertaken in Subzi Mandi (Civil Lines Zone). Safe water supply was lacking. Unlicensed water trolleys were seen operating in the most insanitary conditions. In the same zone, the teams also visited Majnu Ka Tilla and Jahangirpuri, where immunisation programmes against cholera and typhoid were functioning satisfactorily. However, no health education campaigns had been carried out in Jahangirpuri. Open drains were choked and overflowing with wastewater. Exposed cooked food was on sale.

Garbage was littered in the Faiz Road area (Karol Bagh Zone). Restaurants were functioning in insanitary conditions. In Ranjit Nagar, the immunisation programme was yet to begin and exposed food and fruits were seen on sale. Doctors were, however, seen to be imparting health education to the community. In adjacent Baljit Nagar, health education activities and the immunisation programmes were functioning well. However, there was rampant sale of exposed food and cut fruits and vegetables.

In the most congested areas of the old city, garbage heaps were found at Chandni Chowk, Fateh Puri, Khari Baoli and Old Delhi Railway Station (City Zone); the fly index was very high. No publicity materials were seen in the area.

No vaccines had been administered in Harijan Camp, Mehrchand Market (Central Zone). Neither had any health education been carried out. In adjacent Kotla Mubarakpur (Central Zone), no immunisation had taken place. Though people were aware of the outbreak of cholera, no health education campaigns had been undertaken. Water from shallow wells was being used by local food vendors and hotels. Lack of safe piped water supply was also noted. The cholera immunisation programme was progressing satisfactorily in schools and dispensaries in Ali village, but the health education component was lacking.

In Sis Ram Park and Indra Park (Shahdara Zone), vaccination was being provided in camps without disposable needles and syringes. Health education activity was conspicuous by its absence, while the sale of exposed food and cut fruits was widespread. In Fazalpur village, immunisation programmes against cholera and typhoid were found to be satisfactory.

People obtained health education messages only through television. In the colonies around the GTB Hospital (one of the worst-affected areas), immunisation activities were satisfactory. Health education was also progressing satisfactorily through posters, public address systems and group meetings. The immunisation coverage was adequate in Gokulpuri. People were aware of oral rehydration therapy only through the television.

The teams inspected not only those areas that were affected by the epidemic, but several other areas as well. Some of these areas are currently endemic foci for cholera. There was an overbearing emphasis on vaccination, and this vertical strategy functioned reasonably well. Interviews with field workers who had served in the epidemic areas in 1988 revealed that owing to the extraordinary emphasis by policy makers and the adequate provision of vaccination services by provider agencies, a demand for vaccination had been created in the community. There had been instances when neighbours and their relations visited the homes of the vaccinators in the evenings and nights to be vaccinated. Not much attention was paid to environmental and food hygiene. The water tanker fleet was inadequate at that time for providing alternative safe water supplies to the affected areas. Health education, a critical tool for epidemic management, was not given due importance, largely because the field staff were overburdened with vaccination targets.

It was essentially the faulty planning and maintenance of resettlement colonies set up during the Emergency regime that resulted in the cholera epidemic in the capital of India. The rhetoric of providing planned settlements and "happy and tension-free lives" for the urban poor through the resettlement colonies stood demystified.[64] The response of the health services was no better. What started as a planning and engineering failure was further complicated by the failure of health administrators to provide rational management strategies for the epidemic.

DIARRHOEAL DISEASES CONTROL: NEW STRATEGIES

Following the 1988 epidemic, the Delhi government and the MCD started a massive programme to prevent and contain diarrhoeal diseases in Delhi.

Post-1988, the word haija (cholera) came to acquire a special connotation. Politicians and citizens started using the term as a tool to attract attention to the water and sanitation problems of their areas, even in the absence of any outbreak of diarrhoeal diseases. Substantial significance is also attached to this word by the media. At times, it works as an early warning system, while on other occasions talk of haija has functioned like a false alarm. Fear of cholera therefore brought diarrhoeal diseases control into focus. The concerned field staff (the Health Department), in turn, considers cholera (and diarrhoeal diseases) control as their main duty, often at the cost of other communicable diseases.

Disease Surveillance

The reporting system for diarrhoeal diseases was strengthened after the epidemic by introducing a sentinel surveillance system. Thirteen index hospitals located in different parts of the city were selected to ensure geographical representation. The number of these sentinel centres was later increased to 22. Particulars of admission of diarrhoeal diseases are collected daily and analysed at the respective zonal level. At each hospital, a medical officer is assigned the exclusive duty of maintaining records and investigating all diarrhoeal deaths. All dispensaries report diarrhoeal cases daily, but generally without any patient details.

Distribution of Chlorine Tablets and ORS

Chlorine tablets (one tablet being sufficient to disinfect 20 litres of water for 24 hours) were distributed through different agencies in the following areas:

- MCD: in unauthorised colonies without piped water supply
- Urban Basic Services (UBS) Department: in JJ clusters
- Directorate of Social Welfare (Delhi administration): through anganwadi workers in the areas of their operation

Since 1996, only the MCD has continued with this programme, while other agencies have stopped distribution in their respective areas; distribution in those areas has been taken over by the MCD. The UBS programme itself has been defunct over the last five years, and its functions have been taken over to some extent by the erstwhile India Population Project (IPP)-VIII programme of the MCD.

Interviews with field workers revealed that the use of chlorine tablets by communities remains low. In the post-epidemic phase, there were plans to supply chlorine tablets that would last two weeks and would purify the drinking water requirement of an average-sized family; these tablets were to be supplied to households at their doorsteps. Fourteen chlorine tablets (each tablet being sufficient to purify 20 litres of water per day) were packed in a sachet, and were meant to last two weeks for a family. The field worker would thus need to visit every family once a fortnight to maintain the supplies of chlorine tablets. Over the years, the rise in population and the number of settlements lacking access to safe water supply has made it inordinately difficult for MCD field workers to reach the fortnight's supply to each and every home.

The WHO, in association with Population Services International and Sulabh International, started a pilot project in 2002 in selected slums in west Delhi for the social marketing of liquid chlorine for home chlorination, along with the promotion of narrow-mouthed container to prevent domestic-level contamination. This strategy has been implemented in several countries around the world. In Delhi, the partners chosen were Population Services International, for their experience in social marketing of contraceptives, and Sulabh International, for their experience in the sanitation sector and network of community-level workers. The experience of this project was not encouraging, and it was discontinued after the pilot phase. Subsequently, the Health Department became involved in the distribution of liquid chlorine at the household level.

A network for the distribution of ORS packets has been set up through:

- Major hospitals (ORT Corners)
- Dispensaries, colony hospitals and primary health centres
- Maternity and child welfare centres and maternity homes
- Mobile dispensaries
- Field staff

Health education regarding the use of ORS has been imparted to various groups, including schoolchildren. Since 1999, chlorine–ORS depots have been set up within each vulnerable cluster in coordination with local social and political leaders to make these available within the community with the help of community volunteers. About 2,500 such depots were set up. The strategy thus shifted from house-to-house distribution to making supplies available at the community level at chlorine–ORS depots. Despite these programmes, the usage of chlorine tablets remains low among vulnerable communities. The use of ORS is, however, considerably higher.[65]

Food Hygiene

The food hygiene measures implemented, particularly during the vulnerable season,include the following:

- Food items exposed to dust and flies, including cut fruits, are seized and destroyed.
- No hawkers are allowed to sell eatables outside schools.
- Sale of water through unlicensed trolleys is not allowed.
- Sale of ice from unlicensed ice factories is not allowed.
- Sugarcane crushers operating in the open and unlicensed sugarcane crushing shops are removed or closed down.
- Sale of all types of *kulfi*s and *chuski*s (ice candies) is stopped.
- Vendors are prevented from selling various types of drinks from unlicensed factories.
- A watch is kept on ice that is imported from the neighbouring states.

A foodborne outbreak was reported in 1991 from the Delhi Cantonment. There were nine laboratory-confirmed cholera cases. In the absence of environmental risk factors, rectal swabs from all food handlers were tested. Two of them (working in the same mess) were detected to be positive for *Vibrio cholerae* (El Tor, Ogawa).[66] The outbreak was controlled by the isolation and treatment of carriers. In the absence of similar studies from other parts of Delhi, it is difficult to estimate the contribution of carriers and foodborne outbreaks to the endemicity of cholera. A three-month health education campaign using posters and interactive sessions with flip charts reported significant change among 136 foodhandlers in a study conducted by the Department of Community Medicine, Maulana Azad Medical College.[67]

This regulatory role of the programme is extremely lax. Rather than a routine, sustained process, the emphasis is on conducting food hygiene raids and the policing of traders (Figure 4.6). This function is a classic example of the "inspector raj", and is subject to political interference and corruption.

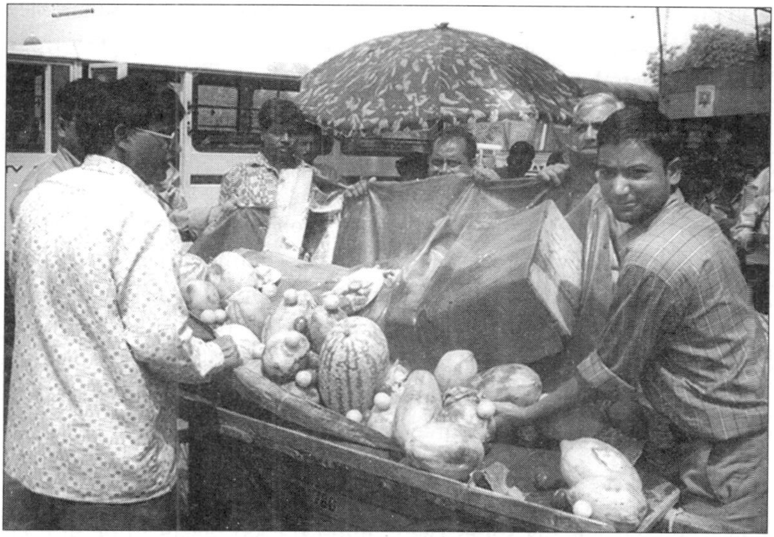

Figure 4.6: Raids on Selling of Cut Fruits by Food Hygiene Squads. Photograph by author.

All open wells whose water is used for drinking are disinfected with bleaching powder twice or thrice a week during the vulnerable season. Wells are a minor source of drinking water and are used mostly in rural areas; a few wells are also operational in the walled city. There are about 250 such wells, but only a small proportion of them are used for drinking purposes. The current emphasis, therefore, is on preventing the breeding of mosquitoes in unused wells by releasing larvivorous fish into them.

Contaminated ice is a major source of waterborne diseases.[58] A large proportion of ice consumed in Delhi is imported from the neighbouring states of Uttar Pradesh and Haryana. Ice from these factories as well as those in Delhi is tested once a year at the time of renewal of licences. There are no mechanisms for regular monitoring of quality. Further, there are unlicensed factories that produce and sell ice. The microbiological quality of ice being sold in Delhi remains suspect, and there is scope for improvement in the regulatory aspects of this source of infection.

The residual chlorine content of the water sold through refrigerated water trolleys at the roadside is checked by health staff to ensure that safe and potable water is supplied to citizens. The quality checks in this trade are better than those for ice.

Health Education

The lack of effective health education strategies during the 1988 epidemic has been highlighted by the VHAI report.[69] Following the epidemic, there was no change in the approach. The authorities continued with more of the same, and handbills and posters remained the mainstay of such campaigns. Their ineffectiveness in the context of vulnerable communities, many of whom cannot read, is obvious. The use of mass media was conspicuous by its absence. The dengue epidemic of 1996 focused attention on the role of health education, and resource allocation on this head also improved considerably.

Audio-visual media began to be utilised in a major way. Cable television and cinema slides (with audio tracks) began to be utilised (Figure 4.7). Film shows began to be conducted within the clusters vulnerable to waterborne diseases. A variety of outdoor media, including Delhi Transport Corporation buses, bus shelters, large hoardings and kiosks on streetlight poles were included. Visual messages were designed for handbills, posters and stickers; the emphasis on written words was reduced. Schoolchildren have shown involvement in the programme; this is a component that needs to be strengthened as schoolchildren constitute a very powerful medium. The emphasis in the messages is on personal hygiene, including washing hands with soap and water after defecation and before having meals;the consumption of water made potable by adding chlorine tablets where piped water supply is not available; avoiding the consumption of food and cutfruits exposed to dust and flies; and promoting the use of ORS and other home-based fluids in case of onset of diarrhoea and vomiting.

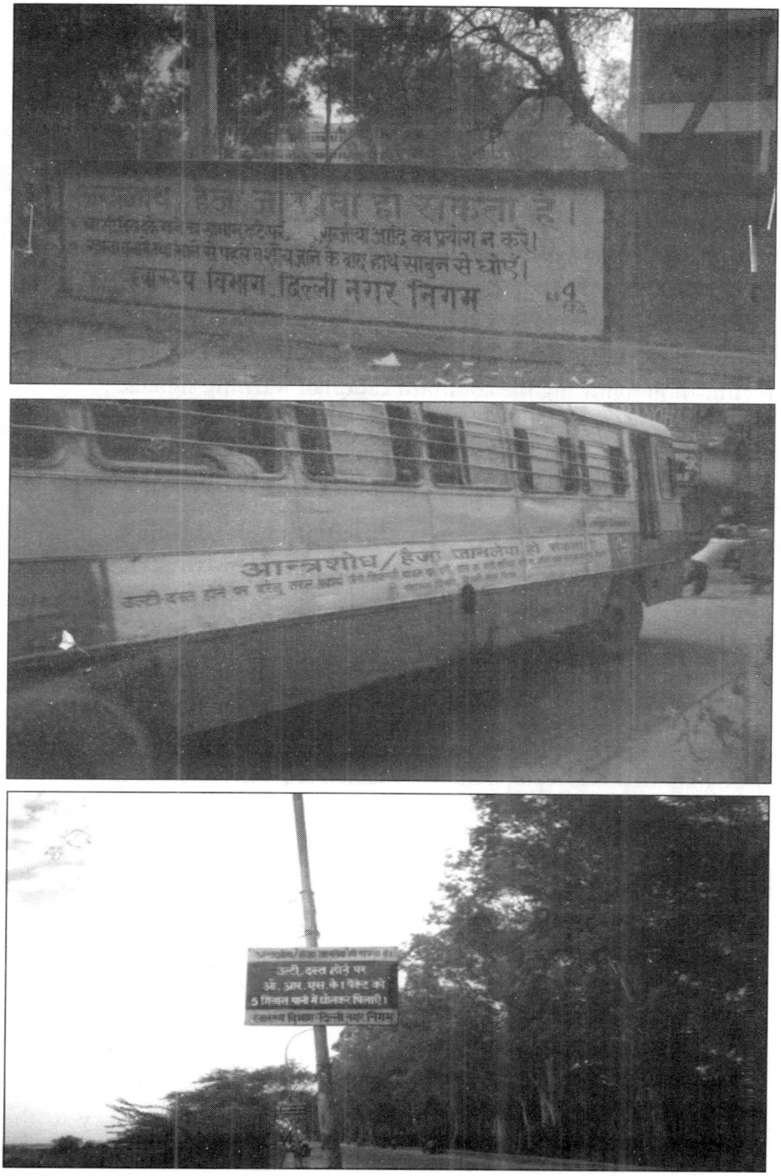

Figure 4.7: Information, Education and Communication (IEC) Campaigns. Photographs by author.

Water Quality Surveillance

Since 1998–99, there has been a special thrust on early detection of contamination of water supply. Each week, surveys are conducted by field workers in their respective areas on the functioning of chlorinators, pipelines passing through drains, residual chlorine in water samples at the consumer end and leakages in pipelines. Information regarding these warning signals are conveyed to the DJB at both local and headquarters levels. Surveys of accumulated garbage, choked, open drains and waterlogging are conducted in coordination with the CSE. These measures have helped build up better intersectoral coordination and facilitated early rectification following the communication of warning signals.

SPECIAL MEASURES AGAINST CHOLERA CASES

Zonal deputy health officers and zonal epidemiologists are required to investigate and take containment measures with regard to all cholera cases, all GE deaths and the clustering of GE cases, i.e., more than three cases in a house or a particular locality. The probable cause has to be identified through epidemiological investigations. Water samples are tested from the affected household from which the cholera case is reported, along with samples from adjacent households. In case of focal contamination of water, the DJB undertakes repairs. Chlorine tablets are distributed, or distribution is intensified in the area; supplies for two weeks are provided to each family at a time. Health education campaigns at the community level are launched or intensified. Correction of insanitary conditions is done by the CSE. Food hygiene raids are conducted in the area to destroy unhygienic food. Antibiotic chemoprophylaxis (doxycycline or tetracycline for adults and furazolidone or cotrimoxazole for children) is given to the family contacts of the cholera cases; this was discontinued in 1999, following a directive from the Union Ministry of Health and Family Welfare.

These measures were implemented rigorously following the epidemic, and the incidence of cholera cases declined briefly. The key to the prevention of diarrhoeal diseases—adequate safe water and safe disposal of excreta—received less attention. There were no major programmes to build up infrastructure in the colonies where it was needed most. In the absence of these two key services, the role of these measures remained peripheral at best. The low incidence rate could not be sustained. From 1990, the incidence rate began rising despite this elaborate programme. With the arrival of the *Vibrio cholerae* O139 strain, incidence rates rose above the 1988 level, and cholera was back on the public health agenda in a major way.

NOTES

1. The first El Tor case was reported in India from Calcutta. Barua, "History of Cholera".
2. Patnaik and Kapoor, *Statistical Review of Cholera Problem in India.*
3. Prepared by the author on the basis of raw data provided in the Appendix.
4. Patnaik and Kapoor, *Statistical Review of Cholera Problem in India.*
5. C. S. Chuttani, "Epidemiological and Clinical Characteristics of Cholera in Delhi", *Indian Journal of Medical Research* 55, no. 8, 1966, 815–24.
6. Pushpa Aggarwal et al., "Current Epidemiological Aspects of Cholera in Delhi", *Journal of Communicable Diseases* 15, no. 1, 1983, 26–31.
7. Prepared by the author on the basis of raw data provided in the Appendix.
8. Varsha Amin et al., "Clinical Profile of Cholera in Young Children: A Hospital Based Report", *Indian Pediatrics* 31, no. 7, 1994, 755–61.
9. K. Rajeshwari et al., "Diarrhoeal Outbreak of *Vibrio cholerae* O1 Inaba in Delhi", *Tropical Doctor* 28, no. 2, 2008, 105–7.
10. Srujuna Mohanty, "Seasonality and Antimicrobial Resistance Pattern of *Vibrio cholerae* in a Tertiary Care Hospital of North India", *Tropical Doctor* 24, no. 4, 2004, 249–51; Shukla Das, Rumpa Saha and Iqbal R. Kaur, "Trend of Antibiotic Resistance of *Vibrio cholerae* Strains from East Delhi", *Indian Journal of Medical Research* 127, no. 5, 2008, 478–82.
11. Prepared by the author on the basis of raw data provided in the Appendix.
12. Voluntary Health Association of India (VHAI), *Civic Neglect and Ill-Health* (Delhi: VHAI, 1988).
13. Avdesh Kumar et al., "An Epidemiological Profile of Gastro-enteritis Deaths in Delhi State", *Journal of Communicable Diseases* 26, no. 2, 1995, 92–99.
14. J. Singh et al., "Prescribing Pattern by Doctors for Acute Diarrhoea in Children in Delhi, India", *Journal of Diarrhoeal Diseases Research* 13, no. 4, 1995, 229–31.
15. J. Singh et al., "Unusual Occurrence of Cholera in Delhi during January 1994: Epidemiological Investigations", *Journal of Diarrhoeal Diseases Research* 14, no. 2, 1996, 107–9.

16. Prepared by the author on the basis of raw data provided in the Appendix.
17. Ibid.
18. Ibid.
19. Sachdeva et al., "Widespread Emergence of *Vibrio cholerae* O139 in India".
20. Data collected from the NICD while conducting the research for this book.
21. Ibid.
22. Ramamurthy et al., "Emergence of Novel Strain of *Vibrio cholerae*".
23. Ibid.
24. Albert et al., "Large Outbreak of Clinical Cholera".
25. Jagvir Singh et al., "Epidemiology and Transmission of *V. cholerae* O1 and *V. cholerae* O139 Infections in Delhi in 1993", *Journal of Diarrheal Diseases Research* 14, no. 3, 1996, 182–86.
26. Jagvir Singh et al., "*Vibrio cholerae* O1 and O139 in Less Than 5 Years Old Children Hospitalised for Watery Diarrhoea in Delhi, 1993", *Journal of Diarrheal Diseases Research* 15, no. 1, 1997, 3–6.
27. Dasgupta, "Cholera Outbreak in Garhi"; Shalu Gupta and M. M. A. Faridi, "Cholera Pattern in Children of Delhi", *Indian Pediatrics* 42, no. 2, 2005, 90–91.
28. N. C. Sharma et al., "Changing Profile of *Vibrio cholerae* O1, O139 in Delhi and Its Periphery (2003–2005)", *Indian Journal of Medical Research* 125, no. 5, 2007, 633–40.
29. Shukla Das and Sunil Gupta, "Diversity of *Vibrio cholerae* Strains Isolated in Delhi, India during 1992–2000", *Journal of Health, Population and Nutrition* 23, no. 1, 2005, 44–51.
30. K. K. Dutta et al., "Epidemiological Features of Cholera Outbreak in Delhi in 1988", *Journal of Communicable Diseases* 25, no. 2, 1992, 57–61.
31. K. K. Khanna et al., "Cholera Outbreak in Delhi in 1988", *Journal of Communicable Diseases* 22, no. 1, 1990, 35–38.
32. A Bharatiya Janata Party fact-finding team claimed that this was a cholera outbreak; that 25 people had died and that 250 were affected. VHAI, *Civic Neglect and Ill-Health.*
33. Report filed with the NICD, New Delhi.
34. VHAI, *Civic Neglect and Ill-Health.*
35. Ritu Priya, "Mr. Pitroda Goes to Sunder Nagari", *Seminar* 354, 1989, 1–4.
36. Data collected from the NICD during the research for this book.
37. It is interesting that during June–July 1968, 47 per cent isolation was reported by Pal and Misra out of a total of 193 diarrhoea admissions. Pal and Misra, "Laboratory Investigation of Cholera Epidemics".
38. Khanna et al., "Cholera Outbreak in Delhi in 1988".

39. Dutta et al., "Epidemiological Features of Cholera Outbreak in Delhi in 1988".
40. Priya, "Mr. Pitroda Goes to Sunder Nagari".
41. VHAI, *Report of the Independent Commission on Health in India* (New Delhi: VHAI, 1997).
42. Dutta et al., "Epidemiological Features of Cholera Outbreak in Delhi in 1988".
43. VHAI, *Civic Neglect and Ill-Health.*
44. Dutta et al., "Epidemiological Features of Cholera Outbreak in Delhi in 1988".
45. Ibid. During the 1988 epidemic, Shahdara constituted a single administrative zone. In the aftermath of the epidemic, one of the many steps taken was to bifurcate Shahdara into Shahdara (North) Zone and Shahdara (South) Zone in 1990, for more effective administration. The entire area on the east bank of the Yamuna was one Shahdara zone. The railway line from the Old Yamuna Bridge to Uttar Pradesh was taken as the line of demarcation between the two zones.
46. Priya, "Town Planning, Public Health and Urban Poor".
47. Ibid.
48. The intermediate sizes of plots recommended by the DDA at various points of time were 80 square yards and 55 square yards.
49. The committee consisted of Mr P. C. Tyagi, Chairman, Central Pollution Control Board, Mr B. P. C. Sinha, Chief Hydrologist, and Dr Mira Shiva, Voluntary Health Association of India. The report was submitted in 1990.
50. VHAI, *Civic Neglect and Ill-Health*; Priya, "Mr. Pitroda Goes to Sunder Nagari".
51. Priya, "Mr. Pitroda Goes to Sunder Nagari".
52. VHAI, *Civic Neglect and Ill-Health.*
53. Priya, "Mr. Pitroda Goes to Sunder Nagari".
54. NEERI and ITRC conducted the tests between 25 July and 3 August 1988.
55. C. P. Baveja et al., "Bacteriological Study of Drinking Water during Epidemic of Cholera in Delhi", *Journal of Communicable Diseases* 21, no. 1, 1989, 59–61.
56. Baveja et al., "Bacteriological Study of Drinking Water"; Report of the three-member committee appointed by the Supreme Court in response to Writ Petitions (Criminal) Nos. 330 and 400 of 1988.
57. WHO, *Guidelines for Drinking-Water Quality*, vol. 3, 2nd ed. (Geneva: WHO, 1997).
58. WHO, *Guidelines for Drinking-Water Quality.*
59. Khanna et al., "Cholera Outbreak in Delhi in 1988".

60. Ibid.
61. VHAI, *Civic Neglect and Ill-Health*.
62. Priya, "Mr. Pitroda Goes to Sunder Nagari".
63. Report of the three-member committee appointed by the Supreme Court in response to Writ Petitions (Criminal) Nos 330 and 400 of 1988.
64. Priya, "Town Planning, Public Health and Urban Poor".
65. Based on informal discussions with Population Services International, which conducted baseline surveys before starting the project on social marketing of liquid chlorine and safe containers.
66. V. W. Tilak, R. Bhalwar and J. S. Ratti, "Epidemiological Study of an Outbreak of Cholera in Delhi Cantonment", *Indian Journal of Public Health* 41, no. 2, 1997, 61–67.
67. R. Malhotra et al., "Evaluation of a Health Education Intervention on Knowledge and Attitudes of Food Handlers Working in a Medical College in Delhi, India", *Asia Pacific Journal of Public Health* 20, no. 4, 2008, 277–86.
68. Koo et al., "Epidemic Cholera in Guatemala".
69. VHAI, *Civic Neglect and Ill-Health*.

5

Vulnerability to Cholera

A Spatial Epidemiological Analysis

Having looked at the broader time trends and the relative shifts in cholera incidence and mortality, the discussion now moves on to an understanding of the macrodeterminants of these trends. Inter-zonal and intra-zonal commonalities and differences determine the epidemiological dynamics of the disease and help identify the determinants of the vulnerability of colonies. The incidence of cholera cases in different municipal zones of Delhi for the period 1994–2000 is analysed and put into relation with the relevant characteristics of the zones. Through the identification of the most-affected colonies, the interplay of social determinantsis deconstructed.

DOES LOCATION MATTER? THE RELEVANCE OF AREA EFFECTS

The socio-economic characteristics of areas have been associated by several scholars with different health outcomes in a wide range of contexts.[1] The social gradient of diseases by their location have been examined by Villermé in his 1826 study using Parisian data, and by Engels in the context of Manchester, England, in 1844.[2] A fairly common contemporary approach is to use regression methods at the level of individual characteristics. The methodology adopted in the present study does not examine individual confounders across categories of area deprivation. The analysis is comparable to that by Breeze et al. in so far as "the combined (as opposed to the 'independent') effects of social class and area deprivation" have been captured.[3] The caution expressed by Diez Roux in this context is significant:

> The assumption is that the people living in the least deprived areas are a good proxy for what the people living in the most deprived areas would be like if they did not live in the most deprived areas. Usually in epidemiological jargon, this implies no residual confounding by measured variables and no unmeasured confounders. The inability to undeniably confirm the validity of this assumption is the crucial limitation of observational analyses.[4]

A fully adequate causal model of public health must therefore be able to explain the disease at the ecological level. In contrast with the universalism of the natural sciences, the ecologism of the biological sciences entails localisation and attention to the bounds that limit generalisations about biological, human and social systems.[5] Ecological constructs try to deal with the true complexity of the biological world.[6] Ecosocial perspectives have thus emerged in order to explain the social, political and economic processes that shape epidemiological patterns.[7] The framework outlined by Krieger is useful in exploring the determinants of vulnerability for cholera-endemic areas.[8] Emphasis is placed on two key concepts:

- A cumulative interplay between exposure, susceptibility and resistance conceptualised at multiple levels—neighbourhood, regional and politico-administrative jurisdictions and in multiple home and public settings
- Accountability and agency in relation to institutions and communities

While emphasising accountability, it is argued that much of the vulnerability stems from "institutional discrimination" transacted through notions of legality and planning in urban spaces, deriving these material pathways at multiple levels. Thus, this approach transcends standard "biological" or "social" analyses and explores a relatively more holistic explanation of vulnerability to waterborne diseases. Cholera has been used as a marker of waterborne diseases since it is closely monitored and laboratory-confirmed data is available.

ZONAL DISTRIBUTION OF CHOLERA CASES, 1994–2000

The years 1994–2000 have been taken as an illustrative period. The incidence rate of cholera cases has been computed per 100,000 population for each zone (Table 5.1). The validity of this data lies in comparative analysis over space (inter-zonal) and time rather than as figures for real incidence rates.

Table 5.1: Incidence Rate of Cholera per 100,000 for 12 Zones, 1994–2000[9]

Zone	*1994*	*1995*	*1996*	*1997*	*1998*	*1999*	*2000*	*Average*
Civil Lines	60.32 (637)	42.90 (472)	18.15 (208)	25.63 (306)	48.71 (606)	24.31 (315)	13.70 (185)	33.39
Narela	57.00 (109)	73.47 (141)	18.64 (40)	10.89 (28)	36.47 (85)	19.40 (51)	8.50 (27)	32.05
Najafgarh	59.64 (225)	46.56 (1,883)	13.68 (56)	8.91 (38)	15.53 (69)	11.66 (54)	8.91 (43)	23.55
Rohini	31.96 (212)	29.67 (205)	13.06 (94)	12.80 (96)	44.54 (348)	15.23 (124)	10.26 (87)	22.50
South	36.82 (225)	21.20 (135)	9.05 (60)	8.10 (56)	11.53 (83)	18.27 (137)	22.40 (175)	18.20
Central	6.94 (85)	20.83 (266)	11.35 (151)	9.31 (129)	10.11 (146)	12.23 (184)	11.55 (181)	12.30
Shahdara (North)	29.70 (281)	16.64 (164)	7.89 (81)	7.20 (77)	10.86 (121)	9.13 (106)	4.63 (56)	11.76
Shahdara (South)	7.82 (89)	9.11 (108)	3.48 (43)	3.27 (42)	6.34 (85)	5.80 (81)	2.48 (36)	5.48
Sadar Pahargunj	11.09 (71)	5.11 (37)	3.24 (27)	2.21 (18)	4.12 (34)	8.14 (61)	4.03 (19)	5.42
Karol Bagh	3.63 (30)	6.03 (52)	2.56 (23)	2.46 (23)	3.49 (34)	6.01 (61)	1.80 (19)	3.71
City	3.30 (28)	3.74 (33)	2.07 (19)	2.61 (25)	3.51 (35)	6.25 (65)	2.31 (25)	3.40
West	2.92 (30)	2.52 27)	1.43 (16)	1.55 (18)	2.81 (34)	1.27 (16)	0.91 (12)	1.91
Total	21.22 (2,022)	18 36 (1,823)	7.91 (818)	7.94 (856)	14.97 (1,680)	10.79 (1,262)	7.30 (889)	12.64

Note: Figures in parentheses indicate number of notified cases.

The zonal incidence of reported cholera cases exhibits a wide range (Table 5.1), from 2.92 per 100,000 to 64 per 100,000 in 1994; during 1998 it ranged from 2.81 per 100,000 to 488.71 per 100,000, and in 2000 it ranged from 0.91 per 100,000 to 22.40 per 100,000. While all zones were markedly affected in 1994–95, Civil Lines and Rohini were the most affected in 1998 and others showed minor increase. Rohini, Narela and Najafgarh Zones demonstrated a downward trend by 2000. Shahdara (North) and Shahdara (South) Zones too showed a similar trend. In contrast, a rising trend is visible in 1999–2000 in the Central Zone, and more so in the South Zone. The zones can thus be grouped into epidemiological patterns, as detailed in the following.

High but Declining Trend

Civil Lines has the highest average incidence rates among the 12 municipal zones (Table 5.1), but a declining trend can be observed, which is also reflected in its contribution to total reported cases (Table 5.2). Narela, Najafgarh and Rohini Zones are similarly high-incidence zones and demonstrate declining time trends. Following a high incidence rate in 1994, there was a sharp decline. The peak in 1998 in all these zones was lower than the level in 1994. The percentage contribution of annual cases showed little variation in the cases of Rohini and Narela Zones. The proportion of cases reported from Najafgarh Zone, however, declined sharply.

Intermediate but Declining Trend

Shahdara (North) Zone, the worst-affected zone during the 1988 epidemic, is situated on the eastern side of the Yamuna. It was an intermediate-level zone during the mid-1990s, but showed a declining trend following a high in 1994. A number of initiatives were taken after the epidemic to improve infrastructure, particularly for the poorer localities. Between 1994 and 2000, the incidence rate declined from 29.70 per 100,000 to 11.76 per 100,000.

Intermediate but Rising Trend

The Central and South Zones are geographically contiguous, but an administrative relocation of certain areas from the South Zone to the

Central Zone occurred during 1994–95. These two zones displayed intermediate levels of incidence in the mid-1990s, but were marked by some of the highest incidence rates by 2000. The incidence rate in Central Zone remained nearly constant over the years, while South Zone has clearly demonstrated a strong consistent upward trend since 1997 (Table 5.1). This difference is not adequately reflected in Table 5.2, because of the transfer of areas and population from the South to the Central Zone. During 1999, the South Zone accounted for nearly 11 per cent of the cases, almost reaching the 1994 level. The year 2000 saw a further rise to almost 20 per cent of the total cases reported for that year. While the rise in the percentage contribution of the Central Zone can be explained in part by the transfer of certain areas from the South Zone, the steady rise in the contribution of the South Zone is significant.

Low but Steady Trend

Sadar Pahargunj, Karol Bagh and City Zones are geographically adjacent zones that reported nearly similar incidence rates per 100,000 cases, averaging about 4–6. The figures for 2000 show the rates in these zones settling down below the previous levels. The incidence rate ranged between one and three cases per 100,000 population.

Low but Declining Trend

Shahdara (South) Zone is adjacent to Shahdara (North) Zone across the river, but has consistently reported lower incidence rates. Even during the 1988 epidemic, this zone was relatively less affected. The declining trend during 1994–2000, however, can be observed here.

Several key questions need to be addressed. Why is it that different zones in Delhi have different incidence rates? What are the factors that have led to a general rising trend? Why do the Sadar Pahargunj and City Zones despite the high population density and varied socio-economic groups have low levels of incidence? What has been the reason for a spectacular decline in the incidence of cholera in Shahdara, the hotspot of cholera during the 1988 epidemic? Why is the incidence rising in the Central and South Zones?

INTER-ZONAL DIFFERENCES

Analysing the relevant characteristics of the zones and the vulnerable colonies helps us identify the determinants of cholera in Delhi. The spatial distribution of cholera cases in each zone (derived from the residential addresses provided in the notification) indicates that there are several areas from which these cases are consistently reported. Another investigation by the NICD during this period, a study of all cases in 1995 analysed by PIN (postal index number) codes found that 10 of the 80 PIN code areas accounted for 57 per cent of all reported cholera cases.[10] Two other studies also recognised that there were endemic areas from which most of the cases were reported in most areas.[11] No other study has attempted to identify the spatial epidemiology of endemicity. The details of cholera cases reported from different vulnerable colonies are reported in Appendix Tables A.16 to A.22. Some of these areas are large tracts of land, while others are smaller settlement units like urbanised villages or JJ clusters. The key issues examined include:

- Settlement types
- Economic patterns and occupational activities
- Provision of civic services
- Population density and predominant activities
- Characteristics of the residents
- State of the infrastructure in the field

All the zones have a similar diversity of settlements, but in varying proportions. Changes in economic activity, occupational patterns and the provision of civic services have affected the zones differentially. The percentage of cases reported from these endemic areas in the total number of cases reported from their respective zones is reported in Table 5.2. The under-reporting of differentials from certain areas and/or subpopulations may be a limitation of this analysis, and it is recognised that more such endemic foci may exist. The mean contribution of cases reported from these endemic pockets to the annual cases of cholera is fairly consistent and works out to 76.85 per cent of the total reported in Delhi, with a standard deviation of 2.67 per cent.

A common pattern of affected settlements (among the vulnerable

Table 5.2: Proportion of Cases from Vulnerable Colonies in Different Zones[12]

Zone	*1994*	*1995*	*1996*	*1997*	*1998*	*1999*	*2000*	*Average*
Civil Lines	88.70	82.63	92.79	81.70	90.76	84.44	87.57	86.94
Narela	79.82	58.87	92.50	46.43	64.71	78.43	11.11	61.70
Najafgarh	64.89	84.70	85.71	92.11	69.57	85.19	34.88	73.86
Rohini	88.21	81.46	79.79	72.92	89.66	83.06	64.37	79.92
Central and South	83.23	79.05	68.72	80.00	73.80	79.44	76.12	77.19
Shahdara (North)	81.14	84.76	85.19	83.12	84.30	87.74	83.93	84.31
Shahdara (South)	78.65	72.22	62.79	85.71	65.88	71.60	83.33	74.31
Sadar Paharganj	42.25	35.14	44.44	22.22	50.00	60.29	63.64	45.43
Karol Bagh	73.33	40.38	43.48	69.57	52.94	72.13	89.47	63.04
City	50.00	51.52	36.84	28.00	42.86	33.85	60.00	43.30
West	0.00	0.00	0.00	0.00	0.00	0.00	0.00	0.00

Note: All figures are in percentages.

colonies) is observed across zones. The socio-economic and infrastructural characteristics of these colonies are similar, suggesting the determinants of vulnerability of the resident populations among whom cholera occurs. The availability of infrastructure is dependent on the settlement type—on its legal status and the existing norms and policies.

Though small in number, the cases occurring during the winter (November to March) are from these vulnerable colonies (Table 5.3). During the peak season (June to August) there is little variation across the years, ranging from 72.4 per cent to 77.8 per cent. There is, however, considerable variation across the years at the beginning and the end of the peak season—during April, May, September and October—reflecting increasing endemicity in the vulnerable colonies.

Table 5.3: Month-wise Proportion (%) of Cases from the Endemic Areas[13]

	1994	*1995*	*1996*	*1997*	*1998*	*1999*	*2000*
Jan	100.00	0.00	0.00	0.00	0.00	0.00	50.00
Feb	0.00	0.00	0.00	0.00	0.00	0.00	100.00
Mar	0.00	0.00	100.00	0.00	0.00	0.00	0.00
Apr	30.77	84.62	79.17	100.00	80.00	63.77	93.94
May	93.20	75.57	75.00	75.00	79.34	69.20	50.34
Jun	78.14	76.43	77.19	78.45	80.15	81.05	73.10
Jul	85.90	74.45	84.06	75.47	81.43	83.01	69.44
Aug	73.29	70.08	77.60	78.05	81.48	80.79	80.91
Sep	78.42	85.64	60.42	64.94	66.96	79.52	71.19
Oct	78.26	57.83	70.37	92.16	81.63	76.79	69.29
Nov	100.00	90.91	50.00	80.00	85.71	92.86	84.54
Dec	100.00	0.00	0.00	100.00	50.00	0.00	100.00
Annual	79.48	76.25	76.16	75.12	79.88	76.70	71.65

Note: All figures are in percentages.

CIVIL LINES ZONE

At 33.39 per 100,000 population per year, this zone has the highest average incidence rate among all 12 zones. The incidence of cases is higher during the monsoon than during the summer (see Appendix, Table A.6). An average of 87 per cent of notified cholera cases were reported from vulnerable colonies. The incidence rate was 85.7 per 100,000 population during the 1988 cholera epidemic, and 60.32 and 42.90 per 100,000 in 1994 and 1995, respectively (with about 60 per cent of the cases caused by the O139 strain). The 1998 incidence level was higher than that in 1995 at 48.71 per 100,000. Despite a marginal decline in infection rates, the potential conditions for transmission remain in place.

Civil Lines is one of the larger zones of the MCD, comprising a mix of all types of settlements. British residents were located in the Civil Lines area before the new capital (New Delhi) was constructed. The Old Secretariat was the seat of the local government. The coronation of Emperor George V was also held in this area. Yet a new site, Raisina Hills, was chosen for the construction of the new capital as the Civil Lines area was considered unhealthy in view of the proximity of the Yamuna. However, habitations have come up in the "unhealthy" areas as well. The older constructed areas now form the Delhi University (and other academic institutions) and the residences of the wealthy.

The Grand Trunk Road and the Delhi–Ambala railway line form the south-western boundary of the zone. Densely populated localities along the main roads and highways have come up through ribbon development.[14] The population density of this zone is about 13,500 per sq km; newer unauthorised colonies have a relatively lower density, while older urbanised villages, trading centres and slum clusters are highly dense. There is intense commercial activity along this axis, including the Azadpur Mandi (fruit and vegetable wholesale markets), which has been expanding over the years, and the industries in the large designated industrial areas that are mostly "manufacturing" in nature. The poorer new migrants working in the *mandi* (market) and industries reside in slums, urbanised villages and resettlement colonies along the G. T. Road. Another large body of vulnerable population is located between the river Yamuna and the G T. Road, north of the Outer Ring Road.

Water supply in this zone is at an average of 274 lpcd.[15] But there are vast areas without piped water supply and sewers. Water supply is mostly from the plants. However, some areas in the north-western part of the zone are supplied through Ranneywells.

The vulnerable colonies in the zone consist of several urbanised villages—Chandrawal, Rajpura, Azadpur, Bharola, Sarai Peepalthala and Bhalaswa; JJ clusters in Lal Bagh, Bara Bagh and adjoining areas and in Wazirpur Industrial Area; Jahangirpuri resettlement colony; and unauthorised colonies adjoining the villages of Jharoda, Burari and Nathupura.

Urbanised Villages

Chandrawal village (also known as New Chandrawal) is a relocated village. The Old Chandrawal village was relocated from the banks of the Yamuna when the first waterworks was set up in 1889. It is now a densely populated urbanised village with commercial and industrial establishments. The adjoining trading areas also provide employment to the large numbers of tenants in this village. Chandrawal, along with the adjoining area of Malkagunj, has a population of approximately

15,000, and the annual incidence rate ranges each year between 30 and 40 per 100,000.

Rajpura village and its adjoining colony of Gur Mandi has a population of about 10,000, and is located right on the Grand Trunk Road. The population density is high. A number of manufacturing units are located in the residential buildings. These colonies are bound on the eastern side by the Najafgarh drain, a large open channel carrying liquid waste from the western areas of Delhi. The subsoil in this area is highly contaminated. These colonies also face water scarcity. The residents of these colonies are socio-economically well off, and many of the households have their own motors to access groundwater. Contaminated groundwater constitutes a major risk factor in this area. These colonies were affected in 1994, 1998 and 1999, with an average incidence rate of 110 per 100,000 per year.

Azadpur village is located at the crossing of the Ring Road and the G. T. Road, and is also next to the Azadpur railway station. Between the original village and the railway line, there is an unauthorised colony (Kaushalpuri) and some jhuggis. These unauthorised settlements first came up in 1977. The village has a population of about 10,000, while the unauthorised components have a total population of about 25,000. With increasing population, water scarcity has accentuated in Azadpur. Though there are public hydrants in the slum clusters and household-level supply in the village, this is not sufficient to meet the requirement; residents are forced to access groundwater through shallow handpumps. The landlords in the village who have rented out small tenements have installed motors (popularly known as "borings") to provide the residents with untreated groundwater. Moreover, on-line boosters, both manual (in the slums) and electrical (in the village), contaminate the piped supply. There are sewers in Azadpur village. But the rest of the population in the area accesses open fields along the railway line. In 1994–95, the annual incidence rate of cholera was 200 per 100,000. Following a downward trend in 1996–97, it peaked in 1998 at 236 per 100,000. The years 1999–2000 saw a sharp decline owing to an augmentation of water supply through tankers.

The two villages Bharola and Sarai Peepalthala are adjacent to the fruit and vegetable wholesale market and its truck terminals. Some JJ clusters are recent additions. While the old villages have a total population of 70,000, the slum population is about 35,000. These villages are densely populated, and a large number of small eating houses and hotels cater to drivers, labourers and traders from the north Indian states. The environmental sanitation is very poor; almost as a rule, the open drains are choked and overflowing. Piped water supply and sewers are available inside the village, but the slum population is dependent on public hydrants and open fields. The average annual incidence rate in 1994–95 was 11.4 per 100,000. There was a decline in 1996–97 and a sharp rise in 1998, following the general trend. The incidence rate in 1998 was 27.6 per 100,000. There was no special effort in these villages, unlike Azadpur. The incidence rate in 2000 peaked to 30.4 per 100,000.

Located between Jahangirpuri and the G. T. Karnal (GTK) Road Bypass, Bhalaswa is a small urbanised village with an estimated population of 40,000. Some dairies from the city were relocated to the other side of the GTK Bypass in 1975; the population of Bhalaswa Dairy has grown over time to about 15,000. Most of the residents of the village and the dairy are poor. They are mostly labourers in the Azadpur Mandi and the Rajasthan Industrial Area opposite Jahangirpuri. Both the village and the dairy are located on low-lying land and are prone to waterlogging. The cholera incidence rate in 1994 was comparable with that of neighbouring Jahangirpuri (32.7 per 100,000). Thereafter, with the general declining trend in Civil Lines Zone, the incidence rate halved.

JJ Clusters

Lal Bagh, Bara Bagh and several other JJ clusters are located on a stretch of railway land between the GTK Road and the Delhi–Ambala railway line behind the GTK Industrial Area. These clusters came into existence in about 1980 when the industrial areas were set up. The combined population of these clusters is about 65,000. The residents are mostly migrants from Bihar and Uttar Pradesh. They are employed in these industrial areas and the nearby Azadpur Mandi. There is an IPP-VIII Centre with health posts inside the clusters to serve this population. Environmental sanitation in these slum clusters is very poor and the garbage dumps (locally called dhalaos) are overflowing. The few community latrines are very poorly maintained. They are connected to septic tanks which are not cleaned/ maintained according to the regulations. As a result, the population generally practises open defecation in a large stretch of wasteland on the other side of the railway line, which in fact is in the Rohini Zone! The children generally defecate in the open near their homes in the drains along lanes or near community latrines. These latrines were maintained at one time by the Sulabh Shauchalaya, but maintenance is now back with the MCD. Water supply in these clusters is through public hydrants. The water pressure is low, and therefore at many places residents who can afford manual (hand-operated) boosters have punctured the water pipelines and installed these boosters. There are a number of shallow handpumps as well. With open defecation being so rampant, the shallow water table is highly contaminated. These clusters were severely affected in 1994–95, with an annual incidence rate of about 104.6 per 100,000; this had halved by 1996–97. There was a resurgence in 1998 to the 1994 levels; thereafter, incidence rates declined sharply up to 2000. The period from June to August accounts for 70–90 per cent of the cases. Augmentation of the water supply through the deployment of a large number of tankers has improved the situation. The tanker strategy worked, as the industrial areas provided wide roads for the tankers. Further, these clusters are long with relatively little breadth; the dwelling units are therefore not inaccessible for the tankers.

The construction of Wazirpur Industrial Area began in 1972, and construction labourers started to set up their huts in the vicinity. The labourers were from Bihar and Uttar Pradesh. Gradually, the clusters expanded along the strip of land between the industrial area and the railway line (a loop line connecting the Delhi–Ambala line with the Delhi–Rohtak line and serving several industrial areas). The current population is estimated at 50,000. The clusters are served by the IPP-VIII. Water is supplied through public hydrants. Defecation is practised generally along the railway lines or in open drains. Environmental sanitation is extremely poor. There are large, open drains that are choked almost as a rule.

Resettlement Colonies

Jahangirpuri Resettlement Colony was set up in 1972–73 on the GTK Road, and has an estimated population of 300,000. Slum dwellers from Karol Bagh and Mayapuri were resettled here. A large proportion of the residents are salaried personnel in the organised and semi-organised sectors. Enterprises located in the Rajasthan Small Industries Area (opposite Jahangirpuri) also provide employment to residents of the colony. The area has several medical institutions of the Delhi government and the MCD, including a newly established general hospital. The resettlement colony has expanded several times beyond its initial plan (and capacity) owing to large-scale expansion in the number of floors. Several slum clusters have also come up in different blocks. Water supply is provided by the DJB, and most households now have individual supplies. The use of manual boosters is, however, quite common. In addition, shallow handpumps have been installed by many households who can afford it. There are no sanitary latrines at the household level. Many families have constructed latrines and connected them to the open drains. Sewers were constructed after about three decades, but many of the sanitary latrines are yet to be connected. There are community latrines attached to septic tanks. The septic tanks are not properly maintained and add to the vulnerability of the population. Over the years, there has been a decline in cholera in Jahangirpuri, particularly after the sewers were commissioned. There were 135 cases of cholera in 1994—an annual incidence rate of 67.5 per 100,000. In 1995 the incidence rate nearly halved, followed by further reductions in 1996–97. In keeping with the general trend, incidence increased sharply in 1998 to the 1995 level. Following the installation of sewers in 1999, the incidence rate decreased to a third of the 1998 level. Cases are now reported largely from the slum clusters that have mushroomed at the periphery of the original resettlement colony. These clusters have limited access to piped water supply (through public hydrants) and sanitary latrines (community latrines).

Unauthorised Colonies

Most of the unauthorised colonies of the Civil Lines Zone are located on the land of four villages—Jharoda, Burari, Nathupura and Ibrahimpur, across the Outer Ring Road on the periphery of the Civil Lines Zone, towards Narela Zone. While the slum clusters were being relocated/resettled from the main city areas to the peripheries, those who had the means purchased land in these areas. The landlords in these villages had become "colonisers" (in local parlance) and property dealers, converting agricultural land to residential plots as demand and prices rose. The initial settlers were from Uttar Pradesh, including the hill districts. Many of them were salaried personnel employed in government organisations.

The entire area has historically been part of the floodplains of the Yamuna, and has witnessed floods regularly along with other similarly placed villages upstream in the Narela Zone. The 1978 flood inundated the entire area and the population had to be rescued by the army and volunteers with the help of boats. The inundation also threatened parts of posh colonies like Model Town on the Ring Road. As a result, a series of steps was taken to strengthen the west bank of Yamuna. The Outer Ring Road was constructed on a high embankment that provided direct access to these areas and protected the Kingsway Camp area from floods. Jharoda (closest to the river)–Burari–Nathupura was thus cordoned off from the river. Land prices shot up and new "colonies", "enclaves" and "vihars" mushroomed with each passing year. The current population of this belt is estimated at about 400,000.

One of the most important factors responsible for the popularity of these unauthorised colonies is the easy access to groundwater. Shallow handpumps can easily tap water at a little depth from the surface.[16] Since 1999, the DJB has augmented tanker supply in these areas; the impact, however, has been limited. Tankers are stationed on the main road only; the lanes are too narrow for them to reach the peripheries. Those living in peripheral parts of the colony often do not prefer to access tanker water. Tankers are available for only a limited time, and their visits are often unscheduled. When the tanker arrives, the residents are in a rush to access the water, opening the lids and putting rubber pipes inside, potentially contaminating the supply.

Many of the dwelling units have sanitary latrines connected to septic tanks, which, more often than not, are not constructed according to specifications. Incompletely treated effluent percolates and contaminates subsoil water. There are no regular sanitation services, since these are unauthorised colonies, and there is no official allocation of manpower and vehicles. The solid waste generated is generally dumped into nearby vacant plots; with the first rains, they contaminate the subsoil water. There are no proper surface drains in many parts of these colonies. Liquid waste has no outfall and enters the soil. For such a large area with a sizeable population, health/medical institutions do not exist, except a malaria clinic and a maternity centre at Burari. These colonies were affected in a major way in 1994, which was an epidemic year, with an incidence rate of about 58.1 cholera cases per 100,000 for the year. In 1998, when there was a resurgence after an overall declining trend, cholera was back in this belt with a similar incidence level. Despite some of the limitations of tanker services, the incidence rate dropped to about 10 per 100,000 following the introduction of tankers.

The vulnerable areas in this zone include large slum clusters in the industrial belt that house the poorest population groups and have a very poor state of infrastructure, and large unauthorised colonies (with relatively better-off socio-economic groups) dependent largely on groundwater accessed through shallow handpumps and lacking sanitary latrines. Despite the continuing high population densities, there was a significant decline in cholera in this zone when water tankers were deployed in a major way in the Lal Bagh, Azadpur and Jharoda–Nathupura areas. Tankers have become a part of the local political agenda, with active demand from the community. Despite the immediate dividends, tankers are not a cost-effective and sustainable solution. In Jharoda village, pipelines have already been laid and limited water supply has begun. Piped water supply is also available in Burari and Nathupura villages. But the benefit is limited only to the village and is not available to the residents of the unauthorised colonies that constitute more than 90–95 per cent of the population in these areas. Jahangirpuri has benefited from the installation of sewers and there has been a decline in the incidence of notified cholera cases.

NARELA ZONE

This zone reported the second-highest average incidence rate during 1994–2000 (33.39 cases per 100,000). During 1995 and 1996, Narela reported the highest incidence rates among all zones. Thereafter, there has been a steady decline in the incidence rate across the years, falling to a low of 8.50 cases per 100,000 during 2000, when Narela was ranked sixth among the zones.

Essentially a rural zone, the resident population is largely indigenous. Several recent changes have impacted on the cholera scenario. With the indigenous population gradually shifting from agriculture, land has been sold as residential plots and several unauthorised colonies (with little infrastructure) have come up. Godowns and industries have been constructed in villages that are close to National Highway 1. All this has led to the influx of migrants.

Consequent to a decision of the Supreme Court in 1998, a large number of industries in residential and non-conforming areas of Delhi were relocated to newly designated industrial areas in Narela Zone, bringing about changes similar to those witnessed in the neighbourhood of other industrial areas throughout Delhi. Several JJ clusters from different parts of Delhi have been relocated to Narela on land acquired from villages. Some of these resettlement colonies have been properly planned and constructed by HUDCO, while, in others, relocated families were allotted land and dumped in the open fields; several outbreaks of waterborne disease occurred. Population density is about 743.38 per sq km, but is increasing as newer colonies are established.

Water is supplied by the DJB at an average of 32 lpcd.[17] The supply is from Ranney wells, which have recently been augmented by additional deep tubewells. The water supply situation in the zone improved after a pumping station was commissioned at Holambi during 1998, and adequate water began to be supplied to Narela (town) and adjacent areas. The entire zone is without sewers. Most of the houses in the villages have septic tanks.

The proportion of annual cholera cases reported from vulnerable colonies averaged 61.70 per cent for the study period. There are wide fluctuations in the proportion of annual cases being reported from vulnerable colonies during the study period. In 1996, as many as 92.5 per cent of the total notified cases reported were from vulnerable colonies. By 2000, there was a sharp drop to only 11 per cent. The vulnerable colonies in this zone are located mostly in the urban agglomerations of Narela, Alipur and Bawana. Lampur village and the brick kilns represent special cases.

Urban Agglomerations

Narela is the largest urban agglomeration in the Narela Zone. It is a congested town and a thriving trading centre for grains and agricultural products. There are designated industrial areas as well. Though the DJB provides piped supply, there are several pockets of water scarcity. Since 1999, several slum clusters have been relocated to this area. As water and sanitation services were deficient in the initial stages of relocation, cholera cases were reported from these resettlement colonies. About 15 to 20 cases are reported each year from Narela, without much variation. In addition to Narela, the two other urban agglomerations of the zone—Alipur and Bawana—also constitute cholera hotspots. Villages located along the Alipur–Narela (Bakhtawarpur, Holambi, Hiranki and Bakoli villages) and Narel–Bawana (Bajeetpur, Ghogha and several other smaller villages) roads reported sporadic cases.

Slum clusters have also been relocated to Holambi; however, these clusters were poorly planned. Plots were allotted, but infrastructure was grossly deficient. The communities that were relocated were left in the open fields; water tankers and mobile latrines were provided. But there was no physical structure to live in till the allottees constructed the dwelling units. Several cholera cases have been reported from these colonies.

Lampur

Lampur is a small village with four "homes" run by the Delhi government—three for beggars and the destitute, and one for foreigners waiting for deportation. Water supply is provided through deep tubewells fitted with chlorinators. Focal outbreaks occur every few years; the cause has generally been traced to faulty chlorinators.

Brick Kilns

The worst-affected communities in 1994 and 1995 were the migrant labourers in the brick kilns that dotted the countryside in Narela. Following a court ruling, these kilns shifted to Haryana in 1996. The living conditions in these kilns were poor, with the community accessing drinking water from shallow handpumps and defecating in adjacent fields. Cholera (and diarrhoeal diseases) would typically occur as small focal outbreaks affecting children and adults. Foodborne outbreaks following community feasts were not uncommon.

There was a decline in clustered and sporadic cases following the operationalisation of the Holambi reservoir in 1998–99. There are several Ranney wells in the Yamuna corridor in Narela Zone. Water is pumped from Ranney wells to the Holambi reservoir, where it is chlorinated and distributed through the piped network. The shifting of the brick kilns from

Delhi to Haryana (following judicial intervention) also contributed to the overall decline in the incidence of cholera in Narela.

NAJAFGARH ZONE

Najafgarh Zone experienced a consistent declining trend in the cholera incidence rate, from 59.64 per 100,000 in 1994 to 8.91 per 100,000 in 2000, with an average annual incidence rate of 23.55 per 100,000 population, the third-highest among the zones.

Najafgarh Zone is rural in large tracts, with no vulnerable pockets in these areas. Most of the growth in terms of settlements and population has occurred along three axes—Nangloi–Mangolpuri–Sultanpuri, Palam–Dabri, and the settlements surrounding the airport complex. The settlements in Nangloi–Mangolpuri–Sultanpuri are resettlement colonies set up during the Emergency (1975–77). These are residential colonies with industrial areas and unorganised trading centres in their vicinity. The Palam–Dabri Road is an important axis in south-west Delhi, where a large number of unauthorised colonies were set up in the early 1980s and regularised over time. The airport and the cantonment are large employers in this zone. Consequently, several urbanised villages in the area have become highly congested and constitute vulnerable areas from which cholera is reported regularly. The average population density in the zone is about 1,126.52 per sq km, with wide variations between highly congested urban areas and the rural areas.

Average water supply in the zone is about 74 lpcd.[18] Some of the rural villages do not have piped water supply. Those that have water supply are serviced through deep tubewells. Sewers are available in the urbanised parts of the zone. The resettlement colonies have community latrines, while unauthorised colonies and rural villages mostly have individual latrines with septic tanks.

In Najafgarh Zone, an average of 73.86 per cent of annual cases were reported from the vulnerable areas during 1994–2000. Between 1996 and 1999, vulnerable colonies in Najafgarh Zone were contributing about 80–90 per cent of the total zonal cases each year. In 2000, this proportion reduced sharply to about 35 per cent. The vulnerable colonies include a group of resettlement colonies in Mangolpuri, Sultanpuri and Nangloi;

unauthorised/regularised colonies in the Palam–Dabri belt; and a group of urbanised villages—Mahipalpur, Rangpuri and Nangal Dewat.

Resettlement Colonies

Mangolpuri–Sultanpuri and Nangloi are located on either side of the Delhi–Rohtak railway line and the Delhi–Fazilka National Highway. Mangolpuri, Sultanpuri and J. J. Colony–Nangloi are resettlement colonies. Slum residents of Minto Road and Delhi Gate were relocated to these colonies. Large portions of these colonies were located on low-lying wasteland; some land was also acquired from Mangolpur Khurd and Nangloi villages. Over time, several JJ clusters have come up in the neighbourhood of these two villages. Several unauthorised colonies have also been "promoted" by the landlords of Nangloi village; some more have mushroomed on the wasteland beyond Sultanpuri. The Mangolpuri Industrial Area and Peeragarhi Industrial Area (near Nangloi) provide employment. Nangloi has always been a traditional trading centre for rural Delhi and adjacent areas of Haryana. Good road transport facilities and a railway station at Nangloi have attracted a large body of tenants employed in different areas of Delhi.

Delhi Jal Board water supply is available in all these localities, except in the unauthorised colonies. However, the quantity of water available is inadequate for the population, which is currently estimated at about 400,000. Shallow handpumps have been sunk on individual initiative and cost; water pipelines are also punctured to install manual boosters. The JJ clusters are dependent on public hydrants, and there is no DJB supply in the unauthorised colonies.

The community sanitary latrines in the resettlement colonies are generally in a poor state of maintenance. Open defecation by children is common in these colonies. Many households, particularly those on the ground floor, have made structures for "sanitary latrines" that open directly into the drains. With water pipelines crossing through these open drains, the risk of contamination is very high. Residents of the JJ clusters either use the community latrines of the resettlement colonies or defecate in the open. Mobile latrines have been stationed in a few clusters, but again, they are often in a poor state of maintenance. The unauthorised colonies have (individual sanitary) latrines connected to dug wells. The annual incidence rate of cholera in 1994 in these colonies was 46.4 cases per 100,000 population. There was a sharp decline after 1996 when the annual incidence rate dropped to 1.27 per 100,000 with further declines over the subsequent years. By 2000, this rate was down to 2.7 per 100,000. Availability of adequate safe water from the Haiderpur plant has made a difference. Cases are now generally confined to the unauthorised colonies.

The contribution of this belt to the total case load of Najafgarh underwent considerable change over the study period. During the peak period of 1994 and 1995, this belt reported 51 per cent and 61 per cent, respectively, of the total cases in the zone. Though the incidence of cholera in Najafgarh Zone had reduced drastically by 1996 and 1997, this belt contributed 68 per cent of the cases in each of these years. The share of this belt in the total cases in the zone declined sharply between 1998 and 2000, from 51 per cent to 26 per cent.

Unauthorised/Regularised Colonies

The Palam–Dabri belt consists of several villages—Palam, Dabri, Nasirpur, Bindapur and Matiala—and unauthorised colonies "promoted" on the land of these villages since the early 1980s. This belt is also adjacent to the airport and the cantonment, and is surrounded on three sides by the Dwarka township. Over the years, these colonies have attracted large populations—particularly those employed by the defence and aviation services. Good transport connections to south Delhi, where the offices of the organised sector are located, have attracted middle-class populations to this belt. The current estimated population of this belt is about 200,000.

Earlier, the only source of water supply was groundwater accessed through shallow handpumps or, in a small proportion of households, through "borings". All houses have sanitary latrines—connected to dug wells or open drains. None of these houses has a proper septic tank. To complicate matters, there is no outfall for the liquid waste and wastewater that flow in the open drains. Vacant plots are used to dump solid waste and, in many cases, liquid waste also flows into such plots. Either way, most of the liquid waste enters the subsoil water—the only water source. Ironically, the famed Sulabh movement has its headquarters on the Palam–Dabriroad at Mahavir Enclave, one of the earliest colonies in this area that was regularised in the late 1980s. Sulabh, despite its national and international acclaim, missed all that was happening in its own backyard. These colonies began to be regularised gradually. With regularisation came piped water supply, roads and paved drains. Some of these colonies are, however, yet to be regularised.

In 1994, the annual incidence rate in these settlements was eight per 100,000 population. Despite a downward trend in Najafgarh Zone, the rate increased to 12.5 per 100,000 in 1995. From 1996, on the initiative of one of the local MLAs (there are two assembly constituencies in the belt), water supply was extended to many more colonies from the Uttam Nagar–Najafgarh Road line. Tankers were deployed in many of the areas. Cases declined to zero in 1997. During 2000, sewers were laid in a few of these colonies; in a repetition of ironies, the sewers had no outfall as they were not connected to the trunk sewers. Water supply without sewers brought about a new problem. The water pipes passed through open, choked drains and were a new route of infection.

Urbanised Villages

Mahipalpur, Nangal Dewat and Rangpuri villages are located on National Highway 8 (Delhi–Jaipur), close to the airport. These villages have become major commercial centres and have dwelling units constructed exclusively for letting out. Each year, on average about four to five cases of cholera are reported, without much variation.

ROHINI ZONE

Rohini Zone has consistently reported one of the highest incidence rates. The incidence rate in Rohini during the monsoon is about 3–3.5 times that during the summer.

Rohini Zone was carved out of Civil Lines and West Zones in 1990. The residential colonies of this zone are largely middle-class in nature. The vulnerable settlements, several large JJ clusters, are located mostly around the GTK Road, including a few urbanised villages and an industrial area. There are a few unauthorised colonies along the Kanjhawala Road. Commercial activity is low, and the land use pattern is largely residential.

The proximity to sanitary landfill (SLF) sites is a critical determinant. Some of these colonies have come up *on* low-lying land that was used for SLF sites earlier. The population density of the zone is about 8,847.83 per sq km.

Though SLF sites remain a major source of infection, the Haiderpur water treatment plant that started functioning from the mid-1990s has played a key role in the reduction of incidence. The average water supply in this zone is about 274 lpcd.[19] Most of the areas are also served by sewers. An average of about 80 per cent of the annual reported cholera cases occur in the vulnerable colonies. They consist of urbanised villages—Shalamar, Haiderpur, Samaipur, Badli, Libaspur—and the JJ clusters around them. In addition, JJ clusters in Sawan Park, unauthorised colonies in Budh Vihar and Wazirpur JJ Colony (a resettlement colony) are also vulnerable colonies in the zone.

JJ Clusters

The most critical vulnerable belt in Rohini Zone is a group of urbanised villages, their extensions and surrounding JJ clusters. These are located around the GTK Road stretching from Shalamar village through Haiderpur village to Samaipur, Badli, Libaspur, Shahbad–Daulatpur and Siraspur villages. Employment opportunities are available in several nearby industrial areas (including one at Badli), in industries in the villages and in the transport industry at the Sanjay Gandhi Transport Nagar. The hallmark of these areas is that, other than the original villages, all the settlements have come up on what were previously sanitary landfill sites. On account of improper waste disposal at these sites, the groundwater in these areas is highly contaminated. While the unauthorised colonies have no water supply or only a "skeletal supply" (through tankers), the slum clusters are supplied through public hydrants. Though household-level water supply is available in the villages, large-scale tenancy has led to conditions of scarcity. The communities are therefore acutely dependent on groundwater. The use of boosters is also high in certain localities.

The slum clusters in these areas came up in 1982 when the industrial areas were being set up. The wholesale market at Azadpur and the truck terminal accelerated the growth of the slums. Many families living in different slum clusters in Delhi shifted to these areas, as the jhuggis were available at cheaper rates. Newer avenues of employment were also available in these areas. The villages of this area underwent commercialisation and industrialisation. In the later phases, unauthorised colonies were promoted by landlords for the economically better-off groups who purchased land to build their own houses.

The estimated population is about 200,000. The environmental sanitary conditions are extremely poor. In addition to domestic solid waste, industrial solid waste is also poorly disposed of, and is often found dumped in these areas; the hazards are different and potentially more serious. The area is low-lying and prone to waterlogging during the rains. Water supply in the JJ clusters, made available through public hydrants, is grossly insufficient and communities are acutely dependent on shallow handpumps. The villages have household-level water supply that often requires boosting. The unauthorised colonies have no other source than groundwater.

Villages have sanitary latrines and sewers. The JJ clusters have community latrines at a few places, but open fields are the commonest places for defecation. The annual incidence rate of cholera in these clusters in 1994 was 71.4 per 100,000—one of the highest in Delhi. The rate reduced to about one-third by 1996 and continued at this level in 1997. Despite an overall low endemicity, this period was marked by an increase in the number of cases in Shahbad, where construction had begun on the campus of the Delhi Engineering College (which was shifting from its previous location at Kashmiri Gate).Cholera cases were reported regularly from among construction labourers and their families, including several deaths related to diarrhoeal disease among infants and children. The construction was over by 1998–99, and these cases subsided. Though 1998 saw an upward spike in cases in each zone and practically each of the localities, for Rohini Zone this was an extraordinary year. The annual incidence rate in Haiderpur was 212 per 100,000 and the zonal annual incidence rate was 44.5 per 100,000. In Samaipur–Badli the rate was 380 per 100,000. In the JJ clusters of Shalimar Bagh, the rate was 214.3 per 100,000. In 1994, this belt accounted for 75 per cent of the cases from the vulnerable areas of Rohini Zone. The situation improved in 1999–2000 with the large-scale deployment of tankers in the affected areas. Despite a general decline, incidence did not decline in Siraspur, as the population in the newly formed unauthorised colonies had increased without any additional infrastructure. In 1998, a landfill was started at a new site, bound on the east by the G. T. Karnal Road, on the west by the Delhi–Ambala railway line, on the south by Outer Ring Road and on the north by Sanjay Gandhi Transport Nagar. It is no secret that the sanitary landfills are not run according to specifications; there is little that is "sanitary" about them. They are merely dumping sites, where there is complete disregard of bio-hazards. A public interest litigation (PIL) filed in the Hon'ble Supreme Court (*B. L. Wadheravs MCD and Others)* detailed the state of affairs in such dumping sites. The PIL argued that the groundwater was highly contaminated, both bacteriologically and chemically.

Sawan Park consists of several small JJ clusters located on the fringes of Ashok Vihar Phases II and III (posh colonies in that part of the city) along the Delhi–Ambala railway line, opposite the Lal Bagh and Bara Bagh slum clusters of the Civil Lines Zone. Water supply is provided through public hydrants and, in the absence of any community latrines, tracts along the railway tracks are used for open defecation. In 1994, the annual cholera incidence rate was 328.6 per 100,000—three times the incidence rate in Lal Bagh and Bara Bagh. The real decline in incidence came in 1999, when tankers were deployed and the public hydrant network was also expanded.

Unauthorised Colonies

Budh Vihar, an unauthorised colony on Kanjhawala Road, is situated on the banks of a major open drain that carries household and industrial liquid waste. The colony was established in the mid-1980s. The initial group of residents were mostly salaried individuals, including some retired personnel from the armed forces. The colony was still developing during 1994. There were few paved roads. The only source of water was shallow handpumps. There were "sanitary latrines" linked to dug wells. Waterlogging was the norm during the monsoons. The solid waste of adjacent households was dumped into vacant plots, and in many cases liquid waste would also flow into such sites. In 1994,the annual cholera incidence rate was 52.5 per 100,000. Phase I of this colony, located on Kanjhawala Road, is the commercial hub, including offices of the property dealers who double up as local politicians. Phase I thus developed faster than Phase II. Delhi Jal Board water was made available through public hydrants from which illegal household connections were later drawn. Tanker supply was also begun by the DJB in 1995. The incidence of cholera decreased in Phase I. Other than the odd, sporadic case, cholera in Budh Vihar became confined to Phase II.

Resettlement Colony

Wazirpur JJ Colony was set up in 1974. The residents of slum clusters in Mayapuri were relocated here. Later, migrants from Haryana, Uttar Pradesh and Bihar moved in. The dead end of an irrigation "canal" lies along the western boundary of the colony, providing water for some of the daily needs of residents. This water is stagnant per se and highly polluted due to liquid waste from the colony draining into it. Slum hutments also dot the bank of this canal. Many residents of these clusters are hawkers selling fruits and salad vegetables in Azadpur and adjacent business areas. The fruit and vegetables hawked locally are washed in this canal. As these items are consumed raw, it is not difficult to imagine that they are sources of infection for cholera and a variety of other waterborne diseases.

Though Rohini is one of the highly endemic zones of Delhi, 1998 was an exceptionally bad year. Haiderpur–Samaipur–Badli–Siraspur constitutes the belt that is highly endemic for cholera. The beginning of a new sanitary landfill area spelled doom for the communities in these areas. Though the situation is "under control" with the help of tankers, this is not a permanent and sustainable solution and there can be a flare-up at any time.

SOUTH AND CENTRAL ZONES

The reasons for considering these two zones together have been explained earlier. The years 1994 and 1995 were peak incidence years following the introduction of *Vibrio cholerae* O139. In 1994, the incidence rate in South Zone was 36.8 per 100,000. The incidence rate in Central Zone for that year was only 6.9 per 100,000. In 1995, the incidence rate was similar in the two zones: 20.8 per 100,000 in Central Zone and 21.2 per 100,000 in South Zone. Between 1995 and 1998, there was little difference in the incidence rates in the two zones. Since 1998, the incidence rate in South Zone has risen compared to Central Zone. During the 1988 cholera epidemic, the incidence rates were much lower than current levels.

The South and Central Zones are among the larger zones of the MCD. They span the area from the Southern Ridge (of the Aravalli Hills) to the River Yamuna. While a few colonies were set up in connection with the rehabilitation of Partition refugees, most of the growth has occurred since the 1970s. Affluent colonies and institutions of the knowledge economy are the hallmark of these zones, along with good roads and public transport. Land for institutions and planned residential colonies was provided by villages. These urbanised villages acquired a lot of wealth in the process, which was invested in household industries and real estate (for sale as office space or tenancy for residences). The tertiary sector boomed in these zones, more so following the liberalisation of the economy in the 1990s.

During this period, construction, financing, insurance, real estate and personal services emerged as the leading growth sectors. Much of this increase can be expected to have occurred in these two zones, given the profile of their economic activity.

Large areas of the South and Central Zones suffer from low per capita supply of water. The DUEIIP puts the availability of water at 29 lpcd in the Mehrauli Zone of the Delhi Jal Board.[20] In the rest of the Central and South Zones, this figure is 148 lpcd against an optimum supply of 150–225 lpcd. Most water treatment plants are located in the northern parts of Delhi, and water has to travel a long distance to the south resulting in loss of pressure; the colonies located at higher elevations in these two zones are thus the worst hit.

The fast-depleting groundwater level in south Delhi is a matter of serious concern. These zones had adequate groundwater, upto about 6 metres, till the late 1980s.[21] The DJB remains the largest extractor of groundwater in these two zones. Of a total of 2,111 DJB deep tubewells in Delhi, 1,409 are located in these two zones. In the unauthorised colonies located in the riverine areas of the Central Zone, there are large numbers of shallow handpumps.[22]

About 76 per cent of the annually notified cases were reported from the vulnerable colonies in these two zones. There are commonalities in the risk factors that make these colonies vulnerable to cholera. Except for the few peripheral unauthorised colonies, the hallmark of the settlements is high population density and overcrowding. The urbanised villages have one-room units (generally with common toilets) built specifically for renting out. There are adequate employment opportunities in industries in the designated industrial areas, unauthorised industries in the urbanised villages, as well as other jobs in the tertiary sector, both formal and informal.

Environmental sanitation conditions are poor in these colonies. Piped water supply is scarce because of an adverse demand–supply situation, particularly in the summers. The colonies situated in the rocky, higher elevations of the Southern Ridge are the worst off, being at the tail end of the piped network. To augment the water supplied from the water treatment plants, the DJB operates a large number of tubewells in these areas. These tubewells are fitted with chlorinators. Ironically, these tubewells are in many instances the source of contaminated water supply. The supply of bleaching powder is irregular. Maintenance of the chlorinators is poor and breakdowns are common. "Contracting" of tubewells and chlorinators by the pump operators (DJB employees) is a common practice. The room (the pump house) is given out on rent and, in return, the tenant merely switches the pump on and off; such tenants are technically incapable of handling the chlorinator. Often, the keys to the pump house are left with local residents, particularly in the urbanised villages, who are also not able to operate the chlorinators. Installation of automatic chlorinating devices in the last few years has nearly eliminated this "risk factor". The rampant use of on-line boosters on the main line is common in the well-to-do areas. The use of manual boosters by puncturing the pipelines is also equally prevalent in the low-income settlements.

Unauthorised colonies lacking piped water supply use different options to access water. Shallow handpumps are the most common source, particularly in the riverine belt. Colonies situated on the rocky belt access groundwater either through Mark II handpumps installed by the DJB or through electric motors installed in individual households by those who can afford it. Water is also purchased by the residents in some colonies (Badarpur area) from private tankers, who in turn draw groundwater through motors. In addition, there are private piped networks whereby an "entrepreneur" draws water through a motor and supplies adjacent households through pipes laid on the surface; there are several such networks in Sangam Vihar and Tughlakabad Extension. There are instances where DJB water is privately sold. Privately owned large storage tanks are filled by DJB tankers, and this water is then sold to the neighbourhood through networks of rubber pipes travelling across lanes and over roofs. Groundwater has been tested from all these sources and has consistently proved unfit for human consumption; this includes the DJB Mark II handpumps also, which, like the shallow handpumps, have been painted red at several places by the DJB as a mark of warning!

Unauthorised colonies have no sewers. Sanitary latrines are connected to septic tanks or dug wells, and wastewater often tracks down to the subsoil. Open defecation is common. Urbanised villages and regularised colonies pose a unique problem. The sewers were installed much later in the narrow lanes and by-lanes. As a result, water pipelines, joints and valves often lie close in the vicinity of sewers; the intermittent supply of water leads to contaminated matter being sucked in when there are minor cracks in the pipes. Use of on-line boosters also leads to contamination when the water pipelines are in contact with sewage.[23] During the summer, owing to the overall lack of water and reduced flow, the probability of contaminated matter being sucked into the water pipelines increases.

The vulnerable colonies of South and Central Zones include resettlement colonies—Ambedkar Nagar, Dakshinpuri, Madangir, Khanpur, Deoli and Tigri; unauthorised colonies—Sangam Vihar and Badarpur area; one regularised colony—Govindpuri; JJ clusters—Govindpuri and Okhla Industrial Areas; urbanised villages—Chiragh Dilli, Garhi, Jamroodpur, Kotla Mubarakpur, Madanpur Khadar, Hauz Rani, Masjid Moth, Mehrauli, Lado Sarai, Neb Sarai and Shahpur Jat.

Resettlement Colonies

The resettlement colonies of the South and Central Zones are Ambedkar Nagar, Dakshinpuri, Madangir, Khanpur, Deoli and Tigri, in one contiguous belt. These colonies were established between 1970 and 1972 to relocate slum populations from INA, R. K. Puram, Ansari Nagar and East of Kailash. Currently, a sizeable proportion of the residents in these colonies are salaried personnel in the government and private sectors. The current population is estimated at 300,000. This includes several slum clusters that have grown in the peripheries of these resettlement colonies.

Also included in this belt are Khanpur, Deoli and Tigri villages, whose land was acquired for these colonies. The annual cholera incidence rate in these colonies was 14.2 per 100,000 in 1994, rising to 23.4 per 100,000 in 1995. Unlike other zones where the incidence of cholera declined in 1995 following a high in 1994, the incidence rose by about 25 per cent in these two zones. Following a decline between 1996 and 1998, incidence rates in 1999 and 2000 were similar to the 1994 level. Scarcity of water continues to be a problem in these colonies. Water pipelines passing through open drains along the lanes and by-lanes render households vulnerable to waterborne infections.

Unauthorised Colonies

Adjacent to these resettlement colonies is Sangam Vihar, one of the largest unauthorised colonies, claimed by local promoters and property dealers as the "largest unauthorised colony of Asia"! This colony is located on rocky terrain, part of the Southern Ridge. The construction of houses began around 1985, and the current population is estimated at about 200,000. The early settlers were migrants from Haryana, Uttar Pradesh, Bihar, Bengal and Kerala who had been residing in Delhi for several years and had accumulated enough capital to buy plots of land and construct their own houses. Almost as a rule, groundwater is the water source. As the terrain is rocky, handpumps have to be sunk deep, a more expensive venture here than in many other areas of Delhi. Water is often purchased, either from individuals who have sunk deep-bore pumps and laid private pipe networks, or from private tankers who sell untreated groundwater. As the colony is unauthorised, there are no provisions for sewers, drains or paved roads. Gradually, some developmental activities have taken place through the utilisation of funds allocated to the MLAs and municipal councillors. Houses located along the Mehrauli–Badarpur Road and other arterial roads have access to public hydrants. The annual incidence of cholera was nearly uniform during 1994–99, with an average annual incidence rate of about 12.5 per thousand. During 2000, the incidence rate was only about 25 per cent of the previous level. Efforts by the DJB possibly explain this improvement—large-scale deployment of water tankers and provisioning of Mark II (deep-bore) handpumps.

Badarpur is located on Mathura Road near the Faridabad (Haryana) border. This is the commercial hub of the entire area, with the Badarpur Thermal Power Station of the National Thermal Power Corporation dominating the skyline. With the power plant and transport industry as major employers, this area has been populated by large numbers of people. They include many who work in the industries of Faridabad. Lands belonging to the villages of Badarpur, Tajpur, Mithapur, Jaitpur, Jasola and Ali were sold off as residential plots, and large unauthorised colonies came up, stretching from Mathura Road (National Highway 2) to the Yamuna. The estimated population in these areas is about 500,000. There is no piped water supply for unauthorised colonies. Groundwater is either accessed by handpumps or bought from private tankers. The unauthorised colonies have "sanitary latrines" with dug wells; alternatively, open fields are used for defecation. Tajpur, located on a portion of the ridge, was the site of a large stone quarry that was mined for building materials; the village is also called Tajpur Pahari. There is no mining activity now, but the abandoned mining pits act as natural drainage for the colonies that are situated on the heights above the pits. The cholera incidence rate was seven per 100,000 in 1994, increasing sharply to 11.4 per 100,000 in 1995. Since 1996, the incidence rate has remained at about eight per 100,000 with little variation across the years.

Regularised Colonies

Govindpuri began as an unauthorised colony while Kalkaji was a planned colony; both were set up in the aftermath of Partition. Later, Govindpuri was regularised. Both these colonies remain essentially residential. Kalkaji benefited from the development programmes of the DDA, while Govindpuri expanded in a haphazard manner. Water and sewer pipelines were installed later in the narrow lanes of the colony, leading to numerous potential points of contamination where the water pipelines passed through sewers.

JJ Clusters

The Okhla Industrial Area, a large industrial area located on the Delhi–Agra railway line, was built on land from Tehkhand village. Employees of these industries generally reside in different colonies of this vulnerable belt; the poorest of them live in several large slums that are located within the industrial area. There are several large slum clusters in Govindpuri also. The Okhla Industrial Area, the Tughlakabad Container Terminal of the Railways and several other large factories provide employment to the residents of these clusters. The DJB piped water supply in these areas is dual. The supply from the Okhla plant has to be augmented with the help of deep tubewells, which brings its own set of problems. Owing to the rocky terrain, there are some water-deficient hotspots (within these vulnerable areas) that are located against the gradient. Tankers of the DJB also augment the water supply.

Urbanised Villages

The urbanised villages in South and Central Zones (Chiragh Dilli, Garhi, Jamroodpur, Kotla Mubarakpur, Madanpur Khadar, Hauz Rani, Masjid Moth, Mehrauli, Lado Sarai, Neb Sarai and Shahpur Jat) are highly vulnerable to cholera. Building activities are unregulated in these urbanised villages. There are large numbers of tenants with very little per capita space and often with one toilet for several families. Open drains are covered to maximise space. There are large numbers of one/two-room industrial-cum-residential units; many of them deal in garments for the export market. These areas are characterised by intense commercial utilisation of space. Environmental sanitation is poor. Street foods and drinks are sold in unhygienic conditions. There is acute shortage of piped water supply, which is provided primarily through DJB deep tubewells with chlorinators and their attendant problems. Deep-bore motors and on-line boosters to augment water supply are used on a large scale. Because of unreliable and inadequate water supply, storage of drinking water is high and domestic contamination is common. Water and sewer lines passing in close proximity or crossing each other in narrow lanes are additional vulnerability factors. The cholera situation in these urbanised villages is best described as endemic with focal outbreaks. The conditions just outlined favour the endemicity of cholera, which is the case for all of these villages. The focal outbreaks are generally due to public health engineering faults, either in the pipelines or in the tubewells.

SHAHDARA (NORTH) ZONE

There was a general decline in the incidence rate of cholera cases in Shahdara (North) Zone between 1994 and 2000. The incidence rate showed a steady decline from 29.7 per 100,000 in 1994 to 7.2 per 100,000 in 1997, and it declined further to 4.6 per 100,000 in 2000. The 1988 epidemic of cholera (with an incidence rate of 55.7 per 100,000) took a major toll in different areas of Shahdara. The peak incidence is during the monsoon—July and August.

Shahdara was traditionally a trading centre before the British arrived in Delhi.[24] The rail link established by the colonial rulers further boosted commercial activities and enabled easy access to the United Provinces (Uttar Pradesh). The zone witnessed an accelerated phase of growth during the 1970s, when the local Member of Parliament, Shri H. K. L. Bhagat, was the Congress Minister of State for Works and Housing. He is considered to have played a major role in both official and unofficial developments in the colonies.[25] The result was that resettlement colonies and unauthorised colonies were set up, housing large numbers of socio-economically weaker groups. A number of small household industries mushroomed. Industrial areas were also set up to provide employment to the increasing numbers of people. The 1988 cholera epidemic hit the resettlement and unauthorised colonies the hardest. Unauthorised colonies and slum clusters had grown along the Yamuna Pushta and the Wazirabad Road. A large number of unregulated and polluting industries in this zone were closed down following the directions of the court during 1998.

The population density of the zone is 17,200 per sq km, with pockets of high population density of socio-economically poor groups in resettlement and unauthorised colonies. The average availability of water in the zone is 130 lpcd.[26] The number of shallow handpumps is high, as poorer communities often do not have the means to afford the piped supply. Large areas of this zone are without sewers. Many of the colonies have community latrine blocks that are operated either by the MCD or the Sulabh Shauchalaya.

Between 1994 and 2000, the proportion of reported cases from vulnerable colonies remained steadily above 80 per cent, with an average of 84.31 per cent. The vulnerable colonies of the zone include several resettlement colonies—Brahmpuri, Gokulpuri, New Seelampur, Seemapuri (Old and New), Nand Nagri and Sunder Nagri; JJ clusters in the Shastri Park area; urbanised villages—Khajuri Khas, Bhajanpura, Dayalpur and Gamri; and unauthorised colonies in Sonia Vihar and Karawal Nagar areas.

Resettlement Colonies

The resettlement colonies of Shahdara (North), including Brahmpuri, Gokulpuri, New Seelampur, Seemapuri (Old and New), Nand Nagri and Sunder Nagri, were set up in 1974. Residents of slum clusters in Jama Masjid, Turkman Gate, Daryagunj, Ajmeri Gate, Minto Road, Kashmiri Gate, Sunder Nagar and Friends Colony were relocated here. The total population of these colonies is currently estimated at about 800,000. The better-off residents of these colonies are skilled wage workers in the government and organised sectors. A sizeable proportion of the population is self-employed. Slum clusters have come up in the fringes of these colonies, and the residents of these clusters are generally employed as labourers in small unregulated industries and the transport/goods sector. The colonies have access to piped water supply, largely in the form of public hydrants, and household-level connections for a smaller proportion of the residents. The quantum of piped water supply is inadequate to meet the demand. Shallow handpumps have been installed on private initiative and at private cost. The superficial table of groundwater is unfit for human consumption without any purification, and constitutes an important risk factor for cholera. Community latrine blocks have been provided but are in a poor state of maintenance. It is not uncommon to come across "sanitary latrines" constructed at the household level. They simply empty into the open drains along the lanes. With water pipelines often crossing these drains, the risk of waterborne diseases (and cholera) is compounded. In addition, open defecation by small children is not uncommon. Open drains are generally in a state of poor maintenance. Environmental sanitation is generally poor, or average at best.

Among these colonies, the incidence rate in Brahmpuri did not decline, in contrast to the general trend of the zone. Though this area received water from the Bhagirathi plant, demand outstrips the supply and the use of shallow handpumps remains high.

In the case of Gokulpuri (and the adjoining area of Mustafabad that consists of unauthorised colonies set up at about the same time), the rate of decline was slower than for the zone as a whole. The real decline started in 1996–97. But in 1998, when there was an upward trend in most areas, the decline in this area continued. A possible reason could be that piped water supply came in later than in many of the other areas in the zone.

Nand Nagri and Sunder Nagri were among some of the most-affected colonies during the 1988 epidemic. In 1994, the incidence rate was about 20 per 100,000 in these two colonies, almost double that of two neighbouring villages—Mandoli and Saboli—and unauthorised colonies around the villages. Incidence rates in the resettlement colonies had halved by the next year. The incidence of cholera cases in Mandoli and Saboli also declined over the period 1994–2000. The decline continued, and in 2000 only two cases were reported from the resettlement colonies in the entire year, and only one from the villages. The improvement in water supply, on account of the Bhagirathi plant, has worked wonders for this area.

The annual incidence rate in Old Seemapuri and New Seemapuri in 1994 was about 73/100,000. The Seemapuri cases were more concentrated in the slum clusters than in the resettlement colony. These slums are among some of the poorest areas in Delhi, with skeletal infrastructure and appalling sanitary conditions in some areas. While annual cases halved in the zone, cases in Seemapuri actually registered a rise in 1995. There was a sharp decline in 1996–97 and, like the Gokulpuri area, there was no rise even in 1998.

New Seelampur area was badly affected in 1994, with an annual incidence rate of about 42.7 per 100,000. There was a steady decline till 1997. In 1998, this area experienced the maximum increase in the number of cases compared to other vulnerable colonies. The incidence rate in 1999 remained at the same level, and declined marginally in 2000. New Seelampur holds a strategic position by virtue of being the gateway to Delhi from the Shahdara side. With excellent transport connections, this colony enjoys a prime position both as a residential and a commercial area. The population density is one of the highest in east Delhi, and hygiene conditions are among the poorest, with the operation of a whole range of unregulated commercial activities, including food trades. The use of shallow handpumps is high, as the piped water supply is inadequate to meet the demand.

Adjacent to New Seelampur is the Shastri Park–Taj Colony vulnerable belt. This belt along the eastern bank (the *pushta* in local terminology) is followed by the Gamri–Dayalpur–Bhajanpura belt, and then across the Wazirabad Road lies the Khajuri Khas–Sonia Vihar belt.

JJ Clusters

During 1974–75, several slum clusters came up on the G. T. Road near the Old Bridge, which gradually grew into a colony called Shastri Park.[27] A little ahead, as one travels along the G. T. Road, another group of slums developed into the Taj Colony. The population of these groups of colonies is about 45,000. The residents of these colonies are migrants from Rajasthan, Gujarat, Bihar and Uttar Pradesh. The population is socio-economically poor, with most of the males working as labourers.

The water supply is provided through public hydrants. The network of these hydrants is confined by and large to the main roads. The clusters slope away from the main road towards the river bed. The peripheral parts of the colony are prone to waterlogging and occasional flooding from the Yamuna. Households that are located away from the main road often do not access the public hydrants, and rely instead on shallow handpumps. Open defecation has led to the contamination of groundwater in these colonies. The sanitation services are also poor, particularly in the peripheral parts of the colonies.

The annual cholera incidence rate in 1994–95 was about 32.5 per 100,000. After a drop in 1996, the incidence rate was back to this level in 1997. In September 1997, Shastri Park was brought under the coverage of water tankers by the Delhi Jal Board; cholera cases declined. When the construction of the Metro rail corridor began, roads were disrupted and the tankers were withdrawn. Shastri Park was particularly badly affected with a high incidence rate of 225 per 100,000. The tankers were brought back and the situation improved in 2000.

Urbanised Villages

Khajuri Khas, Bhajanpura, Dayalpur and Gamri villages, with an estimated population of 35,000–40,000,were cholera-endemic areas. They benefited greatly from the enhanced water supply from the new plant. The incidence rate in this belt declined from 60 per 100,000 in 1994 to only five per 100,000 in 2000. The estimated population in the Maujpur and Ghonda villages is about 35,000. The average annual incidence rate in 1994 in this belt was about 35 per 100,000. There was a rapid decline in the incidence of cholera after 1995, with additional water being available from the new plant. Even during the 1998 spurt in other areas, Maujpur–Ghonda was not badly affected. However, in the last week of May and early June in 1999, there was a focal outbreak in the area owing to contamination on account of leakage in a water pipe. Eight cases were reported in about 16 days. Following repairs, the outbreak was controlled.

Unauthorised Colonies

Within a kilometre of the Wazirabad barrage (on the Yamuna) lies Khajuri Khas village. Since 1977–78, the land of this village has been sold off as residential plots and several unauthorised colonies grew in this area. The Khajuri area is protected by a spur. In between this spur and the previous spur (towards the river), Sonia Vihar, an unauthorised colony, began to come up in the second half of the 1980s. During the 1994 epidemic, the incidence rate in Sonia Vihar was nearly 500 per 100,000, as the colony was still *katchi* (raw/undeveloped, in local parlance), compared with its neighbour Khajuri Khas and its extensions. Sonia Vihar at that time consisted of spread-out houses with a large proportion of available plots still vacant. The current population of Sonia Vihar is about 20,000. The migrants were largely from Bihar, West Bengal and Uttar Pradesh. The only source of water supply was shallow handpumps; defecation, almost as rule, was in the open fields. This low-lying colony on the floodplains of the Yamuna hardly has any outfall for wastewater.

The incidence of cholera was confined to just two months—July and August. The incidence rate had halved by 1995 and cases were spread over four months, June–September. There was a gradual reduction till 1997, and the incidence rate declined to about 200 per 100,000 in 1998; cases were reported from April to October. In 1999, one case was reported in November as well. Cholera became endemic in Sonia Vihar. With the deployment of tankers in 1999–2000, the incidence of cases declined but the environmental situation has remained neglected.

North–north-east of Wazirabad barrage, along the Wazirabad Road, are two villages, Karawal Nagar and Johripur, and their unauthorised extensions. Uttar Pradesh lies on this side of the Wazirabad Road, and there are several colonies in Delhi that have to be accessed through UP, so peculiar and convoluted has been the nature of growth and expansion in this part of Delhi.

The unauthorised colonies in these areas began to be established during the late 1970s and the peak growth took place in the first half of the 1980s. The residents were generally migrants from Uttar Pradesh, including its hill districts. Later, pockets of Bihari and Bengali migrants also developed, particularly in the Karawal Nagar area. Many of them had been working in Delhi for quite some time in salaried positions, including the government and organised sectors. Some of them were small traders. There were entrepreneurs who set up small industrial units, which in turn acted as a "pull factor". With the Wazirabad Road providing bus services to different parts of Delhi, those working in industries in other parts of Delhi and Ghaziabad (UP) have also been shifting to these colonies, living in rented accommodation or purchasing plots and constructing their own houses. The population of Karawal Nagar is about 250,000. A large proportion of the population in these colonies is dependent on groundwater through shallow handpumps. Liquid waste is drained through open drains into several larger drains. Sanitary conditions are poor, and water pipelines passing through choked open drains pose additional risks. The annual incidence rate in 1994 was about 75 per 100,000. The rate had halved by 1995, in tune with the general decline in the zone, and this trend continued till 2000.

SHAHDARA (SOUTH) ZONE

Even during the 1988 epidemic, the areas that at present constitute Shahdara (South) Zone were not much affected. The average incidence rate for the period 1994–2000 was 5.5 cases per 100,000. The annual incidence rate, like Shahdara (North), also showed a steady decline from 7.8 per 100,000 in 1995 to 2.5 per 100,000 in 2000. This zone was carved out of the erstwhile Shahdara Zone following the 1988 cholera epidemic. Large groups of population were rehabilitated after the 1947 Partition near the Old Yamuna Bridge. Later, several resettlement colonies were also located in this zone. Industrial areas were also set up in this zone and adjoining areas of Uttar Pradesh, including NOIDA and Sahibabad, providing employment to large numbers of people. Cooperative group housing societies for the middle class were set up in some parts of the zone, leading to the growth of informal services. The economies of several urbanised villages boomed. All this led to the settling of large populations of poor migrants in settlements that became vulnerable to cholera. The population density of the zone is 20,529.41 per sq km.

Despite the commissioning of the Bhagirathi plant, the average water supply in the zone is about 130 lpcd, and it is not uniformly distributed throughout the zone.[28] Shallow handpumps in large numbers provide water for the poorer communities. Some of the better-off households have their own bore-wells, while group housing societies have deep tubewells. A much larger proportion of areas in this zone is served by sewers compared to its neighbour—Shahdara (North) Zone.

An average of 74.31 per cent of the annually reported cases is reported from the vulnerable colonies. What is of concern in this zone is the fact that there has been an increasing trend in the incidence of cases in the vulnerable colonies from 1998 onwards, with a maximum of 83.33 per cent of cases being reported from vulnerable colonies in 2000. The vulnerable colonies in this zone consist of resettlement colonies—Old Seelampur, Trilokpuri, Kalyanpuri and Khichripur; regularised colonies in Kailash Nagar, Gandhi Nagar, Laxmi Nagar and Shakurpur areas; urbanised villages—Patpargunj, Mandawali; and unauthorised colonies surrounding the Kondli and Gharouli villages.

Resettlement Colonies

Old Seelampur is a resettlement colony that was set up along with other resettlement colonies in Shahdara (North) Zone. This colony was constructed on the agricultural land of Seelampur village. Later, there were unauthorised extensions (called Shanti Mohalla) on the peripheries of the resettlement colony. There are a number of small unregulated industries in these unauthorised settlements. In 1994, the cholera incidence rate was about 18 per 100,000, and most of the cases were reported between June and November. There was a steady decline in the incidence of cases in this colony to zero in 1999. There was no spurt in 1998 either. There was a focal outbreak in two blocks in September 2000.

Trilokpuri, Kalyanpuri and Khichripur are three resettlement colonies that are adjacent to each other. They were established during the Emergency (1975–77). The initial group of settlers comprised those who were relocated from the slums of south Delhi. The picture in these resettlement colonies is no different from that in the other resettlement colonies of this batch. The total population of these colonies is about 70,000. During 1994–97, the average cholera incidence rate was about 15 per 100,000 each year. However, with no improvement in the water sanitation situation, the incidence rate doubled during 1998–2000. Further, over the years, slum clusters have come up in all three resettlement colonies. Most of the reported cholera cases are from the slums lacking piped water supply.

Regularised Colonies

Kailash Nagar and Gandhi Nagar areas were set up after the Partition; migrants of poor socio-economic status from the erstwhile West Punjab settled down here. These colonies are located next to the G. T. Road and the Delhi–Shahdara line at the eastern end of the Old Yamuna Bridge, a double-decker bridge carrying the railway line and the road, constituting the oldest link between Delhi and the eastern states of India. The governmental support that colonies like Lajpat Nagar and Malviya Nagar received was conspicuous by its absence in these parts of Delhi. On account of the bridge and the strategic road and rail links, the embankment was built high, and the wastewater from these colonies had a natural gradient towards the river. Over time, the colonies grew into a vibrant market of readymade garments. With increased wealth and increasing population, four- and five-storeyed buildings came up. Throughout the 1980s, the export of garments to the erstwhile USSR boosted the economy further. Following the collapse of the USSR, the export component declined, but the wholesale market continues to cater to domestic needs. Despite a strong local economy, basic services did not improve much in these colonies, with their big houses along narrow lanes. Each house has piped water supply. The "sanitary latrines" empty into open drains that finally drain into a major drain at the end of the colonies, away from the river, and against the gradient. Untreated liquid waste from this major drain is finally emptied by a pump, without treatment, into the river at a point close to the Old Bridge. Environmental sanitation is poor. Solid waste is lifted and carried outside on buffalo carts. The current population is estimated at 200,000. The annual cholera incidence rate in 1994 was 4.7 per 100,000 population. The year 1995 witnessed a collapse in the drainage system. Cholera cases doubled, but this was only the tip of the iceberg. About 450 cases of viral hepatitis E were identified during house-to-house surveys. Thereafter, there was a slow decline in the incidence of cholera.

Further downstream along the river, Shakurpur and Laxmi Nagar (which started as unauthorised colonies and were later regularised) form a contiguous belt of vulnerable colonies. The population of this belt is about 50,000.Shakurpur and Laxmi Nagar are large business areas, densely populated and with poor sanitary conditions. There has been little fluctuation in the cholera incidence rates.

Urbanised Villages

Patpargunj and Mandawali are urbanised villages that have witnessed phenomenal growth with the development of industries and real estate in the village. The current population is about 150,000. Agricultural land has been sold as residential plots and large colonies have grown since the 1970s. The proximity of this area to the commercial hub of New Delhi, ITO and Connaught Place, has boosted growth. Though basic infrastructure is available in these villages, it is unable to meet the demand. On-line boosters and handpumps are essential to meet the demand for water. The population residing in these villages and colonies are lower-middle-income groups. Some of them are well-to-do traders and entrepreneurs. With no change in the ground conditions, there has been no decline of cholera in these colonies.

Unauthorised Colonies

The 1990s witnessed a spurt in the growth of unauthorised colonies in the quadrangle bounded by NOIDA (Uttar Pradesh), the NOIDA road (running parallel with the Yamuna), the Ghazipur Canal and the National Highway 24 Bypass (to Hapur, Uttar Pradesh). The land in this belt is low-lying, and it costs little to access water through shallow handpumps. The Ghazipur Canal offers an easy way out for (untreated) liquid waste. The industrial and commercial activities of NOIDA, Sahibabad and

Ghaziabad (Uttar Pradesh) are sources of employment for most residents of these colonies. Good roads and efficient road transport have further stimulated growth. The agricultural land of the two villages in this area, Kondli and Gharouli, has been sold off as residential plots. These two villages have also become congested with rise in tenancy and expanding markets. The current estimated population in this belt is about 80,000. The majority are salaried employees, and others are small traders. In 1994, the annual incidence rate was 38.3 per 100,000, and this was the most severely affected belt in the zone. There have been few moves to improve water supply and waste disposal services in these colonies, and thus little decline in cholera.

SADAR PAHARGUNJ ZONE

The average annual incidence in this zone for the period 1994–2000 was 5.7 cases per 100,000 with a high of about 11 per 100,000 in 1994, when a major outbreak occurred at Nabi Karim. August and September were observed to be the peak months. Cases continued to be reported through October as well, though at lower incidence levels. Cases have been reported in November every year since 1998.

The characteristics of this zone are similar to those of its neighbour—the City Zone. This zone is a mix of residential and market areas. The resident population is of comparatively lower socio-economic status than the majority of population in the City Zone. In addition to wholesale markets, there are small manufacturing units. The slaughterhouse was located here till recently, and trades associated with meat, hide, leather and other related products form an important component of the economy. This industry has recorded a decline following the reduction in the number of animals slaughtered at the slaughterhouse as per the stipulations of the high court. The population density is as high as 98,250 per sq km. Average water supply is adequate, at 205 lpcd.[29] There are, however, pockets of water scarcity; shallow handpumps and on-line boosters are present in these areas. The entire zone has sewerage services. The vulnerable area is only one large unauthorised colony, Nabi Karim, which has been regularised.

Regularised Colonies

The population of Nabi Karim is about 10,000. The wholesale business areas, small industrial units and the railway goods yard are located here and are major sources of employment. Nabi Karim began as an unauthorised colony on a graveyard near Lahori Gate Railway Station. The resident population is socio-economically poor. During the past few decades, industries, particularly of bags, suitcases and folding furniture, have grown in this area. The colony is located at a relatively higher elevation, and water does not reach households located on a higher gradient. Further, leaks in old and corroded pipes in these old areas also lead to contamination. The average life of a service pipe is 10–15 years and that of the main lines ranges from 50 to 100 years. The service pipes are rarely changed by the owners unless there is a major problem. On its part, the DJB manages to change about 90–100 km of pipeline annually, against a target of 400 km. In fact, during routine surveillance of water quality, these areas often report the absence of residual chlorine at the consumer end. There are several slum clusters in this area where piped water supply is available only through public hydrants and the communities are dependent on shallow handpumps. These areas were severely affected in 1994, when there was a focal outbreak on account of the old, corroded pipelines. Owing to some urgent action by the DJB, the situation was rectified and cholera was brought under control in this area. The situation worsened in 1999 when availability of water became a problem, with very little allocation for the area even though, ironically, it is situated within 2 km of the Idgah reservoir of the DJB. There were 34 cholera cases in 1999 and 19 in 2000. With acute water scarcity, the majority of the households use booster pumps, thus accentuating water contamination. Shallow handpumps are also in use in a number of households. Pumps have been installed to draw groundwater; some of them function as community sources rather than individual sources. At a few places, the community has installed large overhead tanks which are filled up from these pumps and utilised throughout the day. The groundwater, while it is used extensively, is, however, not treated.

KAROL BAGH ZONE

The average annual incidence for 1994–2000 in the Karol Bagh Zone was 3.7 cases per 100,000, with peak incidence in July. Karol Bagh Zone is a transition between the "old generation" zones (City and Sadar Paharganj) and the "new generation" zones (Rohini, Central and South), and shares some characteristics of both. Historically, the areas where the population spilled over from the walled city comprise the older residential areas of Karol Bagh Zone that have developed into large markets over time. In the peripheral parts of the zone, industrial areas have been established and these have attracted migrants. The Central Ridge (of the Aravalli hills) passes through this zone. The population density of the zone is 33,115.82 per sq km. Water supply is adequate in most parts of the zone, with an average supply of 337 lpcd.[30] In addition to the DJB supply, there are 26 DJB tubewells in Inderpuri, Todapur, Anand Parbat, Baljeet Nagar and Naraina areas. Shallow handpumps are few in number, mostly used in the vulnerable colonies. There are very few unsewered areas in the zone. The colonies situated on the higher elevations constitute some of the vulnerable pockets of the zone. The mean proportion of cases from these endemic pockets was 63.04 per cent. The vulnerable colonies include JJ clusters adjoining the railway line in Daya Basti and Patel Nagar stations; urbanised villages—Shadipur and Naraina; and Baljeet Nagar and Inderpuri resettlement colonies.

JJ Clusters

There are clusters of slum colonies on railway land between Daya Basti and Patel Nagar stations on the Delhi–Rewari line. The annual incidence rate in these slums ranges from 22 to 28 per 100,000. There is another group of clusters along the Najafgarh Road (Shivaji Marg) that runs parallel to the railway line, adjacent to the Najafgarh Road/Rama Road industrial area. The industries along with a number of fringe trades and services are major employers of the population in these areas, about 75,000 in number. These JJ clusters are densely populated; environmental sanitation is very poor with negligible service provided to these areas. Water supply is through public hydrants only in the clusters that lie along the main road. These clusters are at the tail end of the mains that supply this area. Further, the supply is against the gradient, as the land slopes upwards towards Anand Parbat (a portion of the Central Ridge). Per capita availability of water supply is grossly inadequate, and that too at very low pressure. Water pipelines are punctured at regular intervals and rubber pipes are attached to them. The ground is dug out and containers are placed there for filling; the meagre safe supply ends up being contaminated. The local population thus relies largely on shallow handpumps. With open defecation along the railway lines, the groundwater is also highly contaminated.

Urbanised Villages

Shadipur is an urbanised village contiguous with the commercial areas of adjoining Patel Nagar. The village is densely populated, with a large proportion of residents being tenants. The buildings have been haphazardly expanded to create extra space. The rented-out portions are small, one-room units with a common toilet for several families. The available water supply is inadequate, and many houses have installed on-line boosters.

Naraina village is a small, urbanised village located on the Ring Road bordering the Cantonment area and close to affluent areas of south and west Delhi. Like most other urbanised villages, landlords here have constructed one-room units for letting out. Tenants belong to the lower-middle-income group, and are largely from the southern states, mostly civilian employees of the armed forces or of the corporate sector offices of south Delhi. This village, with a population of about 20,000, reported an incidence rate of 0.2 to 0.4 per 100,000 annually.

Resettlement Colonies

Baljeet Nagar, a resettlement colony, was set up in 1977. The residents of slum clusters from Turkman Gate and Matia Khan areas were relocated to this colony. The population of this colony is about 6,000. The incidence rate of cholera ranged from 6–11 per 100,000.

Inderpuri, set up in 1975, adjoins Todapur village, which borders the ridge. The estimated population of these settlements is about 25,000. Like other resettlement colonies, Inderpuri has become overpopulated, considering the initial plans and provision of basic services. A large proportion of residents of this colony are salaried employees in both formal and informal sectors. Some residents work as manual labourers in the adjoining wholesale iron market (Loha Mandi) and the Naraina Industrial Area.

CITY ZONE

The annual incidence rate of cholera in the City Zone (with an average of 3.4 per 100,000 for the period 1994–2000) ranged between 2.7 per 100,000 to 6.2 per 100,000. The peak period was from June to August. This is one of the most densely populated zones of Delhi (80,000 per sq km), and corresponds approximately to the walled city and its extensions. Trade and commerce have flourished in these areas for centuries. There are residential areas as well; overcrowded katras and *havelis* (erstwhile mansions) are unique to this zone. Many trader families moved out over the last several decades as population density increased and newer residential areas developed, particularly in north and west Delhi. Trading is further facilitated by the major railway stations and the inter-state bus terminuses that are also located in this zone. Most areas of the zone have sewers. Open drains are few, and there are hardly any instances of pipelines crossing open drains. Water supply is good at 272 lpcd.[31] There are no tubewell supplies; the entire water supply is from the plants. Owing to the adequate piped water supply, shallow handpumps are also fewer in number. The only major vulnerable area in the City Zone is a group of JJ clusters that stretch along the Yamuna river bank (the Yamuna Pushta). Sporadic cases in the City Zone dominate the overall picture, rather than endemicity in vulnerable colonies.

JJ Clusters

A large number of slum (JJ) clusters were located along the west bank of the Yamuna. They are located virtually on the Yamuna bed. The first settlers of this colony arrived around 1965, and most of the growth took place in the second half of the 1970s, ironically, at a time when slum relocation was undertaken with great vigour (particularly during the Emergency).[32] The initial settlers were from Bihar and Uttar Pradesh, though in the later phases of its growth a significant proportion of the migrants were refugees from Bangladesh, both Hindus and Muslims. The population is estimated at 100,000. These communities are socio-economically among the poorest in Delhi, with most of the males working as rickshaw pullers and labourers in the trading areas of the walled city.

The older parts of the colony are served by public hydrants, and the newer parts (closer to the river) rely on shallow handpumps. These clusters are prone to flooding when the water level in the river rises, which accounts for the high incidence rate of cholera during the monsoons. There are no sanitary latrines and environmental sanitation is very poor. These clusters are a major centre for drug peddling, and there are a large number of drug addicts in the clusters; several NGOs have started providing de-addiction and rehabilitation services. The IPP-VIII programme of the MCD also has a centre serving the cluster. The incidence rate in these clusters was as high as 1.5–1.7 per 100,000 during 1998–2000, a nearly two-fold rise over the incidence in 1994. Despite the presence of the IPP-VIII centre and their outreach family welfare services, there was no positive impact on a disease that affects children. In the current phase of relocation, much of this population has been moved out of this area, to the current generation of resettlement colonies in Narela Zone, nearly 3,040 km away.

WEST ZONE

Cholera cases reported from this zone have been few in number and sporadic in nature. The average incidence rate is 0.91 per 100,000. There are no discernible spatial or temporal trends. There are thus no endemic pockets in this zone. Most settlements in the West Zone are essentially post-independence phenomena. A few colonies came up to rehabilitate the refugees of the Partition. Other colonies were developed by the DDA, including group housing societies and individually owned houses. The resident population in these planned colonies are either salaried employees or businessmen and belong to the middle- and upper-income groups. Schools, hospitals and transport facilities are adequately available in these zones and meet local needs. There are a few urbanised villages and resettlement colonies in this zone. The few unauthorised colonies that came up in the post-independence phase have been regularised, with adequate infrastructure. Slum clusters are confined to the Delhi–Rewari railway line. There are also a few industrial areas in this zone, but no major trading centres or wholesale markets. The population density is 15,192.77 per sq km. Water supply is adequate at an average of 202 lpcd.[33] The group housing colonies have their own private deep tubewell supply. The DJB also provides deep tubewell supplies in several colonies. The zone has sewerage services in most areas.

CONCLUSION

This chapter has discussed in some detail the vulnerability factors that have an impact at the zonal and colony levels. Table 5.4 summarises the key features of each zone.

It is evident that civic services for the less privileged have been inadequate. The provision of housing, water and sanitation facilities has failed to keep pace with the demands of increasing numbers of residents, attracted by the expansion in economic activities and opportunities. The fallout may be seen in the growth of unauthorised colonies, squatter settlements and the extension of laldoras in urbanised villages.[34] These settlements have emerged as endemic areas for cholera in Delhi.

The Civil Lines and Rohini Zones have relatively lower population densities, higher per capita availability of water (274 lpcd), higher coverage of sewers (60–80 per cent), and yet have had high incidence rates of cholera. Though the "averages" in terms of availability of services seem to be on the higher side, there are wide disparities among population groups within the zones, including the level of services available to them. In the 2001 census, the north-west district, which corresponds to the vulnerable belts comprising Civil Lines, Rohini and part of Narela, experienced the second-highest decadal growth rate (+60.12 per cent). Much of this growth involved population groups of low socio-economic status employed mostly in the unorganised and semi-organised sectors. Therein lies the explanation of why 87 per cent and 80 per cent of cholera cases from the Civil Lines and Rohini Zones, respectively, were being reported from the vulnerable colonies in these zones.

Across the river Yamuna, Shahdara (North) Zone experienced similar levels of population growth (+62.5 per cent) during 1991–2001. Shahdara (South) Zone, in contrast, had a growth rate of +41.61 per cent. Per capita

Table 5.4: Determinants of Vulnerability in Delhi's Municipal Zones[35]

Zone	*Average incidence rate (per 100,000)*	*Per cent of cases from vulnerable colonies*	*Predominant economic activity*	*Population density (per sq km)*	*Per capita piped water supply (lpcd)*	*Population having access to sewers (%)*
Civil Lines	33.39	86.94	Small and medium industries, wholesale markets, trading	13,500	274	60
Narela	32.05	61.70	Agriculture, agro-based industries	743	32	Nil
Najafgarh	23.55	73.86	Agriculture, industries, services	1,127	74	25
Rohini	22.50	79.92	Trading, transport, services	8,848	274	90
South	18.20	77.19	Services, small-scale industries, trading	4,237	148	50
Central	11.76			21,486		60
Shahdara (North)	12.30	84.31	Trading, small-scale industries	17,200	130	10
Shahdara (South)	5.48	74.31	Services, trading	20,529		30
Sadar Paharganj	5.42	45.43	Wholesale markets, trading, services, small-scale industries	98,250	205	100
Karol Bagh	3.71	63.04	Wholesale markets, trading, services, industries	33,116	337	90
City	3.40	43.30	Wholesale markets, trading, services	80,000	272	90
West	1.91	0.00	Trading, services, small-scale industries	15,193	202	90

water availability was 130 lpcd, and sewerage services were poorer than in the Civil Lines and Rohini Zones. Yet the cholera incidence rates are much lower. Although the per capita availability of water in absolute terms is lower, lesser disparities within these zones imply that even the poorer sections actually receive far larger quantities of water than in some other zones with higher average availability. The decline of cholera incidence in Shahdara (North) and Shahdara (South) Zones is largely attributable to the commissioning of the Bhagirathi water treatment plant. Sewerage services will need to be augmented to fully reap the benefits of added availability of water.

The City, Sadar Paharganj and Karol Bagh Zones have good availability of services. In particular, the availability of sewerage services is high for all segments of the population in these zones. Despite some of the highest population densities, these zones have actually experienced a decline in the population growth rate during 1991–2001. Against the backdrop of an average growth rate of +46.31 per cent, the central district that corresponds roughly to these three zones recorded a decadal growth rate of –1.91 per cent. The incidence rates of cholera are among the lowest of all the zones.

The two zones that have demonstrated a definite rising trend in incidence rates towards the second half of the 1990s are the South and Central Zones. The apparently low population density of the South Zone is misleading, as nearly two-thirds of the zone comprises rural areas with very low population density. The post-liberalisation period witnessed a remarkable growth of activities based in the tertiary and services sector in these zones. This growth in economic activity corresponded with a high decadal growth rate of population of +50.27 per cent. The vulnerable colonies of these zones comprise urbanised villages and colonies located along the Mehrauli–Badarpur Road. The proportion of vulnerable population is higher in the South Zone than in the Central Zone. The residents of these vulnerable colonies belong to lower-middle socio-economic groups. Along with the high population density in these colonies, there is a high proportion of tenancy. Water scarcity is acute and high levels of contamination occur because of a combination of factors operating at both the colony and the household level. Large disparities exist in the availability of water between these vulnerable colonies and the rest of the zone. The per capita availability of water is only 29 lpcd in these vulnerable colonies, as compared to a zonal average of 148 lpcd.

This chapter has offered a macro-level understanding of the disease and its infrastructural determinants. Causality operates dually, both at the area/population level as well as at the household and individual levels. Some unique vulnerabilities are determined by behavioural factors and practices. While household surveys offer additional insights, analyses at the household level, however, also need to take into account the socio-economic and infrastructure contexts of the residential clusters in which the households are situated. The next chapter uses a primary survey in order to better understand the role of behavioural factors and practices in determining vulnerability at the household level.

NOTES

1. A. V. Diez Roux et al., "Area Characteristics and Individual-Level Socioeconomic Position Indicators in Three Population Based Epidemiologic Studies", *Annals of Epidemiology* 11, no. 6, 2001, 395–405.
2. E. Breeze, D. A. Jones and P. Wilkinson, "Area Deprivation, Social Class and Quality of Life among People Aged 75 Years and Over in Britain", *International Journal of Epidemiology* 34, no. 2, 2005, 276–83. doi:10.1093/ije/dyh328 (accessed 1 March 2012).
3. A. V. Diez Roux, "Estimating and Understanding Area Health Effects", *International Journal of Epidemiology* 34, no. 2, 2005, 284–85. doi:10.1093/ije/dyi020 (accessed 1 March 2012).
4. Diez Roux, "Estimating and Understanding Area Health Effects".
5. Pearce, "Traditional Epidemiology".
6. Ibid.
7. N. Krieger and S. Zierler, "What Explains the Public's Health? A Call for Epidemiologic Theory", *Epidemiology* 7, no. 1, 1995, 107–9.
8. N. Krieger, "Theories for Social Epidemiology in the 21st Century: An Ecosocial Perspective", *International Journal of Epidemiology* 30, no. 4, 2001, 668–77.
9. Based on data collected from the National Institute of Communicable Diseases and Municipal Corporation of Delhi during fieldwork.
10. Jagvir Singh et al., "Endemic Cholera in Delhi, 1995: Analysis of Data from a Sentinel Centre", *Journal of Diarrhoeal Diseases Research* 16, no. 2, 1998, 66–73.

11. S. C. Pal, "A Review of the Studies on Cholera and Gastroenteritis Carried Out at the National Institute of Communicable Diseases, Delhi, 1965–72", *Journal of Communicable Diseases* 4, no. 2, 1972, 219–27; Dutta et al., "Epidemiological Features of Cholera Outbreak in Delhi in 1988".
12. Based on data collected from the National Institute of Communicable Diseases and Municipal Corporation of Delhi during fieldwork.
13. Computed by the author.
14. Nath, "Planning for Delhi and National Capital Region".
15. DUEIIP report, 29.
16. *Times of India* (New Delhi), 10 May 2003, quoting the Central Ground Water Authority, put the water table in this part of Delhi at about 6.5 metres in 2002. It was about a metre during the 1960s and 1970s.
17. A *Times of India* report quoting the Central Ground Water Authority.
18. Ibid.
19. Ibid.
20. Ibid.
21. Ibid.
22. Personal communication, Superintending Engineer, Delhi Jal Board, 7 September 2000.
23. Michael Z. Lahlou, *Water Quality in Distribution Systems.* http://www.nesc.wvu.edu (accessed 12 April 2010).
24. *Delhi—Of Population.* http://www.ofpopulation.co.uk/ (accessed 17 September 2007).
25. Indrani Mazumdar, *Unorganised Workers of Delhi and the Seven Day Strike of 1988.* http://www.indialabourarchives.org (accessed 6 March 2010).
26. DUEIIP report, 29.
27. With the construction of the ISBT bridge and the Delhi Metro, transport and communication facilities for these clusters improved and they expanded rapidly.
28. DUEIIP report, 29.
29. Ibid.
30. Ibid.
31. Ibid.
32. Some clusters from among these were relocated to areas in Shahdara during the Emergency.
33. DUEIIP report, 29.
34. Literally, *laldora* means "red line". Urban/planned Delhi has been constructed largely on agricultural lands acquired from villages. In the earlier phases, the villagers were relocated; later, only their agricultural lands were acquired and

the residential areas were circumscribed by a red line, and thus the term laldora came into use. For a detailed account, see Ministry of Urban Development, *Report of the Expert Committee on Lal Dora* (ECLD) *and Extended Lal Dora in Delhi*, Government of India, New Delhi, 2007. http://urbanindia.nic.in/programme/dd/laldora.pdf (accessed 12 March 2012).

35. Column 2 based on Table 5.1; column 3 based on Table 5.2. The last two columns are based on the DUEIIP report and on a personal communication from the Superintending Engineer, Delhi Jal Board, 7 September 2000, respectively.

6 Making Sense of "Behaviours"

SECONDARY ROUTES

Some researchers have laid emphasis on behavioural factors as the key determinants of diarrhoeal diseases, including cholera. Often described as "secondary routes", the role of behavioural factors in transmission has been considered to be complementary vis-à-vis infrastructural factors like water and sanitation. How do behavioural determinants play out in low-income urban contexts?

A comparative study of the incidence of diarrhoea among children belonging to families of poor socio-economic status in two different environmental situations in Kolkata—one group living in slums and the other residing in relocation projects of the Calcutta Metropolitan Development Authority (CMDA) in multi-storey buildings, did not observe any significant difference.[1] Incidence was high among infants in both groups, but declined sharply in CMDA children at the age of 2. The decline in the case of slum children was observed to take place at the age of 3 years. The provision of running water and sanitary latrines (as common facilities, not at the household level) in CMDA project areas did not reduce diarrhoea to any significant extent as compared to slums.[2] Incidence declined in both groups with increase in mothers' educational status. Partially breastfed children suffered the most among both groups.

In another study, Henry and Rahim examine the transmission of diarrhoea in two crowded areas with different sanitary facilities in Dhaka, Bangladesh.[3] The degree of contamination of each child's drinking water (waterborne) and of the hands of each child (water-washed) was correlated with diarrhoea incidence. Diarrhoea attacks increased significantly for children with more contaminated hands.

Ghosh et al.,[4] through community-based studies, explore the risk behavioural practices of mothers in families residing in slums in Kolkata and Varanasi and in rural areas in Haryana and Hyderabad. They observe that a sizeable proportion of children did not suffer from diarrhoea though they lived in the same area as children with diarrhoea. In Kolkata slums, 53.4 per cent of the children remained diarrhoea-free during the one-year study period with six days a week of active surveillance.[5] The risk behavioural practices of mothers that showed significant association with the presence of a child with diarrhoea in the family included the use of pond water for cleaning child-feeding containers, indiscriminate disposal of children's stool, bottle feeding, non-use of soap for cleaning child-feeding containers, and water storage in wide-mouthed containers.

Bacterial contamination of stored water and stored food was incriminated as a major risk factor for diarrhoeal diseases in a study in West Africa.[6] Factors such as illegal connections of piped water supply, shallow handpumps, high degree of storage, stored food left upto four hours and consumed cold or reheated for short periods, and low breastfeeding among mothers residing in urban slums as compared to rural mothers, were associated with high incidence of diarrhoeal diseases. The study also observed that water quality had no major influence on the standard of food in a community where faecal transmission is high and prolonged food storage is a common practice. In a prospective study, breast milk antibodies against cholera did not appear to protect children from colonisation with *Vibrio cholerae* O1, but did protect against the disease in those who became colonised.[7]

RECOGNISING THE COMPLEXITY

It is generally agreed that the transmission routes of the pathogens of diarrhoea are complex. Considerable emphasis has been laid on intra-household and behavioural factors as key determinants of diarrhoeal diseases, including cholera. In 1984, J. Briscoe pointed out the importance of evaluating multiple routes of transmission and assessing the impact of an individual determinant.[8] While infrastructural conditions constituted the primary routes, the contamination of water within households and other behavioural determinants were considered secondary routes. Briscoe, however, cautioned that it would be erroneous to conclude that improvements in drinking water supply are not an important intervention strategy for controlling diarrhoeal diseases. He advocated that improvements in the secondary routes of transmission can have a dramatic effect on disease incidence only if prior improvements in drinking water quality have been made.[9]

The WHO considers unhygienic transportation and storage of water as a "public health risk" that is behavioural in nature and can be "reduced or eliminated".[10] The importance of secondary routes has been put into proper perspective by some authors who argue that, when drinking water becomes contaminated during collection and storage in the home (as occurs quite commonly in poorer societies), the risk of faecal–oral disease is low.[11] A. Pruss et al. consider various models for the improvement of water supply, sanitation and personal hygiene, but do not take into account the extent to which household behavioural practices are relevant when water and sanitary latrine facilities are poor.[12] They report that the benefits of continuous piped water supply have not been adequately documented. The multi-country study by S. A. Esrey et al. explores the transition between different scenarios when interventions are implemented.[13]

A recent study of eight villages in rural Bangladesh explored the associations of socio-economic variables with the incidence rate of diarrhoeal diseases.[14] The villages were purposively selected to represent areas of high population density. Water samples were drawn from pond water to quantify the load of faecal coliforms. The levels of contamination of all water samples were found to be beyond the permissible limit. The study concluded that faecal coliforms were responsible for the high incidence of diarrhoea. "Surprisingly other SES factors like education, occupation do not have significant impact to decrease the disease incidence, which challenges the theory on 'SES and disease incidence', i.e., higher the SES, lower the incidence of disease."[15] The study acknowledged that there was a "village effect" in the incidence of diarrhoea, and that further ethnographic work was required to complement this exercise. Contrary to conventional public health wisdom, 50 per cent or more of those who used sanitary latrines suffered from high rates of diarrhoea as well. Income was found to be significantly associated with the incidence of diarrhoea at 10per cent level.

A recent meta-analysis by the World Bank argued that hygiene education and water quality improvements were more effective in reducing the incidence of diarrhoeal disease.[16] Point-of-use disinfection of water with chlorine, combined with safe water storage and basic hygiene education, has been considered to provide substantial health benefits at the lowest incremental cost.[17] A system designed by the Centers for Disease Control (CDC) is being socially marketed in order to ensure bacteriologically safe water supply at the household level. The WHO, in association with Population Services International and Sulabh International, started a pilot project in 2002 in selected slums in west Delhi for the social marketing of liquid chlorine for home chlorination, and of a narrow-mouthed container to prevent domestic-level contamination. However, the project was discontinued since the results were poor.[18] Similar results have been reported by an investigation in Mexico, which showed that the existing piped, treated water in the project communities was of good quality, though with suboptimal residual chlorine.[19] Although the project was well intentioned, it was not an appropriate intervention for these communities.

This chapter undertakes a household-level analysis that takes account of the socio-economic and infrastructural context of the residential clusters in which the households are situated. Key determinants and linkages at the micro level are explored. An in-depth study of 300 households was conducted in three selected localities in Shahdara (North) and Shahdara (South) zones, which are endemic for diarrhoeal diseases. These clusters are geographically adjacent to each other. The field work was conducted during May–September 1998. Two slums (JJ) clusters and one resettlement colony were chosen for this field study. A hundred households were chosen in each cluster by random sampling. The detailed methodology is described in the Appendix . The three clusters are:

- Sanjay Amar Colony, JJ Cluster, Shahdara (South) Zone (labelled Cluster 1)
- Taj Colony, JJ Cluster, Shahdara (North) Zone (Cluster 2)
- Welcome Colony, Double Storey, Resettlement Colony, Shahdara (North) Zone (Cluster 3)

A description of the three clusters, detailing their history, population structure, socio-economic characteristics and availability of infrastructure, is followed by details of the incidence rates of diarrhoea obtained from the field survey in these clusters. Thereafter, an analysis of the vulnerability issues, including socio-economic, infrastructural and behavioural factors, is provided.

SANJAY AMAR COLONY

Sanjay Amar Colony in Shahdara (South) Zone is situated near Road No. 67—an important road parallel to the Yamuna, connecting Shahdara to Preet Vihar. Along Road No. 67 flows a large drain carrying liquid waste from residential areas and the adjoining Patpargunj Industrial Area. The construction of the road and the drain began in the mid-1970s. A group of Muslim labourers from Loni, Uttar Pradesh, who were engaged in the construction work, set up a camp at the present site of the JJ cluster in 1978 under the leadership of a priest known as the *mullah pradhan*. The camp expanded gradually and was later renamed Sanjay Amar Colony after the demise of Sanjay Gandhi in 1980. The total population was approximately 26,500.

The JJ cluster is bound on the north by a large block of multi-storey flats (Figure 6.1). On the east, across a congested road, is Bhikam Singh Colony of Vishwas Nagar (an unauthorised colony that was later regularised). The southern and western boundaries of the JJ cluster comprise a large number of important institutions in the most important institutional area of East Delhi. The cluster is located in the backyard of the Shahdara (South) zonal office of the MCD and the District Employment Exchange of the East District of the Government of Delhi. The CPCB is also located in this institutional area, as are other important state institutions like the Directorate of Health Services (DHS), the Subordinate Selection Board and the Karkardooma district courts.

In its present form, the JJ cluster consists of five blocks (A to E). A Block is the largest, with approximately 2,000 dwelling units, followed by B Block with about 1,500 units. C Block is intermediate in size with about 800–900 units. The D and E Blocks are newer and smaller in size with about 250–300 houses each. The residents of the newer blocks are those evicted from another

Figure 6.1: Schematic Layout of Sanjay Amar Colony

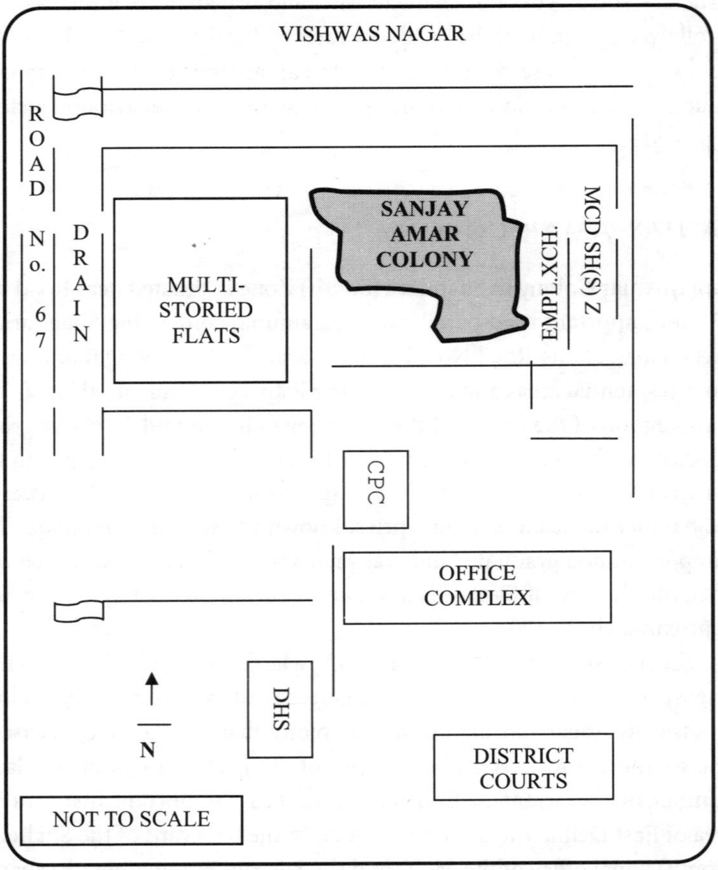

adjacent cluster (also initially set up by a group of construction labourers on the same project) when the block of multi-storey flats came up.

Most houses are made of brick with concrete roofs. Most of the roads and drains inside the cluster are paved. Municipal water supply is made available through public hydrants. In addition, there are a large number of shallow handpumps, with the regulation red paint signifying that it is dangerous to drink the water, but without any written warning to that effect. Each household surveyed had a large number of water containers—ample testimony to water scarcity. The water containers were dirty. The community reported that owing to the shortage of water, the residual water in a container was not wasted, and therefore a container was rarely washed or cleaned.

Ninety-six per cent of the households reported using MCD water from public hydrants as their primary water source; 4 per cent used shallow handpump water. Further, 32 per cent accessed an additional water source that consisted exclusively of handpumps. Eighty-nine per cent of the households reported using MCD piped supply as their source of drinking water, while the remaining 11 per cent used handpump water for drinking. One-third of the public hydrants had continuous supply while the others had interrupted supply

There were no dhalaos (bins) for disposing of solid waste. Garbage was generally dumped in the several "parks", which were not regularly cleaned. While there is large-scale open defecation by children, the adults generally use the two Jan Suvidha complexes (public toilet complexes) of the Slum and JJ Department, on payment. The maintenance of these complexes was reasonably satisfactory. Sixty-three per cent of the households reported using the community sanitary latrines; 36 per cent used open fields for defecation; another 1 per cent used open drains.

Almost every house facing the road on the Vishwas Nagar side has a shop. The vegetable market (*subzimandi*) of Vishwas Nagar is located opposite this cluster, and a number of families are engaged in this trade. D Block has several small manufacturing units producing small machinery parts and bags.

A fair price shop and an MCD primary school are located about a kilometre away in Vishwas Nagar. In 1996, the then health minister (elected from, and a resident of, the adjacent assembly constituency) had laid the foundation stones for a school and a dispensary in the cluster. No progress had taken place after that. The nearest Maternity & Child Welfare (M&CW) Centre of the MCD is about 2.5 km away. There are six registered medical practitioners (RMPs) practising in the cluster and several more in the adjacent colonies of Vishwas Nagar. There is also an "RMP dentist" (exclusively) practising dentistry in D Block. The cluster is also served by the IPP VIII programme of the MCD, with three centres in A, B and D Blocks.

Migrants from Uttar Pradesh constituted the largest group in this cluster. The second-largest group was from Gujarat. It was observed that, among the three clusters, the proportion of those who had shifted recently (less than five years previously) was the highest in Sanjay Amar Colony: 40 per cent. The proportion decreased systematically over subsequent period intervals,[20] to a minimum of 12 per cent for the 16–20 years group. The smallest group, 8 per cent, comprised families who had resided here for more than 15 years.

Occupational status was considered in four categories—labour, service, business and others.[21] The majority of the heads of household in this cluster were labourers. About 80 per cent of them earned less than Rs 1,500 per month. Services constituted the second-largest group. Further, 77.78 per cent of the working women were labourers.

Family income is grouped by dividing the entire income range into 6 percentiles (sextiles). Per capita income in the cluster was Rs 284.05 per month (Table 6.1). More than two-thirds of the families earned less than Rs 1,500 per month. The second-largest occupation group comprised salaried individuals who had family incomes between Rs 2,001 and Rs 3,500 per month. The proportion of heads of household employed in labour decreases for the higher-income categories, and correspondingly the proportion employed in service and petty business activities increases. The proximity to institutional and commercial areas probably explains the relatively higher proportion of salaried personnel.

Responses on education were classified into four mutually exclusive categories—those who were illiterate, those who had attended school, those who had completed school and those who had received higher education. Information was obtained about the educational levels of heads of household, mothers and children. In Sanjay Amar Colony, 59 per cent of the heads of households were illiterate, while 80 per cent of the mothers were illiterate. The proportion of mothers who had attended and completed school was proportionately much lower than the corresponding figure for heads of households. While almost 60 per cent of the children attended school, male attendance was not significantly higher than female attendance.

Table 6.1: Family Income and Occupation in Cluster 1[22]

Family income	Occupation of head of household					Occupation of mother				
	Number of households					Number of households				
	Labour	*Service*	*Business*	*Others*	*Total*	*Labour*	*Service*	*Business*	*Others*	*Total*
<950	6 (85.7)	1 (14.3)	0 (0)	0 (0)	7 (100)	3 (100)	0 (0)	0 (0)	0 (0)	3 (100)
950–1,500	40 (72.7)	8 (14.6)	4 (7.3)	3 (5.4)	55 (100)	3 (75)	0 (0)	0 (0)	1 (25)	4 (100)
1,501–2,000	8 (38.1)	5 (23.7)	4 (19.1)	4 (19.1)	21 (100)	7 (100)	0 (0)	0 (0)	0 (0)	7 (100)
2,001–3,500	2 (25)	6 (75)	0 (0)	0 (0)	8 (100)	1 (33.3)	1 (33.3)	1 (33.3)	0 (0)	3 (100)
3,501–5,500	1 (100)	0 (0)	0 (0)	0 (0)	1 (100)	0 (0)	1 (100)	0 (0)	0 (0)	1 (100)
Total	57 (61.9)	20 (21.7)	8 (8.7)	7 (7.7)	92 (100)	14 (77.8	2 (11.2)	1 (5.5)	1 (5.5)	18 (100)

Note: Figures in parentheses indicate percentages.

TAJ COLONY

Taj Colony, a slum cluster, is literally caught between the symbolic "old" and "new" of Delhi. The Grand Trunk Road and the Metro Rail corridor flank the cluster on either side (Figure 6.2). On the east, there is a large open drain carrying liquid waste, including faecal matter, from the unsewered colonies of Shahdara. Seelampur Station (of the Metro Rail), an interesting piece of architecture, towers over the other bank of this drain. Across the Metro Rail corridor and the railway line (connecting Uttar Pradesh to the Old Delhi Railway Station) lies Old Seelampur. The western boundary of the cluster is a large expanse of wetland. Before the construction of the marginal *bund* (the Yamuna pushta, in local parlance) by the Flood and Irrigation Department, these areas were prone to flooding.

The origin of this JJ cluster is, paradoxically, linked to the clearance of slums in other parts of Delhi. Some displaced Muslim families, who were not "resettled", set up huts in this marshy piece of land during the

Figure 6.2: Schematic Layout of Welcome Double Storey and Taj Colony

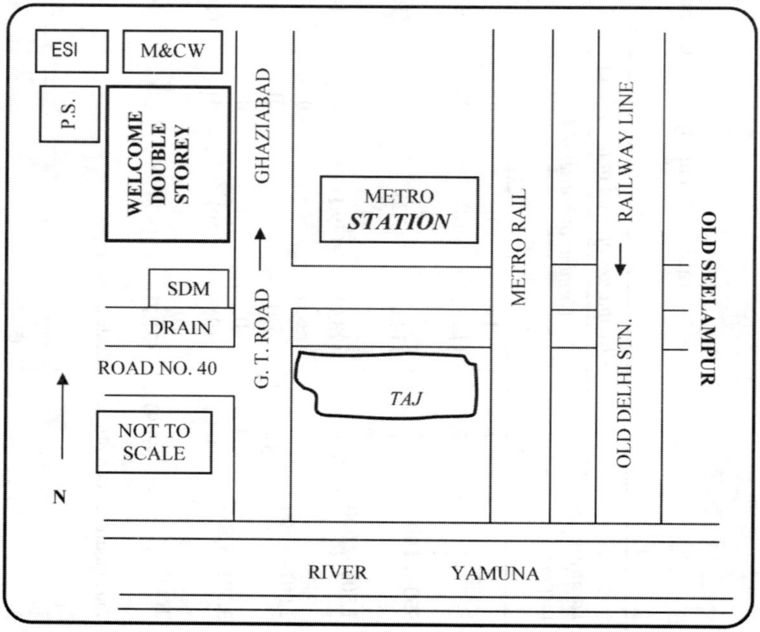

Emergency (1975–77). These victims of the dislocation caused by the then Congress-led government at the centre later supported the local Congress leaders. In the 1984 riots, the residents of this cluster allegedly participated in rioting in a Sikh unauthorised colony—Chauhan Bangar—across the G. T. Road, causing a large number of casualties. In fact, the two most prominent structures on either side of the G. T. Road are a mosque and a gurudwara, mute witnesses to past turbulence.

With an estimated population of 4,000, this small cluster is divided into two blocks. The dwelling units are made of brick, and most have concrete roofs. Some of these units are double-storied. The lanes inside the cluster and the drains are not paved. The drains are full of sullage, with water overflowing at a number of locations. The adjacent drain and the surrounding fields and wetlands are used for defecation. Environmental sanitary conditions are very poor. Of the population, 99 per cent used open fields for defecation and another 1per cent used open drains.

Municipal water supply is provided through public hydrants located along the main lanes of the cluster. Water pressure is low. The height of some the public standposts has been lowered by the residents, or the pipes have been removed completely, leaving only a rubber tube connected to the stump, a sure recipe for contamination.

Fifty-five per cent of the households reported using MCD water from public hydrants as their primary water source; 45 per cent used shallow handpump water. Further, 97.3 per cent reported accessing handpumps as an additional water source. About half the households reported MCD piped supply as their source of drinking water, while the remaining half used handpump water for drinking. Water supply in the public hydrants was reported to be continuous.

The majority of the residents are labourers. The cluster has a market of waste cloth and second-hand garments, with about 30 shops on either side of the main lane. The families engaged in this trade are relatively better off. A school and a fair price shop are about 1.5 to 2 km away. The nearest dispensary and maternity centre (of the MCD), which also has a birth and death registration centre, are about a kilometre away. There is only one RMP practising in the cluster. The adjacent colonies had a large number of RMPs whom the community accessed.

Migrants from Uttar Pradesh constituted the largest group in this

Table 6.2: Family Income and Occupation in Cluster 2[23]

Family Income	*Occupation of Head of Household*					*Occupation of Mother*				
	Number of Households					*Number of Households*				
	Labour	*Service*	*Business*	*Others*	*Total*	*Labour*	*Service*	*Business*	*Others*	*Total*
<950	3 (100)	0 (0)	0 (0)	0 (0)	3 (100)	2 (100)	0 (0)	0 (0)	0 (0)	2 (100)
950–1,500	15 (62.5)	2 (8.3)	6 (25)	1 (4.17)	24 (100)	1 (100)	0 (0)	0 (0)	0 (0)	1 (100)
1,501–2,000	18 (62.1)	3 (10.3)	7 (24.1)	1 (3.45)	29 (100)	7 (100)	0 (0)	0 (0)	0 (0)	7 (100)
2,001–3,500	29 (80.5)	1 (2.8)	6 (16.7)	0 (0)	36 (100)	14 (82.3)	0 (0)	2 (11.8)	1 (5.9)	17 (100)
3,501–5,500	1 (50)	0 (0)	1 (50)	0 (0)	2 (100)	0 (0)	0 (0)	0 (0)	0 (0)	0 (100)
Total	66 (70.2)	6 (6.4)	20 (21.3)	2 (2.1)	94 (100)	24 (88.9)	–	2 (7.4)	1 (3.7)	27 (100)

Note: Figures in parentheses indicate percentages.

cluster; those from Bihar and Rajasthan formed the second-largest group. About 20 per cent of the residents had shifted recently to this cluster. The largest proportion of residents comprised families who had been residing in the cluster for a period of 6–10 years. Like Cluster 1, the smallest group comprised families who had stayed here for more than 15 years: 8 per cent.

Like Cluster 1, the majority of the heads of households in this cluster were labourers (Table 6.2). While services were the second-largest group in Cluster1, business was the second most important category in Cluster 2. Also, 85.71 per cent of the working women in this cluster were labourers. The per capita income of Cluster 2 was Rs 345.71 per month. Though Clusters 1 and 2 were both slum clusters, Cluster 2 was economically better off, with higher levels of income. A higher proportion of families in Cluster 2 were engaged in business, and this accounted for the income differences. It becomes evident from Table 6.2 that the relationship between the proportion of heads of household engaged in labour and increasing income levels is not necessarily an inverse one, as observed in the case of Cluster 1.

This cluster had a higher proportion of illiterates both among heads of households (66per cent) and among mothers (81 per cent), as compared to Cluster 1. The proportion of heads of households who had completed school, and of those had had higher education, was also much lower than in Cluster 1. Surprisingly, attendance in school of male children was marginally lower than that of female children in this cluster.

WELCOME DOUBLE STOREY

The block of double-storied flats of Welcome Colony on G. T. Road is popularly known in the area as "Welcome Double Storey". While G. T. Road forms the cluster's eastern boundary, on the western side lie other blocks of Welcome Colony. To the north lies a string of public institutions, including a maternity and welfare centre of the MCD, an Employees' State Insurance (ESI) dispensary and the Welcome Police Station. The court of the sub-divisional magistrate is to the south of the colony. Beyond it lies a large drain that flows across Taj Colony to Old Seelampur and finally drains untreated liquid waste into the Yamuna, next to the Old Bridge.

The colony was constructed in 1977 as part of the effort to resettle communities living in slum clusters at that time. The allottees were relocated from the Inderlok area in 1978. Welcome had 400 flats, of which 32 had been allotted to the Delhi Traffic Police, who have their offices and residential quarters here. The initial composition of the allottees was one-third Muslims and two-thirds Hindus. Over the last 20 years, the ratio has reversed.

Hindu or Muslim, the common feature among the present lot of residents is the fact that very few of them are the original allottees. Most of these flats have been resold a number of times. Approximately one-third of the original allottees still residing here are Hindus from Punjab who migrated during the Partition, and who now own small factories and businesses in the neighbouring areas of Shahdara. Another third of the owners are Muslim traders who had migrated from Uttar Pradesh in the previous 10–15 years. The rest of the flats are rented out; the tenants generally belong to the service class and are from Uttar Pradesh and Bihar. This cluster largely comprises families who have stayed in Delhi, and also in the cluster itself, for a long period. The proportion of recently shifted residents is about 20per cent, while 32 per cent of the families in this cluster have stayed here for 15 years or more.

This planned colony had access to basic civic amenities. All the flats had household-level connections for municipal water supply. In addition, many of the ground-floor flats had handpumps as an additional source of water. Several houses had tubewells. Most of the households had refrigerators, and drinking water was stored in bottles in the refrigerators. All the households reported using MCD water as their primary water source; 85.1 per cent reported accessing handpumps as an additional water source, while 12.8 per cent used tubewells as the additional source. Despite all the households having individual piped supplies, only 79 per cent reported using it as their source of drinking water. Nineteen per cent used handpump water for drinking, and 2 per cent used tubewell water for this purpose. The municipal water supply was reported to be continuous. Environmental sanitation was found to be satisfactory. All the flats had individual sanitary latrines.

Despite the availability of a M&CW centre in its vicinity and the location of Swami Dayanand Hospital a few kilometres away, the

Table 6.3: Family Income and Occupation in Cluster 3[24]

Family income	Occupation of head of household					Occupation of mother				
	Number of households					Number of households				
	Labour	*Service*	*Business*	*Others*	*Total*	*Labour*	*Service*	*Business*	*Others*	*Total*
1,501–2,000	0 (0)	2 (50)	2 (50)	0 (0)	4 (100)	0 (0)	0 (0)	0 (0)	0 (0)	0 (0)
2,001–3,500	0 (0)	19 (63.3)	11 (36.7)	0 (0)	30 (100)	0 (0)	1 (100)	0 (0)	0 (0)	1 (100)
3,501–5,500	0 (0)	15 (28.3)	37 (69.8)	1 (1.9)	53 (100)	0 (0)	8 (100)	0 (0)	0 (0)	8 (100)
>5500	0 (0)	4 (36.4)	7 (63.6)	0 (0)	11 (100)	0 (0)	2 (66.7)	1 (33.3)	0 (0)	3 (100)
Total	–	40 (40.8)	57 (58.2)	1 (1)	98 (100)	–	11 (91.7)	1 (8.3ss)	–	12 100)

Note: Figures in parentheses indicate percentages.

residents generally accessed the private clinics and nursing homes in Welcome Colony, which were run by and large by qualified medical practitioners.

Cluster 3 is a relatively high-income cluster (Table 6.3). In relative terms, while most households in Clusters 1 and 2 were poor, those in Cluster 3 could be considered middle-class. Of the heads of households in Cluster 3, 58.16 per cent were businessmen and 40.82 per cent were in the services. The majority of working women were also employed in service activities. The per capita income was Rs 879.50 per month. Those running businesses earned more, on an average, than the salaried employees in the cluster. Of the working women in Cluster 3, about 92 per cent were salaried employees, most of them reporting family incomes between Rs 3,501 and Rs 5,500 per month.

This cluster had the highest educational status compared with the other two, with the lowest proportion of illiterate mothers at 9.78 per cent. Only 3 per cent of heads of households were illiterate. In fact, the largest group of mothers (43.48 per cent) and heads of households (78.35 per cent) belonged to the higher education category in this cluster. This is in sharp contrast to the other two clusters, where the majority of both mothers and heads of households belonged to the illiterate category. Correspondingly, school attendance rates for both male and female children were high in this cluster, at 94 per cent and 91 per cent, respectively.

INCIDENCE OF DIARRHOEA

It is important to understand that Clusters 1 and 2 were among the most vulnerable clusters in Delhi, and that the study was conducted during the most critical months from the point of view of diarrhoeal diseases. Incidence rates of diarrhoea for a two-week recall period were computed (Table 6.4). The incidence rates are highest in Cluster 1 for all age groups and recall periods, intermediate in Cluster 2, and lowest in Cluster 3; the exception to this pattern is the incidence rate for under-5 children with a recall period of two weeks, which is highest in Cluster 2.

Table 6.4: Incidence Rate (per 1,000) of Diarrhoea in the Three Clusters[25]

	Cluster 1		*Cluster 2*		*Cluster 3*	
	All Ages	*Under-5 Children*	*All Ages*	*Under-5 Children*	*All Ages*	*Under-5 Children*
No. of cases	42	38	28	21	39	25
Incidence rate (per 1,000)	78.7	157.8	48.0	216.2	18.8	71.4

Bhatnagar and Dosajh[26] report an incidence rate for diarrhoea of 246 per 1,000 among under-5 children residing in the slums of Delhi. The average duration of illness was reported to be 3.9 days per episode. Mehrotra[27] finds an incidence rate of 79/1,000 in Sunder Nagri, a resettlement colony. This figure is comparable to those obtained for Cluster 3 in this study, which is also a resettlement colony situated in the same municipal zone. It is also to be noted that Mehrotra's figures refer to an epidemic period, while the lower figures obtained in the present study relate to endemic levels.

It is interesting to analyse the incidence rate of diarrhoea among different income groups in these clusters (Table 6.5). It is observed that diarrhoea incidence rates are highest for Cluster 1 even by income categories, except for the family income category of Rs 1,501–2,000 per month. There are no unidirectional associations between incidence rates and income levels in any of the three clusters.

Table 6.5: Incidence Rate of Diarrhoea (per 1,000) by Income Group in the Three Clusters[28]

Family Income (Rs/month)	*Cluster 1*	*Cluster 2*	*Cluster 3*
	Incidence Rate per 1,000 (No. of Diarrhoea Cases)		
<950	111.1 (4)	38.4 (1)	–
950–1,500	71.4 (22)	59.7 (8)	–
1,501–2,000	62.0 (8)	64.5 (10)	133.3 (2)
2,001–3,500	132.0 (7)	34.8 (9)	21.5 (3)
3,501–5,500	142.8 (1)	0.0 (0)	90.9 (23)
>5,500	–	–	154.9 (11)

DETERMINANTS OF VULNERABILITY

The correlation coefficient between family income and the educational level of the head of the household (Table 6.6.1) is not significant for any of the clusters at the 5per cent level. The correlation coefficient is marginally higher at 0.06 for Cluster 1 as compared to 0.03 for the other two clusters.

Table 6.6.1: Family Income and Educational Status of Heads of Households[29]

Family income (Rs/month)	*Illiterate*	*Attended school*	*Completed school*	*Higher*
		Cluster 1		
<950	6 (60)	3 (30)	1 (10)	0 (0)
9,50–1,500	35 (60.3)	12 (20.7)	9 (15.5)	2 (3.5)
1,501–2,000	12 (52.2)	6 (27.0)	3 (13.0)	2 (8.8)
2,001–3,500	5 (62.5)	0 (0)	2 (25.0)	1 (12.5)
3,501–5,500	1 (100)	0 (0)	0 (0)	0 (0)
Total	59 (59)	21 (21)	15 (15)	5 (5)
		Cluster 2		
<950	5 (100)	0 (0)	0 (0)	0 (0)
950–1,500	15 (57.7)	10 (38.5)	0 (0)	1 (3.8)
1,501–2,000	20 (66.7)	4 (13.3)	6 (20)	0 (0)
2,001–3,500	25 (67.6)	8 (21.6)	4 (10.8)	0 (0)
3,501–5,500	1 (50)	0 (0)	1 (50)	0 (0)
Total	66 (66)	22 (22)	11 (11)	1 (1)
		Cluster 3		
1,501–2,000	0 (0)	1 (25)	0 (0)	3 (75)
2,001–3,500	3 (9.4)	0 (0)	5 (15.6)	24 (75)
3,501–5,500	0 (0)	3 (5.7)	11 (20.7)	39 (73.6)
>5,500	0 (0)	0 (0)	1 (9.1)	10 (90.9)
Total	3 (3)	4 (4)	17 (17)	76 (76)

Notes: Figures in parentheses indicate percentages. Row totals of percentages equal 100.

In Cluster 1, it is observed that differences in the educational level of the head of the household upto completion of school are not associated with any significant increases in income levels. Within each of the first three educational categories, approximately 70 per cent of the households have income levels below Rs 1,501 per month. It is only for the higher education category that this pattern changes, with 60per cent of the households reporting incomes above Rs 1,501 per month. About 60 per cent of households in each income category have illiterate heads of households. In Cluster 2, the proportion of households in higher income categories increases with increase in educational levels from illiteracy to completion of schooling. It is interesting that 70 per cent of the households earn more than Rs 1,501 per month, of whom 39 per cent earn more than Rs 2,001 per month. However, the proportion of illiterate heads of households is higher than in Cluster 1 for all except one income category. Thus, a positive association between increasing income levels and education is revealed at first glance, but this holds true for only a small number of households within the literate group, since the majority are illiterate. The overall proportion of illiterate heads of households is much lower at 3 per cent for Cluster 3, and all of these households fall in the income category of Rs 2,001–3,500 per month. The same income category also reports the highest proportion of heads of households with higher education in the entire dataset, at 75 per cent. No obvious patterns associating income categories with educational levels are discernible when the data is disaggregated by cross-tabulating income and education.

In Cluster 1, the distribution of households across income categories does not change with changes in the educational levels of mothers (Table 6.6.2). Within each education category, approximately 67 per cent of households had family incomes less than Rs 1,501 per month. The proportion of illiterates within each income category ranges between 75 per cent and 38per cent. In Cluster 2, as in Cluster 1, the majority of households have illiterate mothers. However, the majority of these illiterate mothers are in households with incomes higher than Rs 1,501 per month. The proportion of illiterates within each income category is higher, ranging from 77 per cent to 100per cent. In Cluster 3, the proportion of illiterate mothers is much lower within each income category, and varies from 7 to 14 per cent. The proportion of mothers with higher education was zero in Clusters 1 and 2, but in Cluster 3 this figure is positive for all family income categories, varying between 22 per cent and 53 per cent. However, within the cluster, it is difficult to draw linear associations between increasing income levels and increasing educational levels.

Table 6.6.2: Family Income and Educational Status of Mothers in the Households[30]

Family Income (Rs/month)	*Illiterate*	*Attended School*	*Completed School*	*Higher*
		Cluster 1		
<950	6 (75)	2 (25)	0 (0)	–
950–1,500	44 (81.5)	8 (14.8)	2 (3.7)	–
1,501–2,000	16 (76.2)	5 (23.8)	0 (0)	–
2,001–3,500	7 (87.5)	0 (0)	1 (12.5)	–
3,501–5,500	1 (100)	0 (0)	0 (0)	–
Total	74 (80.4)	15 (16.3)	3 (3.3)	–
		Cluster 2		
<950	5 (100)	0 (0)	0 (0)	–
950–1,500	20 (76.9)	6 (23.1)	0 (0)	–
1,501–2,000	23 (76.7)	4 (13.3)	3 (10)	–
2,001–3,500	29 (85.3)	3 (8.8)	2 (5.9)	–
3,501–5,500	1 (100)	0 (0)	0 (0)	–
Total	78 (81.2)	13 (13.5)	5 (5.2)	–
		Cluster 3		
1,501–2,000	0 (0)	2 (50)	1 (25)	1 (25)
2,001–3,500	2 (6.7)	7 (23.3)	5 (16.7)	16 (53.3)
3,501–5,500	7 (14..3)	8 (16.3)	13 (26.6)	21 (42.8)
>5,500	0 (0)	4 (44.4)	3 (33.3)	2 (22.3)
Total	9 (9.8)	21 (22.8)	22 (23.9)	40 (43.5)

Note: Figures in parentheses indicate percentages. Row totals of percentages equal 100.

In general, across clusters, MCD piped supplies were reported as the primary water source. However, there are exceptions to the pattern within clusters across income groups. The residents of Cluster 1 (Table 6.7.1), in all income categories, accessed MCD piped supply as the primary water source; public hydrants were distributed in a fairly even manner within the slum cluster. In Cluster 2 (Table 6.7.2), the poorer households were situated farthest from the public hydrants, which were located near the road. Thus, 80per cent of the poorest households reported handpumps as their primary source of water. In Cluster 3 (Table 6.7.3), the higher income groups owned individual handpumps and tubewells that were used as additional water sources. Some of the handpumps in Clusters 1 and 2 were installed by the civic authorities. <runon>However, groups of families with higher incomes also pooled their resources to install shallow handpumps for augmenting water supply. In all three clusters, the data reveals a positive association between households with an additional source of water and increasing income levels, particularly with regard to the middle income ranges across clusters.

Table 6.7.1: Water Sources Accessed by Families in Different Income Groups in Cluster 1[31]

Family income (Rs/month)	*Primary water source*			*Additional water source*			*Source of drinking water*		
	Number of households			*Number of households*			*Number of households*		
	MCD	*HP*	*Total*	*MCD*	*HP*	*Total*	*MCD*	*HP*	*Total*
<950	10 (100)	0 (0)	10 (100)	0 (0)	2 (100)	2 (100)	9 (90)	1 (10)	10 (100)
950–1,500	55 (94.8)	3 (5.2)	58 (100)	0 (0)	20 (100)	20 (100)	51 (87.9)	7 (12.1)	58 (100)
1,501–2,000	22 (95.6)	1 (4.4)	23 (100)	0 (0)	9 (100)	9 (100)	20 (87)	3 (13)	23 (100)
2,001–3,500	8 (100)	0 (0)	8 (100)	0 (0)	0 (0)	0 (0)	8 (100)	0 (0)	8 (100)
3,501–5,500	1 (100)	0 (0)	1 (100)	0 (0)	1 (100)	1 (100)	1 (100)	0 (0)	1 (100)
Total	96 (96)	4 (4)	100 (100)	0 (0)	32 (100)	32 (100)	89 (89)	11 (11)	100 (100)

Note: MCD: piped water supply; HP: handpump. Figures in parentheses indicate percentages.

Table 6.7.2: Water Sources Accessed by Families in Different Income Groups in Cluster 2[32]

Family income (Rs/month)	*Primary water source*			*Additional water source*			*Source of drinking water*		
	Number of households			*Number of households*			*Number of households*		
	MCD	*HP*	*Total*	*MCD*	*HP*	*Total*	*MCD*	*HP*	*Total*
<950	1 (20)	4 (80)	5 (100)	0 (0)	1 (100)	1 (100)	1 (20)	4 (80)	5 (100)
950–1,500	19 (73.1)	7 (26.9)	26 (100)	0 (0)	12 (100)	12 (100)	17 (65.4)	9 (34.6)	26 (100)
1,501–2,000	14 (46.7)	16 (53.3)	30 (100)	1 (9.1)	10 (90.9)	11 (100)	13 (43.3)	17 (56.7)	30 (100)
2,001–3,500	21 (56.8)	16 (43.2)	37 (100)	0 (0)	13 (100)	13 (100)	20 (54.1)	17 (45.9)	37 (100)
3,501–5,500	0 (0)	2 (100)	2 (100)	0 (0)	0 (0)	0 (0)	0 (0)	2 (100)	2 (100)
Total	55 (55)	45 (45)	100 (100)	1 (2.7)	36 (97.3)	37 (100)	51 (51)	49 (49)	100 (100)

Notes: MCD: piped water supply; HP: handpump. Figures in parentheses indicate percentages.

Table 6.7.3: Water Sources Accessed by Families in Different Income Groups in Cluster 3[33]

Family income (Rs/ month)	*Primary water source*		*Additional water source*				*Source of drinking water*			
	Number of households		*Number of households*				*Number of households*			
	MCD	*Total*	*MCD*	*HP*	*TW*	*Total*	*MCD*	*HP*	*TW*	*Total*
1,501–2,000	4 (100)	4 (100)	0 (0)	3 (100)	0 (0)	3 (100)	2 (50)	2 (50)	0 (0)	4 (100)
2,001–3,500	32 (100)	32 (100)	0 (0)	14 (93.3)	1 (6.7)	15 (100)	24 (75)	8 (25)	0 (0)	32 (100)
3,501–5,500	53 (100)	53 (100)	1 (4)	20 (80)	4 (16)	25 (100)	44 (83.1)	7 (13.1)	2 (3.8)	53 (100)
>5,500	11 (100)	11 (100)	0 (0)	3 (75)	1 (25)	4 (100)	9 (81.8)	2 (18.2)	0 (0)	11 (100)
Total	100 (100)	100 (100)	1 (2.1)	40 (85.1)	6 (12.8)	47 (100)	79 (79)	19 (19)	2 (2)	100 (100)

Notes: MCD: piped water supply; HP: handpump; TW: tubewell. Figures in parentheses indicate percentages.

Table 6.8: Income Levels and Access to Toilet Facilities[34]

Family income (Rs/month)	*Cluster 1*				*Cluster 2*			*Cluster 3*	
	Open field	*Open drain*	*Sanitary latrine (community)*	*Total*	*Open field*	*Open drain*	*Total*	*Sanitary latrine (individual)*	*Total*
<950	1 (10)	0 (0)	9 (90)	10 (100)	4 (80)	1 (20)	5 (100)	–	–
950–1,500	24 (41.4)	0 (0)	34 (58.6)	58 (100)	26 (100)	0 (0)	26 (100)	–	–
1,501–2,000	8 (34.8)	1 (4.3)	14 (60.9)	23 (100)	30 (100)	0 (0)	30 (100)	4 (100)	4 (100)
2,001–3,500	3 (37.5)	0 (0)	5 (62.5)	8 (100)	7 (100)	0 (0)	7 (100)	32 (100)	32 (100)
3,501–5,500	0 (0)	0 (0)	1 (100)	1 (100)	2 (100)	0 (0)	2 (100)	53 (100)	53 (100)
>5,500	–	–	–		–	–		11 (100)	11 (100)
Total	36 (36)	1 (1)	63 (63)	100 (100)	99 (99)	1 (1)	100 (100)	100 (100)	100 (100)

Note: Figures in parentheses indicate percentages.

In Cluster 1 (Table 6.8), 90 per cent of the households with the lowest family incomes accessed the community sanitary latrines. This proportion dropped to an average of about 60 per cent for the higher income levels. In Cluster 2, there are no provisions for community sanitary latrines. Also, there is no scope for the construction of individual latrines, irrespective of incomes. Dwelling units in Cluster 3 were constructed with individual sanitary latrines. Thus, in these clusters, colony-level factors emerge as more critical than individual income levels in determining access to sanitary latrines, community or individual.

Eleven per cent of the households reported using handpump water for drinking in Cluster 1. Among these families, 73 per cent of the heads of households and 89 per cent of mothers were illiterate (Table 6.9). With improvement in the educational status of both, the use of handpump water for drinking decreased significantly. The trend was similar in Cluster 2 as well. The trend was different in Cluster 3, however. One hundred per cent of the heads of households using tubewell water, and 66.67 per cent of those using handpump water for drinking, belonged to the higher education group; they were also households reporting high incomes. But among mothers belonging to the higher education group, 87.5 per cent were using MCD water for drinking. As the educational status of mothers declined, the consumption of handpump water for drinking increased significantly.

In Cluster 1, the only water sources were three shallow handpumps and six public hydrants. Water samples were collected from all these sources, since these were the only sources accessed by all the households in these clusters. All three handpumps (Table 6.10) had the maximum possible contamination, with counts of 2,400 each. The six public hydrants all passed the test with the best possible quality—a count of zero each.

Like Cluster 1, the only water sources in Cluster 2 were eight shallow handpumps and four public hydrants. Water samples were collected from all these sources, as for Cluster 1, since these were the only sources accessed by all the households in this cluster. The eight handpumps were all found unfit. The MPN counts ranged from a minimum of 75 to a maximum of 2,400. The four public hydrants passed the test, with MPN counts ranging from 0 to 4.9.

Table 6.9: Educational Status of the Head and the Mother of the Household and Source of Drinking Water[35]

Educational Status	*Cluster1*			*Cluster2*			*Cluster3*			
	Number of Households									
	MCD	*HP*	*Total*	*MCD*	*HP*	*Total*	*MCD*	*HP*	*TW*	*Total*
Head										
Illiterate	51 (86.4)	8 (13.6)	59 (100)	34 (51.5)	32 (48.5)	66 (100)	2 (66.7)	1 (33.3)	0 (0)	3 (100)
Attended School	20 (95.2)	1 (4.8)	21 (100)	10 (45.4)	12 (54.6)	22 (100)	3 (75)	1 (25)	0 (0)	4 (100)
Completed School	14 (93.3)	1 (6.7)	15 (100)	6 (54.6)	5 (45.4)	11 (100)	12 (70.6)	5 (29.4)	0 (0)	17 (100)
Higher	4 (80)	1 (20)	5 (100)	1 (100)	0 (0)	1 (100)	62 (81.6)	12 (15.8)	2 (2.6)	76 (100)
Total	89 (89)	11 (11)	100 (100)	51 (51)	49 (49)	100 (100)	79 (79)	19 (19)	2 (2)	100 (100)
Mother										
Illiterate	66 (89.2)	8 (10.8)	74 (100)	39 (50)	39 (50)	78 (100)	4 (44.4)	4 (44.4)	1 (11.2)	9 (100)
Attended School	14 (93.3)	1 (6.7)	15 (100)	7 (53.8)	6 (46.2)	13 (100)	13 (61.9)	8 (38.1)	0 (0)	21 (100)
Completed School	3 (100)	0 (0)	3 (100)	4 (80)	1 (20)	5 (100)	19 (86.4)	3 (13.6)	0 (0)	22 (100)
Higher	–	–	–	–	–	–	35 (87.5)	4 (10)	1 (2.5)	40 (100)
Total	83 (90.2)	9 (9.8)	92 (100)	50 (52.1)	46 (47.9)	96 (100)	71 (77.2)	19 (20.6)	2 (2.2)	92 (100)

Note: Figures in parentheses indicate percentages.

Table 6.10: Results of Bacteriological Tests of Water Sources in the Three Clusters[36]

Cluster	*Sources*							
	Handpump		*MCD (Public Hydrant)*		*MCD (Household)*		*Tubewell*	
	F	*U*	*F*	*U*	*F*	*U*	*F*	*U*
Sanjay Amar Colony	0	100	100	0	n/a	n/a	n/a	n/a
Taj Colony	0	100	100	0	n/a	n/a	n/a	n/a
Welcome D. Storey	0	100	n/a	n/a	100	0	50	50

Note: All figures are in percentages. F: fit; U: unfit; n/a: not applicable.

In Cluster 3, two households used water from tubewells as their source of drinking water. Samples were taken from both these tubewells. One tubewell was found to be fit (MPN count 3.1) while the other the other was found unfit (MPN count 13).

The MCD pipelines supplying these flats entered the colony from two sides. Two samples were taken, one from each side. The rationale was that the supply made available should be evaluated on the basis of the quality of water in the main pipelines, as the responsibility of the provider is upto this level only. Beyond these points, the maintenance of the service pipelines is the responsibility of the consumers (residents). All the MCD samples tested fit. There were 19 households drinking water from shallow handpumps. These were all individually owned handpumps, in contrast to the community handpumps in the other two clusters. Water in all the handpumps tested unfit for drinking.

In order to analyse the relevance of storage practices with regard to diarrhoeal incidence rates, households were classified on the basis of the source of drinking water accessed—MCD and non-MCD. For households that stored water drawn from MCD sources, data was analysed with reference to storage practices. For purposes of comparison, incidence rates of diarrhoea were also computed for households that accessed MCD sources but did not store the water, and for the remaining set of households, namely, those that accessed non-MCD sources. Bacteriological tests revealed that MCD sources (public hydrant and household) were 100 per cent fit (Table 6.10). Thus, in order to isolate the effect of storage practices, after controlling for source contamination, only water stored from MCD sources was considered for the analysis. The impact of the use of a separate utensil to draw water from the storage containers is relevant only in case of those households that stored water in wide-mouthed containers (Table 6.11).

Table 6.11: Storage Practices in the Three Clusters[37]

	MCD Sources					
Cluster 1	*Covered Vessel, Wide Mouth*	*Covered Vessel, Narrow Mouth*	*Uncovered Vessel, Wide Mouth*	*Uncovered Vessel, Narrow Mouth*	*Not Stored*	*Non-MCD*
No. of households	37	39	6	6	1	11
Incidence Rate	63.8 (12)	107.9 (23)	68.9 (2)	64.5 (2)	0 (0)	44.1 (3)
Cluster 2						
No. of households	15	12	21	–	3	49
Incidence Rate	70.4 (5)	27.0 (2)	53.4 (7)	–	62.5 (1)	44.7 (13)
Cluster 3						
No. of households	38	36	2	3	–	21
Incidence Rate	65.4 (11)	104.3 (17)	0.0 (0)	47.6 (1)	–	86.2 (10)

UNDERSTANDING THE DETERMINANTS

Epidemiological wisdom suggests that incidence rates of diarrhoea among households with the best storage practices should be lowest, provided other factors are comparable. In the context of the present dataset, the best storage practice would correspond to households that store water in covered vessels with narrow mouths. The use of a separate utensil to draw water from the storage container also constitutes best practice. However, there are variations in the sources from which water is drawn for storage, and this implies variations in the quality of water being stored by households, as demonstrated earlier through the laboratory results. In

Clusters 1 and 3, the highest incidence rate for diarrhoea was observed in the best practice category, while for Cluster 2 the expected results were obtained. These findings prompt further exploration of the vulnerability factors underlying the apparent paradox.

Analytically, a standard starting point is to explore differences in diarrhoeal incidence rates by age. In analysing the findings obtained, a distinction was made between children under-5 (U-5) years and those in the age group 5–18 years. It is hypothesised that U-5 children who stay at home, particularly where the proportion of working mothers is low, are likely to be under better supervision, and therefore show a lower incidence of diarrhoea. In contrast, children going to school are more likely to consume unsafe water and drinks outside the home.

The proportion of U-5 children in the best practice category of households was lower in Cluster 1 as compared to the other storage categories; diarrhoea incidence was higher among the 5–18 years age group in the best practice category. In Cluster 2, this pattern was reversed, with a higher proportion of U-5 children and a lower incidence of diarrhoea among children in the 5–18 years age group in the best practice households as compared to the other storage category households. In Cluster 3, the pattern of Cluster 1 was observed, with a lower proportion of U-5 children and a higher incidence of diarrhoea in the 5–18 age group for the best practice households.

These findings prompt a further exploration of children in the school-going age, that is, 5 to 18 years. The proportion of children attending school was computed for each cluster. It was found that in Cluster 1, 64.2 per cent children attended school, while 38.2 per cent and 93 per cent attended school in Clusters 2 and 3, respectively. Comparison of these attendance rates with the evidence on incidence rates of diarrhoea discussed earlier leads to the confirmation of the hypothesis that school-going children from households of lower socio-economic status are exposed to greater risk of diarrhoeal diseases because of consuming contaminated water, drinks, and food (mostly from street vendors). In Guatemala, Koo identified ice-based candies prepared with unsafe water as highly contaminated; vibrios survived in these items.[38] It is likely that similar routes of transmission may explain the higher incidence of diarrhoea among school-going children among the poorer communities of Delhi.

It was found that the incidence rates of diarrhoea in households which did not use separate utensils to draw water from storage containers were higher than among those that did so in Clusters 1 and 2 (Table 6.12). These results are as per theoretical expectations. However, in Cluster 3, the incidence rates were higher for homes that used separate utensils. In Cluster 1, 11 water samples were collected from households that stored water from public hydrants. Of these 11 stored samples, six (55 per cent) failed the test and five (45 per cent) were found to be fit for human consumption. Eight water samples were collected from Cluster 2 households that stored water from public hydrants. Of these eight stored samples, five (62.5 per cent) failed the test and three (37.5 per cent) samples were found to be fit for human consumption.

Table 6.12: Use of a Separate Utensil to Draw Water in the Three Clusters[39]

Cluster 1	*Separate Utensil*	*No Separate Utensil*
No. of households	33	10
Incidence Rate	56.81 (10)	97.56 (4)
Cluster 2		
No. of households	26	10
Incidence Rate	41.37 (6)	105.26 (6)
Cluster 3		
No. of households	25	15
Incidence Rate	70.17 (8)	46.87 (3)

A unique feature of Cluster 3 was 100per cent storage, i.e., all 100 households surveyed stored water. Purposive sampling was done to apportion the remaining 16 samples among 19 handpumps (source) and 99 households (rejecting one household where the source—a tubewell—had already been declared unfit). The samples were selected from each category in the ratio of 19:99. This worked out to three samples from handpumps and 13 stored samples. Three handpumps were randomly selected from the 19 shallow handpumps in question. All tested unfit for human consumption, with MPN values of 270 to 2,400. Of the 13 stored samples, one was purposively selected from the household using the tubewell that tested unfit. The other 12 were selected from households with individual

MCD piped supply, as handpump sources had already been found to be unfit. Ten (83 per cent) stored MCD samples were found fit while two (17 per cent) were found to be unfit. A summary of the results is tabulated in Table 6.13.

Table 6.13: Results of Bacteriological Tests of Stored Water in the Three Clusters[40]

Cluster	*Source*					
	MCD (Public Hydrant)		*MCD (Household)*		*Tubewell*	
	F	*U*	*F*	*U*	*F*	*U*
Sanjay Amar Colony	45.4	54.6	n/a	n/a	n/a	n/a
Taj Colony	60	40	n/a	n/a	n/a	n/a
Welcome D. Storey	n/a	n/a	83.3	16.7	50	50

Note: All figures are in percentages. F: fit; U: unfit;n/a: not applicable.

HOW CRITICAL ARE "BEHAVIOURS" AND "PRACTICES"?

It is important to establish the associations between the determinants of diarrhoeal diseases and the incidence rates on a cluster-by-cluster basis. The vulnerability of each cluster is assessed in order to explain the patterns of incidence of reported diarrhoea.

For each age group, Cluster 3 had the lowest incidence rates compared to the other two clusters. Cluster 1 had the highest incidence of disease for all age groups and recall periods, except the under-5 age group and adults (>18 years), the recall period being two weeks in both cases. For all other categories, the incidence rates in Cluster 2 were substantially lower than those in Cluster 1.

Though nearly all households reported accessing MCD water as their primary source of water in Cluster 1, about a tenth did not use it for drinking purposes. Compared to the other clusters, the use of handpumps was lowest in Cluster 1. Despite these relative safety factors, the vulnerability of this cluster lay in the fact that water supply was intermittent. This forced all but one household (located next to a public hydrant) of those surveyed to store MCD water.

Cluster 1 had lower per capita income at Rs 284.05 per head as compared to Rs 345.71 in Cluster 2. The income distribution is skewed towards the lower end in Cluster 1, with 68per cent of the households earning not more than Rs 1,500 per month. In as much as the level of family income is an indicator of vulnerability, capturing the effects of factors not otherwise accounted for (such as the ability to afford better alternatives in a situation of contamination or to adopt better preventive practices), family income levels show that Cluster 1 was at a relative disadvantage compared to the other two clusters, especially Cluster 3.

The educational status of mothers in Clusters 1 and 2 was comparable, with most (over 80per cent) being illiterate. The proportion of literates among heads of households is higher in Cluster 1 than Cluster 2. Illiteracy among the heads of households as well as illiteracy among mothers had a positive association with the consumption of handpump water. A similar association had also emerged between family income levels and consumption of handpump water.

While both income level and illiteracy emerged as vulnerability factors for Cluster 1, educational status in Cluster 2 could potentially be an important factor, indicating aspects of vulnerability such as awareness levels. This is further substantiated by evidence on school attendance by female children, with much higher numbers of female children in the 5-plus age group not attending school in Cluster 2. Combined with the total lack of sanitary latrines and the relatively higher reported usage of handpump water as the primary means of accessing water for household purposes, infrastructural problems combined with educational status to make this particular cluster vulnerable to the incidence of diarrhoeal disease.

Cluster 3 reported the lowest incidence of illness for all age groups and recall periods. This finding also has an obvious correlation with data on several socio-economic characteristics. The per capita income in this cluster, at Rs 879.49 per month, was substantially higher than the other two clusters. While this cluster ranked best in terms of the educational status of the head of the household, the differences are marked in the case of the mothers' educational levels, with less than 10per cent of the mothers being illiterate as compared to over 80per cent in the other two clusters. With 100 per cent households having access to sanitary latrines, Cluster

3 was at an advantage compared to the other two clusters in terms of the vulnerability indicators analysed in this study.

In Cluster 3, as many as 40 per cent of the households reported the use of handpump water as a secondary source of water for household purposes. On the one hand, it is statistically not possible to establish a unidirectional causation between the incidence of illness and the extent of contamination arising from the mere use of a secondary source of water. It would be valid to hypothesise that, with 19 per cent of the households reporting direct consumption of water from handpumps and 40 per cent reporting the use of handpump water as a secondary source to supplement the primary source, the cluster would potentially be vulnerable to diarrhoeal illness, albeit perhaps to a lesser extent than the other clusters, where socio-economic factors would combine to make the situation more complicated.

Among households storing MCD water (proven to be safe at source), adherence to the best storage practices does not translate into lower incidence rates compared to those with relatively unsafe practices. As has been argued earlier, a possible explanation for this lies in factors that are external to the home and largely beyond the control of the affected household members. While information, education and communication (IEC) are important, the relevance of IEC weakens when surrounding infrastructural conditions are unfavourable. The vulnerability of children in schools emerges as a matter of concern. Children from these clusters attended either a municipal primary school or private schools. Both of these lacked basic civic amenities. Street foods are poorly regulated, and the working status of mothers implied that children most often did not carry food from home, instead consuming food outside. Similar findings have been reported by another study of school-going children in Delhi in similar settings.[41] These findings have serious implications for children in general and for diarrhoeal diseases in particular.

NOTES

1. A. K. Chakraborty and J. C. Das, "Comparative Study of Incidence of Diarrhoea among Children in Two Different Environmental Situations in Kolkata", *Indian Pediatrics* 20, no.12, 1983, 907–13.

2. F. J. Henry and Z. Rahim, "Transmission of Diarrhoea in Two Crowded Areas with Different Sanitary Facilities in Dhaka, Bangladesh", *Journal of Tropical Medicine and Hygiene* 93, no. 2, 1990,121–26.
3. Henry and Rahim, "Transmission of Diarrhoea in Two Crowded Areas".
4. S. Ghosh et al., "Risk Behavioural Practices of Rural Mothers as Determinants of Childhood Diarrhoea", *Journal of Communicable Diseases* 29, no. 1, 1997, 7–14.
5. Studies from urban Bangkok and a suburb of Rangoon also failed to detect any significant association between diarrhoea and socio-economic status. K. Vathanophaset al., "The Study of Socioeconomic, Behavioural and Environmental Factors Related to Diarrhoeal Diseases in Children under 5 in Congested Areas of Bangkok Metropolis", *Journal of Medical Association of Thailand* 69, Suppl. 2, 1986, 156–62.
6. K. Mølbak et al., "Bacterial Contamination of Stored Water and Stored Food: A Potential Source of Diarrhoeal Diseases in West Africa", *Epidemiology and Infection* 102, no. 2, 1989, 309–16.
7. R. I. Glass et al., "Protection against Cholera in Breast-Fed Children by Antibodies in Breast Milk", *New England Journal of Medicine* 308, no. 23, 1983,1392–98.
8. Briscoe, "Technology and Child Survival".
9. J. Briscoe, "Intervention Studies and the Definition of Dominant Transmission Routes", *American Journal of Epidemiology* 120, no. 3, 1984, 449–55.
10. WHO, *WHO Chronicle No. 31* (Geneva: WHO, 1997).
11. R. G. Feachem, "Interventions for the Control of Diarrhoeal Diseases among Young Children: Promotion of Personal and Domestic Hygiene", *Bulletin of the World Health Organization* 62, no. 3,1984, 467–76.
12. A. Pruss et al., "Estimating the Burden of Disease from Water, Sanitation and Hygiene at a Global Level", *Environmental Health Perspectives* 110, no. 5, 2002, 537–42.
13. Esrey et al., "Interventions for the Control of Diarrhoeal Diseases".
14. Azizur R. Molla, "Pond Water Contamination and Incidence of Disease in Rural Bangladesh". http://paa2005.princeton.edu/download.aspx?submissionid=51339 (accessed on 19 February 2006).
15. Molla, "Pond Water Contamination and Incidence of Disease".
16. L. Fewtrell and J. Colford, "Water, Sanitation and Hygiene: Interventions and Diarrhoea—A Systemic Review and Meta analysis". Health, Nutrition, and Population Family of the World Bank Human Development Network.http://www1.worldbank.org/hnp/Pubs_Discussion/Fewtrell & ColfordJuly2004.pdf. (accessed 12 December 2005).

17. R. E. Quick et al., "Diarrhoea Prevention in Bolivia through Point-of-Use Water Treatment and Safe Storage: A Promising New Strategy", *Epidemiology and Infection* 122, no. 1, 1999, 83–90.
18. R. Dasgupta, "Mapping Cholera in Delhi: Looking at Micro and Macro Solutions", Proceedings of the Fifth All India People's Technology Congress, Kolkata, 18–20 February 2005.
19. D. S. Lantagne, R. Quick and M. D. Eric, "Household Water Treatment and Safe Storage Options in Developing Countries: A Review of Current Implementation Practices", 2005. http://www.wilsoncenter.org/water (accessed on 7 July 2006).
20. Based on key-informant interviews conducted in the cluster.
21. "Business" in the JJ clusters implied petty businesses and shopkeeping.
22. Based on data collected by the author during a field survey conducted in May–September 1998.
23. Same as Table 6.1.
24. Ibid.
25. Ibid.
26. S. Bhatnagar and U. Dosajh, *Diarrhoeal Disease Morbidity in Children below 5 Years in Urban Slums in Delhi* (New Delhi: National Institute of Health and Family Welfare, 1986).
27. Ritu Priya Mehrotra, *The Gastroenteritis Outbreak and Its Control in Sunder Nagri: An Assessment at Community Level* (New Delhi: Jawaharlal Nehru University, 1988).
28. Same as Table 6.1.
29. Ibid.
30. Ibid.
31. Ibid.
32. Ibid.
33. Ibid.
34. Ibid.
35. Ibid.
36. Ibid.
37. Ibid.
38. Koo et al., "Epidemic Cholera in Guatemala".
39. Same as Table 6.1.
40. Ibid.
41. Dasgupta, "Exploring Intra-household Factors in Diarrhoeal Diseases: A Study in Slums of Delhi, India", *Journal of Water and Health* 6, no. 2, 2007, 289–99.

7

Cholera and Urbanisation

An Ecosocial View

URBAN HEALTH AND THE CSDH REPORT

The Report of the WHO Commission on Social Determinants of Health (CSDH) represents a bold initiative in advocating a concerted public health effort towards evolving a "new global agenda".[1] Remarkable as it is, this document has been received with both optimism and scepticism. Nothing is more moving than labelling social injustice as the killing of people on a grand scale. As the American Indian proverb goes, all who have died are equal. The CSDH report seeks to bring back health equity "in a generation".[2] The perceived lack of clarity regarding complex concepts such as "political will" and "evidence" can be an obstacle to generating a robust global health movement that can "dominate future WHO and national agendas" and successfully counter the "counter-revolution" of selective primary health care (SPHC).[3] Failure on the part of the WHO and national governments to translate the recommendations into action would constitute an unmitigated missed opportunity.

An estimated 3.5 billion people in the world live in urban areas, more than the number of those living in rural areas. Importantly, nearly one billion people live in "life-threatening conditions" in the slums of developing countries.[4] Megacities will increasingly be a problem of developing nations and transition economies.[5] These societies have moved slowly and inevitably to the double burden of communicable diseases—largely among children as well as infections such as TB among adults—along with chronic diseases in ageing populations, albeit with onset at lower age groups. The underlying conditions, ranging from under nutrition to substance abuse, complicate the health of the urban poor. Social gradients are evident in most health conditions; urban populations are no exception, with the urban poor being the most affected and most vulnerable. Recommendations 6.1 to 6.3 of the commission's report call for improved participatory governance, improved housing and living conditions (specifically slum upgradation including water supply, sanitation, electricity and paved streets for all households regardless of the ability to pay), and a multitude of other health-promoting activities (such as physical activity and the reduction of violence and alcohol consumption).

Arguing that urbanisation itself was reshaping population health problems (specifically those of urban poor), the commission calls for a new paradigm of urban health. This would come about through an urgent improvement of living conditions in slums. Upfront, the CSDH sees a clear role for local governments in housing and basic services; a prerequisite for this is the political recognition of illegal settlements and the regularisation of tenureship. Much would depend on progress in the improvement of rural livelihoods and health services.[6]

DELHI'S CONTEMPORARY CHALLENGES

The recent, strenuous attempts to beautify Delhi so as to make it a world-class city have been marked by two contradictory trends. Political and electoral compulsions have led to efforts to regularise, while judicial activism has come down heavily on illegal commercial and trading activities, leading to the sealing of such trades, and occasionally ending in violence.[7] There has been a spate of slum demolitions and relocations in the last ten years.[8] A ten-fold increase in the demolition of slum clusters by the MCD and DDA was estimated for the five years leading up to 2000.[9] During 1990–2003, 51,461 dwelling units were demolished under "slum clearance" schemes, and another 45,000 were demolished between 2004 and 2007.[10] A decline (–21.29 per cent) in the notified slum population as a proportion of the urban population in Delhi is a marker of the exclusionary nature of urbanisation.[11] Based on calorie consumption, urban poverty in Delhi increased from 35 per cent to 57 per cent from 1993–94 to 2004–05. This may be explained at least in part by the deterioration in urban employment rates and the increasing privatisation of the supply of utilities, transport and healthcare, along with the reduction of subsidies in these sectors, leading to the substantial increase of non-food costs.[12]

The Khanna Committee in 2006 argued that the DDA master plans had failed to deliver and that the MCD had failed to regulate; it was only natural that violations had crept in that needed to be regularised. It estimated that about half of Delhi's population was residing in unauthorised settlements or slums. The recommendations have been critiqued for blatantly favouring the violators by regularising illegal commercial activity and businesses, rather than outlining any tangible efforts for the urban poor.[13] The actual regularisation process of the 1,600-odd unauthorised colonies continues to be fraught with problems, as there is difficulty in agreeing on regularisation and development charges.[14] The Master Plan of Delhi 2021 continues to bolster commercial activities by lowering the bar, neither paying adequate attention to basics such as providing for sewage treatment plants and effective garbage wastage disposal, nor making any assessment of community needs.[15] There was little hope of augmenting water supply save by drilling 75 more tubewells in the Yamuna bed.

In an effort to avoid "top-heavy urbanisation", India has formulated regional plans for major metropolises in order to divert migrants to peripheral townships.[16] The National Capital Region (NCR) seeks to achieve that end for Delhi. Infrastructural projects, particularly transport connectivity, are gradually being geared towards this objective.

The Bhagidari scheme of the Government of Delhi has been hailed as an innovative form of convergence across agencies as well as for fostering a decentralisation process. In an interview, the Delhi chief minister (credited with the scheme) outlined it as

> a faster method of taking decisions and implementation . . . a process of delivery of solutions arrived at through dialogue between the citizens, resident welfare associations [RWAs], non-government organisations, traders associations, civic agencies such as the New Delhi Municipal Council, the Municipal Corporation of Delhi and public utility services.[17]

Residents' Welfare Associations (RWA) thus emerged as the new avatar of decentralisation, albeit with weak institutional accountability and the tendency to disproportionately benefit the large middle and upper middle class where these associations were institutionalised.[18] Residents' welfare associations have acquired a legitimacy of their own, taking up issues that concern localities rather than individuals. The model has been replicated in overwhelmingly middle-class cities such as Bengaluru.[19] The colonies of the urban poor, however, form a study in contrast. Such institutional niceties as RWAs have not yet reached these communities; instead, coping mechanisms include the private buying of public goods (such as water), private expenditure on public infrastructure (for example, the construction of drains), relying on and/or sharing resources with neighbours (generally on the basis of caste/regional affinities) and taking recourse to gendered labour.[20] There are instances where the RWAs have used the "nuisance law" in petitioning for the removal and eviction of slum dwellers, and the courts have responded by taking blatantly anti-slum positions invoking "cleanliness" as an "environmental good", giving rise to a new "nuisance discourse".[21]

In the last decade, there has been a penchant for making things "world-class". [22] The Jawaharlal Nehru National Urban Renewal Mission (JNNURM) also strives to make Indian cities world-class. These cities are expected to act as engines of growth, catering to the needs of a fast-urbanising India as well as addressing the Millennium Development Goals (MDGs). The mission does have some provisions for the urban poor—for instance, internal earmarking within local bodies' budgets for basic services to the urban poor and the provision of these services, including security of tenure, at affordable prices to these poor.[23] There is also an increasing realisation of the need to make growth inclusive. Are the models being adopted in JNNURM exclusionary vis-à-vis the urban poor? Funding for the mission is subject to elaborate reforms conditionalities. Land tenure is closely linked to the Urban Land Ceiling and Regulation Act, which the JNNURM seeks to repeal; this act has been construed as having a limiting effect on the provision of basic services to the urban poor. There is also an apprehension that City Development Plans are not adequately inclusive of grassroots representation (i.e., they are not a bottom–up model), and therefore will not address the felt needs of the marginalised.[24] With the increasing contractualisation and informalisation of labour, stresses on and insecurities among the working class are on the rise. The crisis is not one of lack of infrastructure, but of lack of local self-governance and the increasingly accepted notion (across sectors) that "the Centre knows best!"[25]

The water crisis is very real, and has an impact across classes. Those who are better off manage to cope, largely by accessing groundwater and partly by augmenting storage space (which in turn pushes up the demand). As demands have soared, piped supply has not been able to keep pace. This is attributable to a large extent to the lack of scope for augmenting the supply from the Ganga and Yamuna rivers to any great extent. The effective management of the Delhi Jal Board has been no less a challenge. The body was transformed from an undertaking under the MCD to a department of the Government of Delhi at a time (in the 1990s) when autonomy and decentralisation were the reigning flavours. This is attributable to the turf war between the MCD and the state government. Subsequently, the Delhi government made efforts to outsource the management to private companies. On the face of it, this strange arrangement defies any logic. It has been estimated that operational costs would escalate and tariffs would need to be raised by up to six times, thus excluding those who need the services the most.[26] A study published at this time found that even the poor were willing to pay (for augmenting public hydrant supplies) if services were assured; however, this form of private sector participation was not committed to providing such assurance.[27] It was emphasised that the type of ownership had no bearing on efficiency and that, in the context of Delhi, the role of the state was crucial in providing for the infrastructurally disadvantaged. As groundwater declines at an alarming pace, those without piped supplies will find it more expensive to access water.[28] Delhi is not new to the water crisis. Earlier innovations such as *baolis* (wells) have served their time, and new solutions, such as rainwater harvesting, will have to be deployed to keep up with the astronomical demands that are depleting an estimated 250 times more than what is replenished per year.[29]

There was a lull in the action on sanitation following the International Water Supply and Sanitation Decade. The MDGs have brought the focus back on to sanitation. The Central Rural Sanitation Programme, now transformed into the Total Sanitation Campaign, has been taken up with some seriousness within the National Rural Health Mission.

The JNNURM committed to 100 per cent sanitation coverage in urban areas. The National Urban Sanitation Policy (NUSP) was announced in October 2008. According to this document, 51 per cent of non-notified slums are without latrines, and so are 17 per cent of notified slums.[30] Thirty-seven per cent of the total human excreta produced is unsafely disposed of. Importantly, the discharge of untreated domestic/municipal wastewater was estimated to have resulted in the contamination of 75 per cent of all surface water across the country. The NUSP reiterated the MDG target of improving sanitation for at least half the urban population by 2015, and providing 100 per cent access by 2025.[31] In May 2010, the NUSP published a ranking of Indian cities by sanitation, based on both primary data collection through field visits and secondary data such as the census.[32] Chandigarh received a maximum score of 73.480. Only four cities/local bodies featured in the "blue" category, the fourth position (with a score of 68.265) going to New Delhi Municipal Committee. Delhi Cantonment, ranked fifth, received a score of 61.367. Urban MCD ranked 168 (among the 423 bodies surveyed) with a score of 36.963. The NUSP, like the JNNURM, has prepared an elaborate gridiron for funding and implementation of sanitation "projects". It bears remembering, however, that "experience has shown that sanitation programmes are successful when they have technologies that are simple and environment-friendly enough to let the community maintain them (a sense of ownership is important), and are interwoven with other health, education and income-generation facilities".[33]

An estimated 6.2 per cent of the urban population in India fell below the poverty line on account of out-patient and in-patient expenditure.[34] While the recently launched Rashtriya Swasth Bima Yojana (RSBY) was meant to take care of catastrophic expenditure and prevent outcomes such as these, Berman et al. comment that RSBY was strong on assumption but weak on evidence.[35]

LEARNINGS FROM THIS STUDY

The present study has taken a holistic epidemiological approach, locating biological, environmental and behavioural factors within a structural framework to understand and analyse the time trends of cholera and its determinants in Delhi. The social determinants framework has been deployed to arrive at a nuanced understanding of the disease in an urban context. Historical methods have proved to be of great relevance in understanding the issues relating to population vulnerability, which act as determinants of waterborne diseases in general and of cholera in particular. Cholera has been viewed as a complex phenomenon that represents the interface between the biomedical, environmental, social and political domains. This study has explored the broad epidemiological trends beginning from the colonial period, moving on to the early post-independence phase and then to the contemporary period, conducting a population analysis for cholera prevalence and its determinants in each period. For the period from 1994 onwards, zonal and household-level analyses have been conducted to construct a holistic picture.

The analysis of time trends brings out some very important features. Beginning with the first pandemic of cholera in 1818, Delhi was affected several times till the sixth pandemic, which ended in the 1920s. Infection generally reached Delhi either from Punjab or from the United Provinces. Unlike in several adjacent states, cholera did not become endemic in Delhi. The experience in Delhi was thus one of periodic outbreaks with years of quiescence in between. In the context of the seventh (current) pandemic that began in 1964, Delhi reported its first El Tor cases in 1965. Since then, along with few other states, Delhi has emerged among the frontrunners in terms of the endemicity of cholera. In the post-independence period (1965–2000), there has been a rising trend in the incidence of cholera (and gastroenteritis), accompanied by a steady decline in deaths; zero mortality was attained during the 1990s.

Another feature that emerges is the seasonality of cholera. During the earlier pandemics, the peak incidence of cholera in northern India was reported during the two monsoon months of July and August. The analysis of the contemporary period establishes that three clear seasonal trends have emerged in Delhi:

- A rising trend during summer
- A steady state during the monsoon
- Since 1994, a rising trend during winter, coinciding with the introduction of the O139 strain

Nineteenth-century scholars observed that cholera did not occur during the summers and winters in northern India. The linkage between rain and cholera in Bengal and the onward transmission of the disease affected Punjab and Delhi. In the transformation from an epidemic to an endemic disease, cholera in Delhi has undergone significant changes in seasonality; it now occurs in the winter months as well.

The broad time trends of cholera in India generally correspond with the global trends till the 1920s. Within these broad trends, the history of the epidemiology of cholera in India may be seen to be a history of epidemics, generally attributed to events such as religious fairs and famines. The British administration during the second half of the nineteenth century concentrated on containing cholera among the troops. In fact, the sanitary commissioners focused on wider public health measures only when it was realised that the sanitary and medical security of the military could not end at the gates of the cantonments, and that such measures needed to be extended into adjacent urban and rural areas. The implementation of such sanitary measures, including water supply and sewage services, resulted in a sharp decline in cholera mortality in Presidency towns such as Calcutta, Bombay and Madras. However, slum dwellers in these towns hardly benefited from such measures. Small towns and villages were not covered by such services, and continued to remain vulnerable to cholera. It was only in the first half of the twentieth century that provision of piped water supplies began to reach the small towns. The benefits were evident, particularly in Bengal and the United Provinces. Significantly, the hallmark of the epidemiological trend during the first half of the twentieth century was the story of declining deaths.

The cholera pandemics that had their origins in the Indian subcontinent and their widespread dissemination became a symbol of fear in the west. Religious pilgrimages were identified as a critical determinant of the origin of epidemics in India. Mass bathing at the Kumbh and Ardh Kumbhmelas at Hardwar and Allahabad, the ritual sipping of water and the pilgrims' practice of bringing back Ganga water were hypothesised as being responsible for propagating the infection. Though epidemic increases in the number of cases have been sought to be correlated with these melas in the literature, careful scrutiny of available data reveals that all fairs did not inevitably result in epidemics. Some of the increases can be attributed to the import of infection from Bengal. There were exceptional years when fairs were held but the incidence of cholera remained low. Colonial health administrators held the poor pilgrims on par with slum dwellers of the industrial towns of Europe in so far as the reservoir and transmission of diseases were concerned. Till the beginning of the twentieth century, cholera was considered inevitable in fairs and pilgrimages, and the role of the state was not given due consideration. With the institution of sanitary measures at the fairs, cholera declined. Simultaneously, with the independence movement acquiring steam, the colonial administration refrained from associating the fairs with the epidemics for political reasons.

There have been epidemic years in Punjab that do not correlate with fairs. These can be correlated with famine years, in line with Zurbrigg's correlation of famines and deaths due to malaria. Famines and cholera have been closely associated in several epidemics in other parts of India, notably Madras Presidency in 1887 and Bengal in 1942. The absence of major famines has been considered one of the crucial causes of the reduction in cholera in the early decades of the twentieth century. Cholera disappeared from Europe after 1925, but continued to occur regularly in several Asian countries. In India, a declining trend was achieved during the 1950s with dramatic decreases in mortality.

With the arrival of the El Tor strain, a new pattern began emerging in the country. In the early phase of this seventh pandemic, cholera outbreaks began to be reported among slum dwellers and the poorer populations of industrial towns. Lack of basic amenities was incriminated as the principal cause in a series of investigations. Delhi along with several other states became new endemic foci and urban centres began to emerge as the new hotspots. India and Bangladesh were affected in a major way on account of the introduction of a new strain, *Vibrio cholerae* O139, and an eighth pandemic was forecasted. It was hypothesised that O139 would replace El Tor in the same manner that El Tor had replaced the classical biotype. This did not happen, and the threat of O139 gradually abated.

Following the first El Tor cases in Delhi in 1965, though there was a general rising trend for the next two decades, there were no epidemics. The first Master Plan of Delhi (MPD-I) aimed at the planned development of Delhi, and the Delhi Development Authority was visualised as the engine of change. The MPD-I was a land management plan that adopted different strategies for particular areas, aiming to channelise the growth of Delhi. It projected a population of five million by 1981, and set urbanisable limits for 1981. The MPD-I was reviewed in 1972–73 and found to be non-responsive to real needs. The 1981 census reported a population of 6.2 million. The housing deficit was put at 380,000, up from 150,000 in 1961. Slum population was estimated at one million. Extensive unauthorised construction had taken place and commercial activities had infiltrated residential areas. The ridge and the green belt were also compromised and environmental pollution had increased. There was a preoccupation with higher-income residential areas and with the beautification of Delhi, while low-cost housing was neglected.

Great emphasis was placed on slum clearance and the relocation of these population groups. The DDA set up 27 resettlement colonies for relocating slum populations from different parts of the city during the Emergency in 1975–77. These resettlement colonies were among the most-affected settlements in the 1988 epidemic, which was a landmark in the contemporary phase of the history of cholera in Delhi. The immediate cause of the epidemic is generally considered to be a breakdown in service provision during the transitional phase as these colonies were being handed over from the DDA to the Municipal Corporation of Delhi. However, there were several intrinsic deficiencies in the resettlement colonies that not only rendered them vulnerable to the epidemic, but have meant that they remain endemic areas for cholera till date. These colonies are generally located at the periphery of the city on low-lying wastelands, often along drains and ditches, in areas unsuitable for human habitation. In contravention of the caution cited in the master plan, many colonies were set up in the trans-Yamuna area without developing adequate drainage systems. Over the years, the size of the plots was lowered from the initial recommendation of 89 square yards to 12.5 square yards. The colonies lacked reliable and adequate piped water supply. The minimum standard of public latrines was fixed at one seat for 20–50 persons, but in actual practice this often worked out to one seat per 150 persons. Disposal of solid and liquid wastes in these colonies was grossly inadequate, and led in turn to the contamination of groundwater. The parallel with earlier historical evidence of cholera being prevalent among poor and infrastructure-deficient groups is obvious.

Following the epidemic, a series of public health and engineering measures were undertaken. At about the same time, the second Master Plan of Delhi (MPD-II) was adopted in consonance with the Regional Plan 2001 that envisaged developing the National Capital Region. Both plans targeted regulation of the growth of commercial activities and population in Delhi by diverting the growth to priority towns within the NCR. The decade of the 1990s was marked by large-scale in-migration, the further growth of industries, the proliferation of slums and unauthorised colonies, shortage of water and electricity and pollution of air and water. The review of MPD-II pointed out the lack of a housing policy and the resultant shortage in housing, leading to the growth of slums and unauthorised colonies. Between 1957 (when the DDA was formed) and 2000, Delhi's population increased from three million to about 14 million. The 11 million increase consisted of about 5.5 million people in the higher income groups, plus economically weaker sections, and another 5.5 million people in the poverty group. During this period, the DDA had provided for one million dwelling units, and the private sector (both formal and informal) provided for another one million units. The shortfall in housing thus stood at 342,000 units by 2002. The review went on to espouse the cause of the private sector; but little reform has taken place. The relocation of slum clusters again received a boost during the second half of the 1990s, but again the process of relocation and resettlement was not improved by any stretch of the imagination.

Inadequacies of safe water supply in vulnerable colonies, the potential contamination of sources and the community's reliance on alternative sources of water, most of which was contaminated groundwater, have emerged as critical issues. The state of the chlorinators of the DJB forces one to conclude that, to a significant extent, cholera in the colonies supplied by DJB tubewells (to which these chlorinators are attached) is man-made. This being evidently a managerial failure, there is scope for correction and consequent reduction in the disease burden of cholera. While piped water supplies of the DJB are generally safe, illegal tappings and poor maintenance of service pipes often lead to focal contamination. Attempts to enhance household-level supply through individual initiatives, such as use of on-line booster pumps, further aggravate the risks of contamination.

It is interesting that the DJB has arbitrary standards for calculating the requirement of different types of colonies—270 lpcd for planned colonies, 153 lpcd for regularised colonies and 50 lpcd for unauthorised colonies and other areas. This constitutes a gross violation and undermining of WHO norms right at the planning stage, with further inadequacies and inequities when it comes to actual distribution. According to estimates made by the DJB, 90 per cent of the population is currently covered by piped water supply. The crucial question is, what proportion of the demand of this 90 per cent population is met by piped sources of water? The Delhi Urban Environment and Infrastructure Improvement Project report observed that 10 per cent of the population has no piped water supply and 30 per cent has grossly inadequate access. In essence, poverty, coupled with poor infrastructure conditions in settlements, has implied that at least half the population of Delhi does not have access to more than 25 lpcd, and some have even less. Per capita consumption of water in Delhi ranged from 313 lpcd in affluent households to 140 lpcd in relatively less well-off households, and a meagre 16 lpcd in slum households. The Delhi Cantonment Board and New Delhi Municipal Committee emerge as the most privileged areas with per capita supplies of 509 and 462 lpcd, respectively; at the other end of the spectrum, Mehrauli Zone of the DJB has a per capita supply of 29 lpcd only.

Open defecation and/or improperly constructed sanitary latrines in JJ clusters and unauthorised colonies, coupled with an acute dependence on untreated groundwater, have been crucial to the emergence of these settlements as highly endemic areas of cholera. The strong association established between sanitary landfill sites and the high incidence of cholera in the localities that surround them has ominous implications that must be taken into account in future planning processes. Further, about half of the urban population is being served by the sewer system. Most of the trunk sewers are heavily silted and non-functional at places due to poor maintenance. Sewage therefore cannot reach the treatment plants.

The availability of civic services has been worse than inadequate for the less privileged. There was inadequate provision of housing, water and sewerage facilities for large numbers of people who were attracted by the growth of opportunities in the expanding economy of Delhi, particularly in the post-liberalisation phase. The growth of the formal sector in Delhi, accompanied by an expanding informal sector, has implied tremendous in-migration. The majority of migrants belong to the lower socio-economic category, and cannot afford housing in planned settlements. It is precisely these population groups that are rendered vulnerable to cholera.

It is in the light of these factors that the trends and issues of vulnerability should be examined. For the period 1994–2000 for which detailed disaggregated data was available, it was possible to conduct an extensive analysis of the causal complexity of cholera. Even within this short time interval, distinct upward or downward trends in the incidence of cholera have been demonstrated among the 12 municipal zones of Delhi. Analysis of the spatial distribution of notified cholera cases leads to the identification of endemic areas/localities within each of these zones. These are localities that have consistently reported cholera cases and contributed significantly to the case load of the respective zones.

The determinants of diarrhoeal diseases are complex and intertwined. Analysis of distinct zonal trends provides pointers towards the identification of key factors for vulnerability to cholera, including:

- Settlement types
- Economic patterns and occupational activities
- Provision of civic services
- Population density and predominant activities
- Characteristics of the residents
- The state of the infrastructure in the field

Civil Lines and Rohini Zones have relatively lower population densities, higher per capita availability of water (274 lpcd), higher coverage of sewers (60–80 per cent), and yet report high incidence rates of cholera. Wide disparities in access to services exist among settlements inhabited by different socio-economic classes. Therein lies the explanation of why 87 per cent and 80 per cent of the cholera cases from Civil Lines and Rohini Zones, respectively, are being reported from the vulnerable colonies of these zones, which comprise largely population groups of low socio-economic status. Across the Yamuna, Shahdara (North) Zone and Shahdara (South) Zone demonstrate a strong declining trend in the incidence of cholera. This decline is largely attributable to the commissioning of the Bhagirathi water treatment plant. Per capita water availability is 130 lpcd, but lesser disparities within these zones imply that even the poorer sections actually receive far larger quantities of water than in some other zones with higher average availability. However, sewerage services will need to be augmented to fully reap the benefits of added availability of water.

The two zones that have demonstrated a definite rising trend in incidence rates are the South and Central Zones. In the post-liberalisation period, there has been unprecedented growth of tertiary and services sector activities in these zones. Vulnerable areas in these zones include urbanised villages and unauthorised colonies. The residents of these vulnerable colonies belong to lower-middle socio-economic groups, many of them being tenants. Large disparities exist in the availability of water, with these vulnerable colonies getting about one-tenth the supply of the rest of the zone. Acute water scarcity and high levels of contamination because of a combination of factors operating at both the colony and household levels have contributed to the rising trend.

Household-level studies confirmed that low-income households in unplanned settlements were the worst-affected group. Though the majority had access to piped water supply, mostly at public hydrants, reliance on a second source to meet gaps in water demand was significant. Most importantly, the additional source was almost invariably water from shallow handpumps, which has conclusively proved unfit for human consumption. Delhi Jal Board tankers have, in recent years, been deployed in large numbers in some of the vulnerable colonies; the benefits of this in terms of decline in the incidence of cholera have been evident. This is not, however, a cost-effective and sustainable solution. Increasing income has been found to be correlated with access to or ownership of an additional water source, sewerage services and water storage. In the aggregate, a large proportion of households store water, although there is no significant difference in the decision to store water between households that have continuous supply and those with intermittent water supply.

It has been recognised that the transmission routes of the etiological pathogens of diarrhoea are complex. The debate on evaluating multiple routes of transmission versus assessing the impact of an individual determinant continues. Differences of opinion exist on whether the critical determinants are engineering/infrastructural or socio-economic/ behavioural in nature. The literature on diarrhoeal diseases has placed considerable emphasis on secondary routes of transmission. The contamination of stored water has been incriminated as a major risk factor for diarrhoeal diseases across countries. Though it is recognised that all these factors are highly intertwined, intervention strategies have often focused on behavioural issues rather than tackling the larger, capital-intensive infrastructural problems.

In the light of this debate, the household-level component of the present study aimed at exploring the relative strengths of neighbourhood and behavioural factors for households located in a given socio-economic setting towards explaining the incidence of diarrhoeal diseases. One hundred households each were surveyed in three clusters in Shahdara (North) and Shahdara (South) Zones, two of which were JJ clusters and one a resettlement colony. The infrastructure conditions in the three clusters studied conformed to similarly placed settlements in vulnerable colonies elsewhere. In effect, households had little choice with regard to safe water sources and toilet facilities in these clusters, since the provision of these is determined by the legal status of the settlement. Thus, the water and toilet facilities being accessed by households are invariant to socio-economic factors such as income and educational levels. With increasing income, households do invest in additional water sources; however, owing to a lack of options for investing in a safe source, they invariably acquire a handpump, or a tubewell (in better-off households), which are sources of contamination. The practice of storage is higher in higher-income households, and the incidence of diarrhoea is higher among households that store water. Despite the availability of a laboratory-proven safe source of piped water supply and theoretically correct storage practices, diarrhoea incidence rates were found to be high in some clusters. Higher incidence rates among school-going children in these clusters indicate that exposure is higher outside the home. The analysis leads to the conclusion that household-level behavioural factors such as storage practices cannot be analysed in isolation as determinants of diarrhoeal illness, when pitted against stronger neighbourhood and external determinants that are beyond the control of the individual household.

This study assumes importance and relevance in the context of the third Master Plan of Delhi (MPD-III), whose guidelines were published recently. Intense debates are on as to the possible impact of MPD-III on the already stretched infrastructural services. Stress is being laid on providing efficient infrastructure and adequate growth opportunities in the towns of the NCR as a way of decongesting Delhi. The new proposed floor area ratios are going to add to the increasing population density. The proposed regularisation of industries in residential areas is bound to have adverse environmental health impacts.

Contemporary epidemiological literature underscores the idea that location matters. Currently, more people in the world reside in urban than in rural areas. About a billion people reside in slums and informal settlements. Megacities, once the pride of developed nations, are increasingly emerging as a challenge for developing countries. Urban-centric growth models and competitive entrepreneurism among cities have become the norm. This has implications for the out-migration of rural populations and increase in urban poor communities living and working in highly vulnerable conditions. Contemporary urban health considerations focus around issues of trauma, substance abuse and climate change, marking an epidemiological shift. Ushering in a "new urban health", the WHO Commission on Social Determinants of Health glosses over the issue of communicable diseases, focusing instead on post-transition conditions. The proposed National Urban Health Mission (NUHM) in India, along the lines of the flagship National Rural Health Mission (NRHM), now stands postponed to the 12th Five-Year Plan. There are indications that the NUHM is increasingly preoccupied with conditions such as diabetes and cancer. The unfinished agenda of water and sanitation, and therefore of acute diarrhoeal diseases including cholera, is a forgotten urban health issue. Increasing informalisation and casualisation of urban workforces and weakening of public health systems are leading to greater vulnerability of the urban poor. The new mantra of urban renewal needs to look beyond high-visibility projects and address the basics as well.

NOTES

1. WHO CSDH (Commission on Social Determinants of Health), *Closing the Gap in a Generation: Health Equity through Action on Social Determinants of Health,* Final Report of the CSDH (Geneva: WHO, 2008), 26.
2. WHO CSDH, *Closing the Gap in a Generation*, 1.

3. Sanjoy Bhattacharya, "World Health Organization and the Social Determinants of Health", in *Social Determinants of Health: Assessing Theory, Policy and Practice*, ed. Sanjoy Bhattacharya (New Delhi: Orient BlackSwan, 2010), 3, 7.
4. WHO CSDH, *Closing the Gap in a Generation*, 60.
5. Darshini Mahadevia, "NURM and the Poor in Globalising Mega Cities", *Economic and Political Weekly* 41, no. 31, 2006, 3399–403.
6. WHO CSDH, *Closing the Gap in a Generation*, 63.
7. *EPW, "Delhi: Regulating a City", Economic and Political Weekly* 46, no. 39, 2006, 4097.
8. Veronique Dupont, "Slum Demolitions in Delhi since the 1990s: An Appraisal", *Economic and Political Weekly* 43, no. 28, 2008, 79–87.
9. Asher D. Ghertner, "Analysis of New Legal Discourse behind Delhi's Slum Demolitions", *Economic and Political Weekly* 43, no. 20, 2008, 57–66.
10. Gautam Bhan, "This Is No Longer the City I Once Knew: Evictions, the Urban Poor and the Right to the City in Millennial Delhi", *Environment and Urbanization* 21, no. 1, 2009, 127–42.
11. Prem Kumar, "Declining Number of Slums: Nature of Urban Growth", *Economic and Political Weekly* 45, no. 41, 2008, 75–77.
12. Utsa Patnaik, "Trends in Urban Poverty under Economic Reforms: 1993–94 to 2004–05", *Economic and Political Weekly* 45, no. 4, 2010, 42–53.
13. Ashok Kumar, "Condoning Unplanned Development: Reviewing the Khanna Committee Report", *Economic and Political Weekly* 41, no. 39, 2006,4105–8.
14. *Indian Express*, "Panel Set Up to Decide Development Charges", 18 January 2011, http://www.indianexpress.com/news/panel-set-up-to-decide-development-charges/738856/ (accessed 18 January 2011).
15. *EPW*, "Delhi Master Plan: Good on Paper", Editorial, *Economic and Political Weekly* 42, no. 11, 2007, 900–901.
16. Amitabh Kundu, "Exclusionary Urbanisation in Asia: A Macro Overview", *Economic and Political Weekly* 44, no. 48, 2009, 48–58.
17. *Frontline*, "Privatisation Not Just for the Sake of It", *Frontline* 19, no. 10, 2002.http://www.hinduonnet.com/fline/fl1910/19100920.htm (accessed 22 December 2009).
18. Marie-Helene Zerah, "Middle Class Neighbourhood Associations as Political Players in Mumbai", *Economic and Political Weekly* 42, no. 47, 2007, 61–68.
19. J. O. Beal, "From Social Networks to Public Action in Urban Governance: Where Does Benefit Accrue?" *Journal of International Development* 13, no. 7, 2001, 1015–21.
20. Madhvi Gupta and Pushkar, "Ethnic Diversity and the Demand for Public

Goods: Interpreting the Evidence from Delhi", *Economic and Political Weekly* 45, no. 43, 2010, 64–72.

21. Ghertner, "Analysis of New Legal Discourse"; Awadhendra Saran, "In the City, Out of Place: Environment and Modernity, Delhi 1860s to 1960s", *Economic and Political Weekly* 47, no. 25, 2006, 4905–11.
22. R. Priya et al., "Operationalising the CMP", *Economic and Political Weekly* 39, no. 27, 2004, 2971–74.
23. Mahadevia, "NURM and the Poor in Globalising Mega Cities".
24. Ministry of Urban Development, "Whither Indian Cities: Urban Reforms", Report of the National Consultation on Jawaharlal Nehru Urban Renewal Mission, Government of India. http://www.hazardscentre.in/hazards_publications/urban_governance_resistance.html (accessed 11 September 2008).
25. Partha Mukhopadhyay, "Whither Urban Renewal?" *Economic and Political Weekly* 41, no. 10, 2006, 879–84.
26. Amit Bhaduri and Arvind Kejriwal, "Reforming the Reformers", *Economic and Political Weekly* 40, no. 53, 2005, 5543–45.
27. P. Dasgupta and R. Dasgupta, "Economic Value of Safe Water for the Infrastructurally Disadvantaged Urban Household: A Case Study in Delhi in India", *Water Resources Research* 40, 2004, W11401.
28. P. S. Vijay Shankar, Himanshu Kulkarni and Sunderrajan Krishnan, "India's Groundwater Challenge and the Way Forward", *Economic and Political Weekly* 66, no. 2, 2011, 37–45.
29. "The Groundwater UP Project", http://www.groundwaterup.com/?page_id=112 (accessed 14 January 2011).
30. Ministry of Urban Development, *National Urban Sanitation Policy, 2008* (New Delhi: Government of India, 2008), http://www.indiaurbanportal.in (accessed 28 July 2009).
31. Ministry of Urban Development, *National Urban Sanitation Policy.*
32. Ministry of Urban Development, "Rank of Cities on Sanitation, 2009–2010: National Urban Sanitation Policy". Government of India, New Delhi, http://pib.nic.in/archieve/others/2010/may/d2010051103.pdf (accessed 17 October 2010).
33. *EPW*, "The Sanitation Challenge", Editorial, *Economic and Political Weekly* 44, no. 4, 2009, 6.
34. Peter Berman, Rajeev Ahuja and Laveesh Bhandari, "The Impoverishing Effect of Healthcare Payments in India: New Methodology and Findings", *Economic and Political Weekly* 45, no. 16, 2010, 65–71.
35. Berman et al., "The Impoverishing Effect of Healthcare Payments".

Appendix

METHODOLOGY

Diarrhoea is defined as the passage of loose, liquid or watery stools. These liquid stools are passed more than three times a day. It should be emphasised that recent changes in the consistency and character of stools are more important than the number of stools. When blood is visible in watery stools, the condition is defined as dysentery. The term gastroenteritis is often loosely used to describe acute diarrhoea. This is not strictly accurate, as the term gives no indication of the causative agent. Only laboratory examination can confirm the microbiological aetiology, and this is not a routine procedure in the clinical management of diarrhoea in the majority of medical institutions of Delhi. It is not cost-effective to routinely undertake microbiological testing of stool samples in each case of diarrhoea.

The division between acute and chronic diarrhoea is arbitrary. Acute diarrhoea is defined as an attack of sudden onset, which usually lasts from three to seven days but may last up to 10–14 days. Diarrhoea lasting for three weeks or more is labelled as chronic.

Incidence rate is defined as the number of new cases occurring in a defined population during a specific period of time. It is calculated by the following formula:

$$\frac{\text{Number of new cases of a specific disease during a given period}}{\text{Population at risk during that period}} \times 1000$$

Incidence rates have been calculated for a recall period of two weeks for the general population and for children under 5 years of age. The associations between household-level vulnerability factors and the incidence of diarrhoea are examined through assessing the distribution of incidence over different types of households.

For the cross-sectional study, water samples were tested from the main sources accessed and from storage containers in the household. Bacteriological tests for water quality surveillance included the following tests:

- Presumptive coliform test (most commonly performed)
- Tests for the detection of faecal streptococci and *Clostridium perfringens*
- Colony count

The presumptive coliform test is the most relevant one for purposes of the present study and is described here in detail. This test is based on the most probable number (MPN) of coliform organisms in 100 ml of water. The test is carried out by inoculating measured quantities of the sample water—0.1, 1.0, 10 and 50 ml—into tubes of McConkey's Lactose Bile Salt Broth with Bromcresol Purple as indicator. The tubes are incubated for 48 hours. From the number of tubes showing acid and gas, an estimate of the MPN of coliform organisms in 100 ml of the sample can be obtained from standard tables. This result is known as the "presumptive coliform count"; the presumption being that each tube showing fermentation contains coliform organisms. The reaction may, however, occasionally be due to the presence of some other organisms or combination of organisms.

Based on the guidelines for drinking water quality recommended by the WHO in 1996, the International Organization for Standardization (ISO) (IS 10500) prescribes that the coliform count of a drinking water sample should be less than or equal to 10 per 100 ml of water. The WHO recommendation for drinking water quality lays down the primary standards as prescribed limits that must never be exceeded in water meant for drinking purposes.

The "coliform organisms" include all aerobic and facultative anaerobic gram-negative, non-sporing, motile and non-motile rods capable of fermenting lactose at 35°C–37°C in less than 48 hours. The coliform group includes both faecal and non-faecal organisms. The classic example of the faecal group is *E. coli*, and that of the non-faecal group is *Klebsiella aerogens.* As a working rule, it is assumed that all coliform organisms are of faecal origin unless non-faecal origin can be proved.

For the purposes of sampling, a total of 60 water samples were collected, i.e., samples were collected from 20 per cent of the 300 households that were surveyed. This ensured that epidemiologically sensitive results were obtained for deriving conclusions about exposure to contamination through the water that was being accessed by these 300 households.

The term water source is defined with reference to the means by which water is accessed. The means of access play the most important role in influencing as well as indicating the quality of water being consumed by a particular household. The word "source", therefore, is used to characterise water available at the point of access throughout the study. Points of access having similar characteristics and implications for water contamination are clubbed together and labelled as a particular source. Thus, for example, shallow handpumps are one source, as distinguished from deep-bore tubewells which are considered as another distinct source.

A two-stage sampling was conducted. In the first round, all the community sources were tested. Based on the results, stored household samples were lifted to test the extent of contamination at the domestic level. If a certain source failed the test, water samples were not tested for households storing drinking water from that source. Only households storing water from sources that had passed the initial screening test were further sampled.

Table A.1: Cholera Cases and Deaths in Delhi, 1965–2000[1]

Year	*Cases*	*Deaths*
1965	55	5
1966	164	3
1967	154	2
1968	333	15
1969	314	9
1970	63	1
1971	192	8
1972	315	16

1. All tables in the Appendix are based on data collected by the author during field work conducted in 2000–03.

Year	Cases	Deaths
1973	261	4
1974	157	3
1975	183	6
1976	162	7
1977	296	4
1978	194	4
1979	144	6
1980	574	22
1981	446	5
1982	265	3
1983	457	3
1984	306	3
1985	596	9
1986	327	1
1987	287	1
1988	1,693	8
1989	197	1
1990	538	0
1991	536	0
1992	1,070	0
1993	689	0
1994	2,226	0
1995	1,989	0
1996	906	0
1997	956	0
1998	1,903	0
1999	1,396	0
2000	959	0

Table A.2: Population Estimates in Delhi, 1965–2000

Year	Population
1965	
1966	3,468,911
1967	3,654,406
1968	3,845,706

Year	*Population*
1969	4,040,570
1970	4,240,524
1971	4,065,698
1972	4,287,498
1973	4,473,618
1974	4,667,819
1975	4,870,449
1976	5,081,876
1977	5,302,480
1978	5,532,661
1979	5,772,835
1980	6,023,434
1981	6,220,406
1982	6,582,500
1983	6,866,600
1984	7,161,600
1985	7,467,700
1986	7,785,100
1987	8,114,000
1988	8,454,700
1989	8,806,900
1990	9,170,900
1991	9,420,644
1992	9,756,500
1993	10,223,200
1994	10,587,700
1995	10,965,200
1996	11,736,000
1997	12,282,000
1998	12,856,000
1999	13,418,000
2000	13,964,000

Table A.3: Month-wise Cholera Cases in City Zone, 1994–2000

	1994	*1995*	*1996*	*1997*	*1998*	*1999*	*2000*
January	0	0	0	0	0	0	0
February	0	0	0	0	0	0	0
March	0	0	0	0	0	0	0
April	2	1	1	0	0	19	0
May	0	6	0	0	0	15	1
June	14	5	4	5	6	10	6
July	4	8	2	5	7	8	4
August	8	8	10	6	6	10	3
September	0	5	2	7	10	2	6
October	0	0	0	1	5	1	5
November	0	0	0	1	1	0	0
December	0	0	0	0	0	0	0
Total	28	33	19	25	35	65	25

Table A.4: Month-wise Cholera Cases in Sadar Pahargunj Zone, 1994–2000

	1994	*1995*	*1996*	*1997*	*1998*	*1999*	*2000*
January	0	0	0	0	0	0	0
February	0	0	0	0	0	0	0
March	0	0	0	0	0	0	0
April	1	0	0	0	0	1	3
May	6	6	1	1	3	10	0
June	18	4	1	1	7	22	12
July	19	8	8	5	7	8	0
August	17	10	8	4	9	5	3
September	9	5	4	6	7	6	2
October	1	4	5	1	0	3	7
November	0	0	0	0	1	1	6
December	0	0	0	0	0	0	0
Total	71	37	27	18	34	68	33

Table A.5: Month-wise Cholera Cases in Karol Bagh Zone, 1994–2000

	1994	*1995*	*1996*	*1997*	*1998*	*1999*	*2000*
January	0	0	0	0	0	0	0
February	0	0	0	0	0	0	0
March	0	0	0	0	0	0	0
April	0	0	0	0	0	2	1
May	5	8	3	1	1	18	1
June	7	12	3	4	10	10	2
July	10	8	3	10	11	12	4
August	4	16	6	3	1	11	0
September	3	6	7	2	8	4	6
October	1	2	0	3	3	3	2
November	0	0	1	0	0	0	3
December	0	0	0	0	0	1	0
Total	30	52	23	23	34	61	19

Table A.6: Month-wise Cholera Cases in Civil Lines Zone, 1994–2000

	1994	*1995*	*1996*	*1997*	*1998*	*1999*	*2000*
January	0	0	0	0	0	0	1
February	0	0	0	0	0	0	0
March	0	0	1	0	1	0	0
April	3	2	1	1	2	17	9
May	35	32	24	27	78	48	7
June	93	68	26	33	112	69	30
July	250	74	59	89	186	62	34
August	199	136	56	83	106	69	33
September	50	127	32	60	82	32	37
October	2	30	9	10	25	15	19
November	0	3	0	3	13	3	15
December	5	0	0	0	1	0	0
Total	637	472	208	306	606	315	185

Table A.7: Month-wise Cholera Cases in Shahdara (North) Zone, 1994–2000

	1994	*1995*	*1996*	*1997*	*1998*	*1999*	*2000*
January	0	0	0	0	0	0	0
February	0	0	0	0	0	0	0
March	0	0	0	0	0	0	0
April	0	1	0	0	1	3	1
May	3	9	3	3	2	24	9
June	29	21	16	15	18	21	9
July	130	25	24	18	35	20	7
August	104	37	19	11	30	24	17
September	15	61	19	22	37	3	5
October	0	7	0	5	7	3	7
November	0	3	0	2	1	8	1
December	0	0	0	1	0	0	0
Total	281	164	81	77	121	106	56

Table A.8: Month-wise Cholera Cases in Shahdara (South) Zone, 1994–2000

	1994	*1995*	*1996*	*1997*	*1998*	*1999*	*2000*
January	0	0	0	0	0	0	0
February	0	0	0	0	0	0	0
March	0	0	0	0	0	0	0
April	1	0	0	0	0	3	0
May	1	5	2	6	5	23	3
June	13	17	14	5	18	20	9
July	17	20	7	11	17	5	9
August	32	28	6	10	12	7	3
September	23	22	13	6	17	6	8
October	1	13	1	4	11	10	2
November	1	3	0	0	5	7	2
December	0	0	0	0	0	0	0
Total	89	108	43	42	85	81	36

Table A.9: Month-wise Cholera Cases in Central Zone, 1994–2000

	1994	*1995*	*1996*	*1997*	*1998*	*1999*	*2000*
January	2	0	0	0	0	0	0
February	0	0	0	0	0	0	0
March	0	0	1	0	1	0	0
April	4	8	17	0	4	48	16
May	16	82	46	23	12	36	64
June	18	47	24	16	19	32	26
July	12	28	30	32	36	29	7
August	17	56	19	19	31	21	8
September	9	36	10	22	17	4	8
October	7	8	4	14	19	10	28
November	0	1	0	3	5	3	22
December	0	0	0	0	2	1	2
Total	85	266	151	129	146	184	181

Table A.10: Month-wise Cholera Cases in South Zone, 1994–2000

	1994	*1995*	*1996*	*1997*	*1998*	*1999*	*2000*
January	0	0	0	0	0	0	1
February	0	0	0	0	0	0	1
March	0	0	0	0	1	1	0
April	2	7	5	1	2	30	3
May	54	39	16	9	2	44	41
June	47	22	7	8	22	12	21
July	33	13	13	7	27	12	2
August	60	39	7	13	13	17	9
September	16	10	9	11	10	8	18
October	10	4	2	6	3	4	26
November	3	1	1	1	3	3	42
December	0	0	0	0	0	6	1
Total	225	135	60	56	83	137	175

Table A.11: Month-wise Cholera Cases in West Zone, 1994–2000

	1994	*1995*	*1996*	*1997*	*1998*	*1999*	*2000*
January	0	0	0	0	0	0	0
February	0	0	0	0	0	0	0
March	0	0	0	0	0	0	0
April	0	0	0	0	0	1	0
May	0	5	0	3	0	9	1
June	2	7	4	7	3	4	2
July	3	1	2	2	13	1	2
August	10	11	0	2	10	1	3
September	5	3	9	4	6	0	3
October	0	0	0	0	2	0	0
November	0	0	1	0	0	0	1
December	0	0	0	0	0	0	0
Total	30	27	16	18	34	16	12

Table A.12: Month-wise Cholera Cases in Rohini Zone, 1994–2000

	1994	*1995*	*1996*	*1997*	*1998*	*1999*	*2000*
January	0	0	0	0	0	0	0
February	0	0	0	0	0	0	0
March	0	0	0	0	0	0	0
April	0	0	0	0	1	1	0
May	9	19	1	2	9	11	2
June	23	11	5	10	40	26	17
July	58	51	28	19	136	23	29
August	95	74	34	31	119	44	15
September	24	36	23	23	23	13	12
October	1	14	3	6	16	3	8
November	1	0	0	5	4	2	4
December	1	0	0	0	0	1	0
Total	212	205	94	96	348	124	87

Table A.13: Month-wise Cholera Cases in Najafgarh Zone, 1994–2000

	1994	*1995*	*1996*	*1997*	*1998*	*1999*	*2000*
January	0	0	0	0	0	0	0
February	0	0	0	0	0	0	0
March	0	0	0	0	0	0	0
April	0	7	0	0	0	0	0
May	18	33	7	4	5	11	4
June	68	29	6	6	19	11	10
July	36	21	16	9	20	12	5
August	74	61	17	13	11	15	11
September	29	32	7	6	7	3	10
October	0	0	2	0	6	1	2
November	0	0	1	0	0	1	1
December	0	0	0	0	1	0	0
Total	225	183	56	38	69	54	43

Table A.14: Month-wise Cholera Cases in Narela Zone, 1994–2000

	1994	*1995*	*1996*	*1997*	*1998*	*1999*	*2000*
January	0	0	0	0	0	1	0
February	0	0	0	0	0	0	0
March	0	0	0	0	0	0	0
April	0	0	0	0	0	1	0
May	0	18	1	1	4	14	12
June	24	20	4	6	13	11	1
July	38	17	15	5	22	14	5
August	39	52	10	10	30	5	5
September	7	33	9	5	13	2	3
October	0	1	1	1	1	3	1
November	1	0	0	0	2	0	0
December	0	0	0	0	0	0	0
Total	109	141	40	28	85	51	27

Table A.15: Month-wise Cholera Cases in MCD Areas, 1994–2000

	1994	*1995*	*1996*	*1997*	*1998*	*1999*	*2000*
January	2	0	0	0	0	1	2
February	0	0	0	0	0	0	1
March	0	0	2	0	3	1	0
April	13	26	24	2	10	138	33
May	147	262	104	80	121	263	145
June	366	263	114	116	267	248	145
July	610	274	207	212	517	206	108
August	659	528	192	205	378	229	110
September	190	376	144	174	227	83	118
October	23	83	27	51	98	56	127
November	6	11	4	15	35	28	97
December	6	0	0	1	4	9	3
Total	2,022	1,823	818	856	1,680	1,262	889

Table A.16: Cholera Cases in Vulnerable Areas of the Zones, 1994

1994	*J–M*	*A*	*M*	*J*	*J*	*A*	*S*	*O*	*N*	*D*	*T*
CITY ZONE											
Nizamuddin				2	2	1					5
Sarai Kale Khan											0
Yamuna Pushta JJ				2	3	4					9
	0	0	0	4	5	5	0	0	0	0	14
S. P. ZONE											
Nabi Karim–Paharganj			4	11	4	1					20
Sadar Bazar			1	3	1	5					10
	0	0	5	14	5	6	0	0	0	0	30
K. B. ZONE											
Anand Parbat–Dev Nagar			1			1	1				3
Baljeet Nagar			1		1	1					3
Inderpuri–Todapur–Loha Mandi			1		1						2
Naraina Village			2		1	2					5
Zakhira–Shadipur			1	1	4	2	1				9
	0	0	6	1	7	6	2	0	0	0	22

1994	*J–M*	*A*	*M*	*J*	*J*	*A*	*S*	*O*	*N*	*D*	*T*
C. L. ZONE											
Azadpur			3	7	20	14	5				49
Bhalswa Village & Dairy			1	2	6	7	2				18
Bharola–Sarai Peepalthala				3	6	2					11
Burari–Nathupura–Ibrahimpur–Jharoda		1	9	30	53	42	23			2	160
Camp–Dhaka–Dhirpur–Malikpur	0	0	13	12	26	15	7	0	0	2	75
Chandrawal–Malkagunj											0
Jahangirpuri			9	14	62	40	9			1	135
Lal Bagh & other JJ			2	15	28	18	3	2			68
Mukandpur				2	8	13	2				25
Rajpura–Gur Mandi				2	4	2					8
Wazirabad–Jagatpur			1	3	2	2	1				9
Wazirpur Industrial Area (JJ)				1	2	4					7
	0	1	38	91	217	159	52	2	0	5	565
SH (N) ZONE											
Bhajanpura–Dayalpur–Gamri			2	2	7	6	4				21
Brahmpuri				1	2	1					4
Johripur				3	4						7
Karawal Nagar			1		20	13	2				36
Loni Road				2	3	1					6
Mandoli–Saboli			1	4	10	5					20
Maujpur–Ghonda				1	5	3	1				10
Mustafabad–Gokulpuri				2	13	5	2				22
Nand/Sunder Nagri				8	6	6					20
New Seelampur–Jaffrabad			1	4	13	9	5				32
Seemapuri				2	7	2					11
Shastri Park–Usmanpur–Taj Colony				2	4	3					9

1994	*J-M*	*A*	*M*	*J*	*J*	*A*	*S*	*O*	*N*	*D*	*T*
Sonia Vihar/Khajuri Khas					13	17					30
	0	0	5	31	107	71	14	0	0	0	228
SH (S) ZONE											
Gandhi Nagar/ Kailash Nagar					3	3	1				7
Kondli–Gharouli–MV3				6	5	6	6				23
Old Seelampur				2		5	1		1		9
Patpargunj Village–Mandawali Village			1	1	2	3	1				8
Shakurpur–Laxmi Nagar					2	3					5
Trilokpuri–Kalyanpuri–Khichripur					2	4	5				11
Vishwas Nagar				2	2	1	2				7
	0	0	1	11	16	25	16	0	1	0	70
CENTRAL & SOUTH ZONE											
Amb Nagar–Dakshinpuri–Madangir			6	2	2	4			2		16
Badarpur–Molar Bandh–Mithapur–Jaitpur		1	1	3	10	6	1	3			25
Chattarpur					3		2				5
Chiragh Dilli			5					1			6
Garhi–Lajpat Nagar–Sri Niwaspuri			10	11	3	5	2	3			34
Govindpuri–Kalkaji	2		7		5	6	1	2			23
Harkesh Nagar–Jasola–Ali			4	2		3		1			10
Jamroodpur			3	1					1		5
Khanpur–Deoli–Tigri			4	2	4	2	3	1			16
Kilokri–Sunlight Colony–Ashram			1		1	1					3
Kotla Mubarakpur		1	1	2		3	1	1			9
Madanpur Khadar–Sarita Vihar			1	5	4	2					12

1994	*J-M*	*A*	*M*	*J*	*J*	*A*	*S*	*O*	*N*	*D*	*T*
Malviya Nagar–Savitri Nagar–Hauz Rani–Khirki		1	4			2	1				
Masjid Moth–Gautam Nagar				3	1	1		1			6
Mehrauli–Lado Sarai–Neb Sarai			2	2	13	5					22
Okhla Industrial Area–Tehkhand			4	5	6	4		1			20
Okhla Village–Jamia Nagar–Abul Fazal Enclave				3	1	1	1				6
Sangam Vihar			3	3	2	7	2				17
Shahpur Jat				6		2	1				9
Tughlakabad			4	1	2	4	2	1			14
	2	3	60	51	57	58	17	15	3	0	258
ROHINI ZONE											
Budh Vihar			1	6	4	12	3				26
Haiderpur				2	3	18	5				28
Rithala–Vijay Vihar					2	1	2				5
Rohini			2		3	6	1			1	13
Samaipur–Badli			5	5	12	17	2	1	1		43
Sawan Park				2	9	6	6				23
Shahbad Daulatpur/ Dairy				1	6	5	1				13
Shakurbasti–Rani Bagh					4	1					5
Shalimar Bagh (JJ) & Village					5	8	3				16
Siraspur					1	1					2
Wazirpur JJ–Nimri Village–Wazirpur Village				2	2	6	3				13
	0	0	8	18	51	81	26	1	1	1	137
NAJAFGARH ZONE											
Mahipalpur–Nangal–Rangpuri				2	1	3	2				8
Mangolpuri–Sultanpuri			5	18	15	26	10				74

1994	*J–M*	*A*	*M*	*J*	*J*	*A*	*S*	*O*	*N*	*D*	*T*
Nangloi			2	10	6	18	6				42
Palam–Dabri			2	5	3	6					16
Pappan Kalan/Dwarka			3	3							6
	0	0	12	38	25	53	18	0	0	0	146
NARELA ZONE											
Alipur			1	1	4	3	1				10
Bakhtawarpur–Palla			1		2	3	2				8
Bawana					4	2					6
Brick Kilns				3		1					4
Holambi					1						1
Lampur					8						8
Narela				1	10	7	1		1		20
Prem Nagar–Kirari				22	5	3					30
	0	0	2	27	34	19	4	0	1	0	87

Table A.17: Cholera Cases in Vulnerable Areas of the Zones, 1995

1995	*J–M*	*A*	*M*	*J*	*J*	*A*	*S*	*O*	*N*	*D*	*T*
CITY ZONE											
Nizamuddin			2		1						3
Sarai Kale Khan			1			1	1				3
Yamuna Pushta JJ			1	1	5	3	1				11
	0	0	4	1	6	4	2	0	0	0	17
S. P. ZONE											
Nabi Karim–Pahargunj				1	1	3		2	1		8
Sadar Bazar					2	1	2				5
	0	0	0	1	3	4	2	2	1	0	13
K. B. ZONE											
Anand Parbat–Dev Nagar						1	2				3
Baljeet Nagar				1	2						3
Inderpuri–Todapur–Loha Mandi			1			2		1			4
Naraina Village											0
Zakhira–Shadipur			1	9	2	8	1				21
	0	0	2	10	4	11	3	1	0	0	31

1995	*J-M*	*A*	*M*	*J*	*J*	*A*	*S*	*O*	*N*	*D*	*T*
C. L. ZONE											
Azadpur			1	6	8	14	16	1			46
Bhalswa Village & Dairy				1		6		1			8
Bharola–Sarai Peepalthala				2	3	3	4				12
Burari–Nathupura–Ibrahimpur–Jharoda		0	9	12	15	41	53	2	1		133
Camp–Dhaka–Dhirpur–Malikpur			7	10	8	9	8	5			47
Chandrawal–Malkagunj			2		1		1				4
Jahangirpuri		1	7	12	10	18	14	5	2		69
Lal Bagh & other JJ		1	3	7	4	16	9				40
Mukandpur				3	2	8	6				19
Rajpura–Gur Mandi											0
Wazirabad–Jagatpur				2	1	3	2				8
Wazirpur Industrial Area (JJ)				1		2	1				4
	0	2	29	56	52	120	114	14	3		390
SH (N) ZONE											
Bhajanpura–Dayalpur–Gamri				2	1	5	4	1			13
Brahmpuri				1		2					3
Johripur			1	5	1						7
Karawal Nagar				2	3	7	9				21
Loni Road											0
Mandoli–Saboli				1			3				4
Maujpur–Ghonda		1		2	1	1	3				8
Mustafabad–Gokulpuri				3		4	12				19
Nand/Sunder Nagri				1	2	3	4				10
New Seelampur–Jaffrabad			1	2	3	4	3		1		14
Seemapuri			2	2	1	5	2	2			14
Shastri Park–Usmanpur–Taj Colony			1	1	1	1	8				12
Sonia Vihar/Khajuri Khas				1	2	3	8				14
	0	1	5	23	15	35	56	3	1		139

1995	*J–M*	*A*	*M*	*J*	*J*	*A*	*S*	*O*	*N*	*D*	*T*
SH (S) ZONE											
Gandhi Nagar/Kailash Nagar			1	1	3	1	3	4	1		14
Kondli–Gharouli–MV3				5	5	4	4	2			20
Old Seelampur			2	1	1	1			1		6
Patpargunj Village–Mandawali Village			1	2	2	1	6	3			15
Shakurpur–Laxmi Nagar					1	1	2				4
Trilokpuri–Kalyanpuri–Khichripur				3		1	5				9
Vishwas Nagar					1	5	3		1		10
	0	0	4	12	13	14	23	9	3	0	78
CENTRAL & SOUTH ZONE											
Amb Nagar–Dakshinpuri–Madangir		4	14	1	2	8	4	2			35
Badarpur–Molar Bandh–Mithapur–Jaitpur		1	12	11	4	8	8	4			48
Chattarpur				2	3		1				6
Chiragh Dilli			1			1	1				3
Garhi–Lajpat Nagar–Sri Niwaspuri			7	4	6	8	3	3			31
Govindpuri–Kalkaji		1	14	7	3	5	2	1	1		34
Harkesh Nagar–Jasola–Ali			3	2	1	1	2				9
Jamroodpur						1					1
Khanpur–Deoli–Tigri		1	2	2	2	10	2		1		20
Kilokri–Sunlight Colony–Ashram			1	2		2					5
Kotla Mubarakpur		1	6	1		2	8				18
Madanpur Khadar–Sarita Vihar			4		1	3					8
Malviya Nagar–Savitri Nagar–Hauz Rani–Khirki		1	5		1	8	1	1			17
Masjid Moth–Gautam Nagar				1		1	1				3

1995	*J-M*	*A*	*M*	*J*	*J*	*A*	*S*	*O*	*N*	*D*	*T*
Mehrauli–Lado Sarai–Neb Sarai			3	3		2	1	1			10
Okhla Industrial Area–Tehkhand			6	8		6	2				22
Okhla Village–Jamia Nagar–Abul Fazal Enclave			4	3	3	2	1				13
Sangam Vihar			10	9		1	3	2			25
Shahpur Jat						1					1
Tughlakabad		2	3	1	2						8
	0	11	95	57	28	70	40	14	2		317
ROHINI ZONE											
Budh Vihar			1	4	1	4					10
Haiderpur					19	12	4	1			36
Rithala–Vijay Vihar			3		1		2				6
Rohini					1	3	1				5
Samaipur–Badli			4	2	7	16	7	2			38
Sawan Park			1		6	13	5	1			26
Shahbad Daulatpur/ Dairy			1	1	1	3	1				7
Shakurbasti–Rani Bagh						7	2	1			10
Shalimar Bagh (JJ) & Village			2		3	2	7				14
Siraspur				1	2						3
Wazirpur JJ–Nimri Village–Wazirpur Village			2	1	4	3	2				12
	C	0	14	9	45	63	31	5	0	0	167
NAJAFGARH ZONE											
Mahipalpur–Nangal–Rangpuri			3	1	2		1				7
Mangolpuri–Sultanpuri			4	2	10	35	14				65
Nangloi			9	10	12	9	7				47
Palam–Dabri		6	5	4	1	3	6				25
Pappan Kalan/Dwarka		1	7			1	2				11
	0	7	28	17	25	48	30	0	0	0	155

1995	*J–M*	*A*	*M*	*J*	*J*	*A*	*S*	*O*	*N*	*D*	*T*
NARELA ZONE											
Alipur			1				6				7
Bakhtawarpur–Palla		1	1	1	3	4	1				11
Bawana			1	2		2	3				8
Brick Kilns			12	7							19
Holambi											0
Lampur											0
Narela			1		1	2	2				6
Prem Nagar–Kirari			1	2	9	11	9				32
	0	1	17	12	13	19	21	0	0	0	83

Table A.18: Cholera Cases in Vulnerable Areas of the Zones, 1996

1996	*J–M*	*A*	*M*	*J*	*J*	*A*	*S*	*O*	*N*	*D*	*T*
CITY ZONE											
Nizamuddin							1				1
Sarai Kale Khan											0
Yamuna Pushta JJ				2	1	2	1				6
	0	0	0	2	1	2	2	0	0	0	7
S. P. ZONE											
Nabi Karim–Pahargunj			1		2	1	2	1	1		8
Sadar Bazar					2	2					4
	0	0	1	0	4	3	2	1	1	0	12
K. B. ZONE											
Anand Parbat–Dev Nagar						1					1
Baljeet Nagar					1						1
Inderpuri–Todapur–Loha Mandi											0
Naraina Village				1			1				2
Zakhira–Shadipur				2	2	1	1				6
	0	0	0	3	3	2	2	0	0	0	10
C. L. ZONE											
Azadpur			2	3	8	7	1				21
Bhalswa Village & Dairy							1				1

1996	*J–M*	*A*	*M*	*J*	*J*	*A*	*S*	*O*	*N*	*D*	*T*
Bharola–Sarai Peepalthala						4		2			6
Burari–Nathupura–Ibrahimpur–Jharoda	1		10	7	9	14	10	4			55
Camp–Dhaka–Dhirpur–Malikpur		1	6	9	6	6	5	1			34
Chandrawal–Malkagunj			1		2		1				4
Jahangirpuri			3		4	4	3				14
Lal Bagh & other JJ				2	23	17	3	2			47
Mukandpur			2				1				3
Rajpura–Gur Mandi											0
Wazirabad–Jagatpur			2	3	1	1	1				8
Wazirpur Industrial Area (JJ)											0
	1	1	26	24	53	53	26	9	0	0	193
SH (N) ZONE											
Bhajanpura–Dayalpur–Gamri			1	2	3	3	2				11
Brahmpuri					1						1
Johripur											0
Karawal Nagar				1	5	1					7
Loni Road					2						2
Mandoli–Saboli					1	1					2
Maujpur–Ghonda						2	2				4
Mustafabad–Gokulpuri				4	4	2		1			11
Nand/Sunder Nagri				2	1	2					5
New Seelampur–Jaffrabad				2	3	1	2				8
Seemapuri			2		1	1					4
Shastri Park–Usmanpur–Taj Colony				2		2	2				6
Sonia Vihar/Khajuri Khas				3	2	2	1				8
	0	0	3	16	23	17	9	1	0	0	69
SH (S) ZONE											
Gandhi Nagar/Kailash Nagar			1	3	1	1					6

1996	*J-M*	*A*	*M*	*J*	*J*	*A*	*S*	*O*	*N*	*D*	*T*
Kondli–Gharouli–MV3						1					1
Old Seelampur				3			1				4
Patpargunj Village–Mandawali Village						1	1				2
Shakurpur–Laxmi Nagar					1		2				3
Trilokpuri–Kalyanpuri–Khichripur			1	4	2	1	1				9
Vishwas Nagar				1	1						2
	0	0	2	11	5	4	5	0	0	0	27
CENTRAL & SOUTH ZONE											
Amb Nagar–Dakshinpuri–Madangir		1	4			1	1	1			8
Badarpur–Molar Bandh–Mithapur–Jaitpur		5	5	2	4	1	1	1			19
Chattarpur				1	2	1	1				5
Chiragh Dilli		1	2		1						4
Garhi–Lajpat Nagar–Sri Niwaspuri		2	5	4	4	2	2				19
Govindpuri–Kalkaji		2	4	1	9	1					17
Harkesh Nagar–Jasola–Ali				1	1	2					4
Jamroodpur									1		1
Khanpur–Deoli–Tigri			1		2						3
Kilokri–Sunlight Colony–Ashram						1					1
Kotla Mubarakpur			3		1	1					5
Madanpur Khadar–Sarita Vihar					1			1			2
Malviya Nagar–Savitri Nagar–Hauz Rani–Khirki			1								1
Masjid Moth–Gautam Nagar				1			2				3
Mehrauli–Lado Sarai–Neb Sarai				1	1						2
Okhla Industrial Area–Tehkhand			5	2	1	1	3				12

1996	*J–M*	*A*	*M*	*J*	*J*	*A*	*S*	*O*	*N*	*D*	*T*
Okhla Village–Jamia Nagar–Abul Fazal Enclave			3	1	2	2					8
Sangam Vihar		4	4	2	5		3	1			19
Shahpur Jat					1	2					3
Tughlakabad	1	2	4			1		1			9
	1	17	41	16	35	16	13	5	1	0	145
ROHINI ZONE											
Budh Vihar					1		1				2
Haiderpur				1	3	8	3	1			16
Rithala–Vijay Vihar						1					1
Rohini					2	1	1				4
Samaipur–Badli					2	2	4				8
Sawan Park					3	4	3				10
Shahbad Daulatpur/ Dairy					6	5	5				16
Shakurbasti–Rani Bagh					1						1
Shalimar Bagh (JJ) & Village					5	3					8
Siraspur					1		2				3
Wazirpur JJ–Nimri Village–Wazirpur Village			1	2		3					6
	0	0	1	3	24	27	19	1	0	0	75
NAJAFGARH ZONE											
Mahipalpur–Nangal–Rangpuri				1		2	1				4
Mangolpuri–Sultanpuri		1		4	7	7	2				21
Nangloi			2	1	1	7	5	1			17
Palam–Dabri			1	1	1				1		4
Pappan Kalan/Dwarka			1	1							2
	0	1	4	8	9	16	8	1	1	0	48
NARELA ZONE											
Alipur				1	4	1		1			7
Bakhtawarpur–Palla					2	1	1				4
Bawana											0

1996	*J-M*	*A*	*M*	*J*	*J*	*A*	*S*	*O*	*N*	*D*	*T*
Brick Kilns				3							3
Holambi											0
Lampur											0
Narela					5	1	3				9
Prem Nagar–Kirari				1	6	6	1				14
	0	0	0	5	17	9	5	1	0	0	37

Table A.19: Cholera Cases in Vulnerable Areas of the Zones, 1997

1997	*J-M*	*A*	*M*	*J*	*J*	*A*	*S*	*O*	*N*	*D*	*T*
CITY ZONE											
Nizamuddin					1						1
Sarai Kale Khan					1						1
Yamuna Pushta JJ				1	1	1	2				5
	0	0	0	1	3	1	2	0	0	0	7
S. P. ZONE											
Nabi Karim–Pahargunj						1		1			2
Sadar Bazar					1		1				2
	0	0	0	0	1	1	1	1	0	0	4
K. B. ZONE											
Anand Parbat–Dev Nagar											0
Baljeet Nagar			1	1				1			3
Inderpuri–Todapur–Loha Mandi											0
Naraina Village				1	1		1				3
Zakhira–Shadipur				3	4	1		2			10
	0	0	1	5	5	1	1	3	0	0	16
C. L. ZONE											
Azadpur		1	3	5	3	4	9	3			28
Bhalswa Village & Dairy						5					5
Bharola–Sarai Peepalthala					1	2	1	1			5
Burari–Nathupura–Ibrahimpur–Jharoda			5	10	20	17	8	1			61
Camp–Dhaka–Dhirpur–Malikpur			7	7	13	5	4	1			37

1997	J–M	A	M	J	J	A	S	O	N	D	T
Chandrawal–Malkagunj				2		2	1	1			6
Jahangirpuri			1	3	12	8	4		1		29
Lal Bagh & other JJ			5	3	15	19	7	1	2		52
Mukandpur			1		6	4	4	1			16
Rajpura–Gur Mandi				1		1					2
Wazirabad–Jagatpur					1	2	3				6
Wazirpur Industrial Area (JJ)				1		2					3
	0	1	22	32	71	71	41	9	3	0	250
SH (N) ZONE											
Bhajanpura–Dayalpur–Gamri			1		1		1				3
Brahmpuri					1		2				3
Johripur					1						1
Karawal Nagar				4	4	3	1		1		13
Loni Road				1	1						2
Mandoli–Saboli					2	1					3
Maujpur–Ghonda				1			1		1		3
Mustafabad–Gokulpuri				2	2	2					6
Nand/Sunder Nagri				3	2		2				7
New Seelampur–Jaffrabad					1	1					2
Seemapuri			2	3	1						6
Shastri Park–Usmanpur–Taj Colony					2	1	5	2		1	11
Sonia Vihar/Khajuri Khas				1		1	2				4
	0	0	3	15	18	9	14	2	2	1	64
SH (S) ZONE											
Gandhi Nagar/Kailash Nagar			2	2	3	4	1	1			13
Kondli–Gharouli–MV3			2				2	2			6
Old Seelampur					1	1					2
Patpargunj Village–Mandawali Village				2	1	1	2				6
Shakurpur–Laxmi Nagar					2						2

1997	*J–M*	*A*	*M*	*J*	*J*	*A*	*S*	*O*	*N*	*D*	*T*
Trilokpuri–Kalyanpuri–Khichripur			1	1		1	1	1			5
Vishwas Nagar				1		1					2
	0	0	5	6	7	8	6	4	0	0	36
CENTRAL & SOUTH ZONE											
Amb Nagar–Dakshinpuri–Madangir			4	1	1	2			1		9
Badarpur–Molar Bandh–Mithapur–Jaitpur			1	5	9	3	5	2			25
Chattarpur					2		2	3			7
Chiragh Dilli			1			1					2
Garhi–Lajpat Nagar–Sri Niwaspuri				2	4	2	3	2	1		14
Govindpuri–Kalkaji			5	2	3	2	1				13
Harkesh Nagar–Jasola–Ali			1		2		1				4
Jamroodpur			1			1					2
Khanpur–Deoli–Tigri			1		3		1	1			6
Kilokri–Sunlight Colony–Ashram			1		1			1			3
Kotla Mubarakpur								1			1
Madanpur Khadar–Sarita Vihar						1	1	2			4
Malviya Nagar–Savitri Nagar–Hauz Rani–Khirki				2	2		1	2			7
Masjid Moth–Gautam Nagar						1	2				3
Mehrauli–Lado Sarai–Neb Sarai						1		1			2
Okhla Industrial Area–Tehkhand			3	1	2		2		1		9
Okhla Village–Jamia Nagar–Abul Fazal Enclave			2	1							3
Sangam Vihar		1	2		3	7	2	5			20
Shahpur Jat					1	2					3

1997	*J–M*	*A*	*M*	*J*	*J*	*A*	*S*	*O*	*N*	*D*	*T*
Tughlakabad			2	2	1		4	1	1		11
	0	1	24	16	34	23	25	21	4	0	143
ROHINI ZONE											
Budh Vihar				1	1	2	4				8
Haiderpur			2	2	3	7					14
Rithala–Vijay Vihar					3						3
Rohini					2	4		1	1		8
Samaipur–Badli				1	2	6	4	1			14
Sawan Park					4	1					5
Shahbad Daulatpur/ Dairy						3	2	2	2		9
Shakurbasti–Rani Bagh						1					1
Shalimar Bagh (JJ) & Village						1	1				2
Siraspur						1					1
Wazirpur JJ–Nimri Village–Wazirpur Village					1	1		3			5
	0	0	2	4	16	27	11	7	3	0	70
NAJAFGARH ZONE											
Mahipalpur–Nangal–Rangpuri					1	1	3				5
Mangolpuri–Sultanpuri				2	2	9	3				16
Nangloi			3	1		3	3				10
Palam–Dabri											0
Pappan Kalan/Dwarka				3	1						4
	0	0	3	6	4	13	9	0	0	0	35
NARELA ZONE											
Alipur						1	2				3
Bakhtawarpur–Palla					1						1
Bawana											0
Brick Kilns				1							1
Holambi											0
Lampur							1				1
Narela											0
Prem Nagar–Kirari				2		5					7
	0	0	0	3	1	6	3	0	0	0	13

Table A.20: Cholera Cases in Vulnerable Areas of the Zones, 1998

1998	*J–M*	*A*	*M*	*J*	*J*	*A*	*S*	*O*	*N*	*D*	*T*
CITY ZONE											
Nizamuddin				2							2
Sarai Kale Khan				3			1	2			6
Yamuna Pushta JJ					1	2	1	3			7
	0	0	0	5	1	2	2	5	0	0	15
S. P. ZONE											
Nabi Karim–Pahargunj			1	1	2		2				6
Sadar Bazar					2	6	3				11
	0	0	1	1	4	6	5	0	0	0	17
K. B. ZONE											
Anand Parbat–Dev Nagar					1			1			2
Baljeet Nagar				1	2						3
Inderpuri–Todapur–Loha Mandi				1	1		1				3
Naraina Village					2						2
Zakhira–Shadipur				3	4		1				8
	0	0	0	5	10	0	2	1	0	0	18
C. L. ZONE											
Azadpur			4	20	22	2	8	3			59
Bhalswa Village & Dairy				4	7	4	1				16
Bharola–Sarai Peepalthala				4	6	5	11	2	1		29
Burari–Nathupura–Ibrahimpur–Jharoda		2	47	33	54	45	18	3	2		204
Camp–Dhaka–Dhirpur–Malikpur			5	11	11	10	9				46
Chandrawal–Malkagunj			1	1			1	2			5
Jahangirpuri			4	4	17	9	14	2	7		57
Lal Bagh & other JJ			2	11	33	10	7	8			71
Mukandpur			5	5	11	11	3	1	1		37
Rajpura–Gur Mandi				3	1	2	1				7
Wazirabad–Jagatpur				5	6	1	2				14

1998	*J–M*	*A*	*M*	*J*	*J*	*A*	*S*	*O*	*N*	*D*	*T*
Wazirpur Industrial Area (JJ)			3		2						5
	0	2	71	101	170	99	75	21	11	0	550
SH (N) ZONE											
Bhajanpura–Dayalpur–Gamri				4	7	2	3				16
Brahmpuri					3						3
Johripur								1			1
Karawal Nagar				5	5	7	5	1			23
Loni Road						1					1
Mandoli–Saboli				1				1			2
Maujpur–Ghonda					3	2	2				7
Mustafabad–Gokulpuri					2	1	1				4
Nand/Sunder Nagri					3	2		2			7
New Seelampur–Jaffrabad				1	2	2	4	1			10
Seemapuri				1		2	2				5
Shastri Park–Usmanpur–Taj Colony				1	2			1			4
Sonia Vihar/Khajuri Khas		1	1	2	3	5	6	1			19
	0	1	1	15	30	24	23	8	0	0	102
SH (S) ZONE											
Gandhi Nagar/Kailash Nagar				1	1	2			1		5
Kondli–Gharouli–MV3				3	3	1	1	1	2		11
Old Seelampur							3				3
Patpargunj Village–Mandawali Village				1	1		2	3			7
Shakurpur–Laxmi Nagar				1	3			1			5
Trilokpuri–Kalyanpuri–Khichripur			2	6	4	4	4	1	1		22
Vishwas Nagar				1			2				3
	0	0	2	13	12	7	12	6	4	0	56

1998	*J–M*	*A*	*M*	*J*	*J*	*A*	*S*	*O*	*N*	*D*	*T*
CENTRAL & SOUTH ZONE											
Amb Nagar–Dakshinpuri–Madangir	2	1	1	6	2	1	2				15
Badarpur–Molar Bandh–Mithapur–Jaitpur				5	10	8	2		2		27
Chattarpur					1	2	1	3			7
Chiragh Dilli					1						1
Garhi–Lajpat Nagar–Sri Niwaspuri				2	3	2	1	3	2	2	15
Govindpuri–Kalkaji		1	1	2	1	6	2	7	3		23
Harkesh Nagar–Jasola–Ali			2	2							4
Jamroodpur						1					1
Khanpur–Deoli–Tigri				1	2			1	1		5
Kilokri–Sunlight Colony–Ashram					2	1					3
Kotla Mubarakpur					2	1		1	1		5
Madanpur Khadar–Sarita Vihar						2	2				4
Malviya Nagar–Savitri Nagar–Hauz Rani–Khirki					2	1	2				5
Masjid Moth–Gautam Nagar					1		1				2
Mehrauli–Lado Sarai–Neb Sarai			1		2	2	1				6
Okhla Industrial Area–Tehkhand			2		1	1	1	3			8
Okhla Village–Jamia Nagar–Abul Fazal Enclave				2	1	1		3			7
Sangam Vihar		2	1	4	5	6	2	1			21
Shahpur Jat					1						1
Tughlakabad				2	4		1	2			9
	2	4	8	26	41	35	18	24	9	2	169
ROHINI ZONE											
Budh Vihar				1	7	4	2				14

1998	*J–M*	*A*	*M*	*J*	*J*	*A*	*S*	*O*	*N*	*D*	*T*
Haiderpur			3	6	38	49	9	1			105
Rithala–Vijay Vihar				2		3	1	1			7
Rohini				3	4	6	3				16
Samaipur–Badli				12	34	20	3	5	2		76
Sawan Park		1	2		11	3	2				19
Shahbad Daulatpur/ Dairy			4	1	3	11					19
Shakurbasti–Rani Bagh			1		5	3		1	1		11
Shalimar Bagh (JJ) & Village				2	7	4	2				15
Siraspur					5	2					7
Wazirpur JJ–Nimri Village–Wazirpur Village				4	3	9	1	4	1		22
NAJAFGARH ZONE											
Mahipalpur–Nangal–Rangpuri					2	1		1			4
Mangolpuri–Sultanpuri			2	2	7	8	4	1			24
Nangloi				1	6	3	1				11
Palam–Dabri					3	2		1			6
Pappan Kalan/Dwarka				1	1	1					3
	0	0	2	4	19	15	5	3	0	0	48
NARELA ZONE											
Alipur			1	6	1		4				12
Bakhtawarpur–Palla				3	1						4
Bawana					3	1	1				5
Brick Kilns				1							1
Holambi				1							1
Lampur											0
Narela				2	6	6	2		1		17
Prem Nagar–Kirari					6	5	3		1		15
	0	0	1	13	17	12	10	0	2	0	55

Table A.21: Cholera Cases in Vulnerable Areas of the Zones, 1999

1999	*J–M*	*A*	*M*	*J*	*J*	*A*	*S*	*O*	*N*	*D*	*T*
CITY ZONE											
Nizamuddin			1				1				2
Sarai Kale Khan		1				2					3
Yamuna Pushta JJ		2	2	6	2	4	1				17
	0	3	3	6	2	6	2	0	0	0	22
S. P. ZONE											
Nabi Karim–Pahargunj		9	3	10	4	1	5	2			34
Sadar Bazar			1	3	2			1			7
	0	9	4	13	6	1	5	3	0	0	41
K. B. ZONE											
Anand Parbat–Dev Nagar			1		2	3	2				8
Baljeet Nagar			1		2	2		2			7
Inderpuri–Todapur–Loha Mandi			2	1	3				1		7
Naraina Village			1	1	2						4
Zakhira–Shadipur		1	4	5	4	4					18
	0	1	9	7	13	9	2	2	1	0	34
C. L. ZONE											
Azadpur			3	7	2	5	4	1			22
Bhalswa Village & Dairy		1	1	2	3	4					11
Bharola–Sarai Peepalthala				7	4	1					12
Burari–Nathupura–Ibrahimpur–Jharoda		3	10	10	15	10	6	4			58
Camp–Dhaka–Dhirpur–Malikpur		2	15	5	3	4	5				35
Chandrawal–Malkagunj							1		1		2
Jahangirpuri		3		12	5	5	2	1			28
Lal Bagh & other JJ		3	1	2	20	21	3	5	2		57
Mukandpur			4	4	4	8	3	1			24
Rajpura–Gur Mandi			1	4		3		1			9
Wazirabad–Jagatpur			1		1			1			3

1999	*J-M*	*A*	*M*	*J*	*J*	*A*	*S*	*O*	*N*	*D*	*T*
Wazirpur Industrial Area (JJ)		1			2		3				6
	0	13	36	53	59	61	27	14	3	0	266
SH (N) ZONE											
Bhajanpura–Dayalpur–Gamri			1	3	1	1					6
Brahmpuri					1			1			2
Johripur											
Karawal Nagar		1	2	1	5	5	1				15
Loni Road					1						1
Mandoli–Saboli					1						1
Maujpur–Ghonda			5	3		1			1		10
Mustafabad–Gokulpuri			3	1			1				5
Nand/Sunder Nagri				1	1	1					3
New Seelampur–Jaffrabad		1	4	2	2	3			1		13
Seemapuri					4	2		2			8
Shastri Park–Usmanpur–Taj Colony			1	3	2	4			4		14
Sonia Vihar/Khajuri Khas			4	3	2	4	1		1		15
	0	2	20	17	20	21	3	3	7	0	103
SH (S) ZONE											
Gandhi Nagar/Kailash Nagar			3	1		3	1	1			9
Kondli–Gharouli–MV3			3	2	2	1		5			13
Old Seelampur											
Patpargunj Village–Mandawali Village			2	5	1	2					10
Shakurpur–Laxmi Nagar			1	1			1		1		4
Trilokpuri–Kalyanpuri–Khichripur			8	4	3						15
Vishwas Nagar			1					1	5		7
	0	0	18	13	6	6	2	7	6	0	58
CENTRAL & SOUTH ZONE											
Amb Nagar–Dakshinpuri–Madangir		3	12	11	1	3	1	2	3		41

1999	*J–M*	*A*	*M*	*J*	*J*	*A*	*S*	*O*	*N*	*D*	*T*
Badarpur–Molar Bandh–Mithapur–Jaitpur		3	8	5	7	6	1				30
Chattarpur					1						1
Chiragh Dilli		3	3	1	2						9
Garhi–Lajpat Nagar–Sri Niwaspuri		3	2	3	3	2	2				15
Govindpuri–Kalkaji		15	5	15	3	1	1	2			42
Harkesh Nagar–Jasola–Ali		1	4	2	1	3					11
Jamroodpur		4	4								8
Khanpur–Deoli–Tigri		3	3		1	3					10
Kilokri–Sunlight Colony–Ashram		1		1	1	1					4
Kotla Mubarakpur		7	1		2	1					11
Madanpur Khadar–Sarita Vihar		1			2						3
Malviya Nagar–Savitri Nagar–Hauz Rani–Khirki				1	2			1			4
Masjid Moth–Gautam Nagar			1			2	2				5
Mehrauli–Lado Sarai–Neb Sarai		3	5	1		2	2		1		14
Okhla Industrial Area–Tehkhand		4	2	2	1				1		10
Okhla Village–Jamia Nagar–Abul Fazal Enclave			4		1			1			6
Sangam Vihar		3	8	4	1	1					17
Shahpur Jat			1								1
Tughlakabad		1	2	5	3	1			1		13
	0	60	65	51	32	26	9	6	6	0	253
ROHINI ZONE											
Budh Vihar					1	3	1				4
Haiderpur			1	3	12	21	2		1		40
Rithala–Vijay Vihar							3	1			4
Rohini				2		3	1	1			7

1999	*J-M*	*A*	*M*	*J*	*J*	*A*	*S*	*O*	*N*	*D*	*T*
Samaipur–Badli			1	3		4	1				9
Sawan Park				4	2	1	1				8
Shahbad Daulatpur/ Dairy			1	5			2				8
Shakurbasti–Rani Bagh					1	2			2		5
Shalimar Bagh (JJ) & Village			3	2	4	1	1	1			12
Siraspur						1					1
Wazirpur JJ–Nimri Village–Wazirpur Village				1	1	2					4
	0	0	6	20	21	38	12	3	3	0	103
NAJAFGARH ZONE											
Mahipalpur–Nangal–Rangpuri			1	3	3						7
Mangolpuri–Sultanpuri			1	3	1	7					12
Nangloi			2	4	3	5	2	1			19
Palam–Dabri			3			1	1		1		6
Pappan Kalan/Dwarka			2		1		1				4
	0	0	9	10	8	13	4	1	1	0	46
NARELA ZONE											
Alipur				6				1			7
Bakhtawarpur–Palla			1	1	2	3					7
Bawana											
Brick Kilns			1								1
Holambi					1						1
Lampur											
Narela			2	3	2						7
Prem Nagar–Kirari			8	1	4	1		3			17
	0	0	12	11	9	4	0	4	0	0	50

Table A.22: Cholera Cases in Vulnerable Areas of the Zones, 2000

2000	*J–M*	*A*	*M*	*J*	*J*	*A*	*S*	*O*	*N*	*D*	*T*
CITY ZONE											
Nizamuddin						1					1
Sarai Kale Khan			1	1				2	1		5
Yamuna Pushta JJ				3	3	1	2				9
	0	0	1	4	3	2	2	2	1	0	15
S. P. ZONE											
Nabi Karim–Pahargunj		1		5		1	3	3	6		19
Sadar Bazar						1		1			2
	0	1	0	5	0	2	3	4	6	0	21
K. B. ZONE											
Anand Parbat–Dev Nagar											0
Baljeet Nagar				1			1		1		3
Inderpuri–Todapur–Loha Mandi					1		1	1			3
Naraina Village											0
Zakhira–Shadipur		1	1	2	1		3		3		11
	0	1	1	2	1	0	3	0	3	0	11
C. L. ZONE											0
Azadpur	1				1	4	8	1	1		16
Bhalswa Village & Dairy			1		4	3		1			9
Bharola–Sarai Peepalthala		2		8	11	5	1	1	4		32
Burari–Nathupura–Ibrahimpur–Jharoda		6	2	5	6	5	6	5	4		39
Camp–Dhaka–Dhirpur–Malikpur				1		2	2	1			6
Chandrawal–Malkagunj		2	1			3					6
Jahangirpuri			1	6	7	1	3	2	2		22
Lal Bagh & other JJ						5	12	6			23
Mukandpur						1	1				2
Rajpura–Gur Mandi			1								1
Wazirabad–Jagatpur					1	1		1			3

2000	*J–M*	*A*	*M*	*J*	*J*	*A*	*S*	*O*	*N*	*D*	*T*
Wazirpur Industrial Area (JJ)							2		1		3
	1	10	6	20	30	30	35	18	12	0	162
SH (N) ZONE											
Bhajanpura–Dayalpur–Gamri						1		1			2
Brahmpuri			1	3	1						5
Johripur											0
Karawal Nagar			1		1	2					4
Loni Road			1			1					2
Mandoli–Saboli				1							1
Maujpur–Ghonda			1		1						2
Mustafabad–Gokulpuri			3	2		2					7
Nand/Sunder Nagri				1				1			2
New Seelampur–Jaffrabad					3	5	1	1			10
Seemapuri					1	2	1		1		5
Shastri Park–Usmanpur–Taj Colony								3			
Sonia Vihar/Khajuri Khas			2	2	1	2					7
	0	0	9	9	8	15	2	6	1	0	47
SH (S) ZONE											
Gandhi Nagar/Kailash Nagar			1	2	1			1	1		6
Kondli–Gharouli–MV3							1				1
Old Seelampur					1		1				2
Patpargunj Village–Mandawali Village				1	2		2				5
Shakurpur–Laxmi Nagar					3	4					7
Trilokpuri–Kalyanpuri–Khichripur			1	1			1	1			4
Vishwas Nagar			1	2			2				5
	0	0	3	6	7	4	7	2	1	0	30

2000	*J–M*	*A*	*M*	*J*	*J*	*A*	*S*	*O*	*N*	*D*	*T*
CENTRAL & SOUTH ZONE											
Amb Nagar–Dakshinpuri–Madangir			6	24			1	10	1		42
Badarpur–Molar Bandh–Mithapur–Jaitpur		6	6	1	1	1	1	3	1		20
Chattarpur			4	2							6
Chiragh Dilli							1		2	1	4
Garhi–Lajpat Nagar–Sri Niwaspuri			3	2				5	2	1	13
Govindpuri–Kalkaji		1	1			1	1	4	5	1	14
Harkesh Nagar–Jasola–Ali			1	1	2			1	1		6
Jamroodpur		2	2	1		2	1	4			12
Khanpur–Deoli–Tigri	1	2	2	3	1		1		8		18
Kilokri–Sunlight Colony–Ashram			1					1	1		3
Kotla Mubarakpur				1		1		4	4		10
Madanpur Khadar–Sarita Vihar		2	7	1	1	1			1		13
Malviya Nagar–Savitri Nagar–Hauz Rani–Khirki		2	4	3					5		14
Masjid Moth–Gautam Nagar			8	2			7	3	1		21
Mehrauli–Lado Sarai–Neb Sarai			2			6					8
Okhla Industrial Area–Tehkhand		2	2		1			2	1		8
Okhla Village–Jamia Nagar–Abul Fazal Enclave						2			1		3
Sangam Vihar							4				4
Shahpur Jat				9	10	3		5	19		46
Tughlakabad			1					4	1		6
	1	17	50	50	16	17	17	46	54	3	271
ROHINI ZONE											
Budh Vihar					1						1

2000	*J-M*	*A*	*M*	*J*	*J*	*A*	*S*	*O*	*N*	*D*	*T*
Haiderpur				1	3	1	2	2	2		11
Rithala–Vijay Vihar											0
Rohini			1		2	2		1	1		7
Samaipur–Badli				3	5	2	4	2			16
Sawan Park								1			1
Shahbad Daulatpur/ Dairy						2		1			
Shakurbasti–Rani Bagh				1	1		1				3
Shalimar Bagh (JJ) & Village						2	1				3
Siraspur			1	1		3					5
Wazirpur JJ–Nimri Village–Wazirpur Village			1		5	1		1	1		9
	0	0	3	6	17	13	8	8	4	0	56
NAJAFGARH ZONE											
Mahipalpur–Nangal–Rangpuri											0
Mangolpuri–Sultanpuri						4	3				7
Nangloi					3		1				4
Palam–Dabri							2	1			3
Pappan Kalan/Dwarka						1					1
	0	0	0	0	3	5	6	1	0	0	15
NARELA ZONE											0
Alipur											0
Bakhtawarpur–Palla											0
Bawana						1					1
Brick Kilns											0
Holambi								1			1
Lampur											0
Narela							1				1
Prem Nagar–Kirari											0
	0	0	0	0	0	1	1	1	0	0	3

Bibliography

Adlakha, Arjun. "Population Trends: India". 1997. http://www.census.gov/ipc/prod/ib-9701.pdf (accessed 23 February 2002).

Aggarwal, Pushpa, R. Sarkar, J. P. Gupta, S. Ahuja, K. Ray and A. N. Rai Chowdhuri. "Current Epidemiological Aspects of Cholera in Delhi". *Journal of Communicable Diseases* 15, no. 1, 1983, 26–31.

Ahrens, W., and I. Pigeot, eds. *Handbook of Epidemiology*. Berlin: Springer, 2005.

Albert, John M., A. K. Siddique, M. S. Islam, A. S. Faruque, M. Ansaruzzaman, S. M. Faruque and R. B. Sack. "Large Outbreak of Clinical Cholera Due to *Vibrio cholerae* Non-O1 in Bangladesh". *Lancet* 13, no. 341, 1993, 704.

Amato, Paul R., and Jiping Zuo. "Rural Poverty, Urban Poverty, and Psychological Well-Being". *Sociological Quarterly* 33, no. 2, 1992, 229–40.

Amin, Varsha, A. K. Patwari, Girish Kumar, V. K. Anand, Neena Diwan and Sunil Peshin. "Clinical Profile of Cholera in Young Children: A Hospital Based Report". *Indian Pediatrics* 31, no. 7, 1994, 755–61.

Anderson, Anne-Marie Nybo. "Life-Course and Social Epidemiology, the Biological Fig Leaf and Bob Dylan". *International Journal of Epidemiology* 36, no. 3, 2007, 540–41.

Arnold, David. *Colonizing the Body: State Medicine and Epidemic Disease in Nineteenth-Century India*. Delhi: Oxford University Press, 1993.

___. "Social Crisis and Epidemic Disease in the Famines of Nineteenth-Century India". *Social History of Medicine* 6, no. 3, 1993, 385–404.

Arora, R. R., and B. S. Misra. "Epidemiological Features of Outbreaks of Cholera in India: A Review". *Journal of Communicable Diseases* 7, no. 2, 1975, 84–89.

Asian Development Bank. Water Utilities Data Book, 1993. http://www.adb.org/documents/books/second_water_utilities/second_water_utilities.pdf (accessed 4 March 2012).

Banerjea, A. C. "Note on Cholera in the United Provinces". *Indian Journal of Medical Research* 39, 1951, 17–40.

Barah, B. C., V. Sipahimalani and P. Dhar. "Urban Water Supply and Sanitation". In Sankar and Mathur, *Economic Instruments for Environment Sustainability* 53–65.

Barua, D., and William Greenough III. *Cholera*. New York: Plenum Medical Book Company, 1992.

Barua, Dhiman. "History of Cholera". In Barua and Greenough, *Cholera*, 1–36.

Baveja, C. P., D. Chattopadhyaya, S. Kumari, K. K. Dutta and S. Sehgal. "Bacteriological Study of Drinking Water during Epidemic of Cholera in Delhi". *Journal of Communicable Diseases* 21, no. 1, 1989, 59–61.

Beal, J. O. "From Social Networks to Public Action in Urban Governance: Where Does Benefit Accrue?" *Journal of International Development* 13, no. 7, 2001, 1015–21.

Bell, David. "The Hospitable City: Social Relations in Commercial Spaces". *Progress in Human Geography* 31, no. 1, 2007, 7–22.

Benjamin, E. *Cholera in Bombay Province*. Bombay, 1949.

Ben-Shlomo, Y. "Rising to the Challenges and Opportunities of Life Course Epidemiology". *International Journal of Epidemiology* 36, no. 3, 2007, 481–83.

Berman, Peter, Rajeev Ahuja and Laveesh Bhandari. "The Impoverishing Effect of Healthcare Payments in India: New Methodology and Findings". *Economic and Political Weekly* 45, no. 16, 2010, 65–71.

Bernier, Francois. *Travels in the Mogul Empire*, trans. Archibald Constable. Reprint. Delhi: Low Price Publication, 1989.

Bhaduri, Amit, and Arvind Kejriwal. "Reforming the Reformers". *Economic and Political Weekly* 40, no. 53, 2005, 5543–45.

Bhan, Gautam. "This Is No Longer the City I Once Knew: Evictions, the Urban Poor and the Right to the City in Millennial Delhi". *Environment and Urbanization* 21, no. 1, 2009, 127–42.

Bharat Sevak Samaj. "Slums of Old Delhi", 1958. http://openlibrary.org/works/OL11148815W/Slums_of_Old_Delhi (accessed 12 May 2001).

Bhatnagar, S., and U. Dosajh. *Diarrhoeal Disease Morbidity in Children below 5 Years in Urban Slums in Delhi*. New Delhi: National Institute of Health and Family Welfare, 1986.

Bhattacharya, S. K., G. B. Nair, D. Dutta, A. Deb, T. Ramamurthy, S. Garg, P. K. Saha, P. Dutta and A. Moitra. "Clinical Profile of Acute Diarrhoea Cases Infected with the New Epidemic Strain of *Vibrio cholerae* O139: Designation of the Disease as Cholera". *Indian Journal of Medical Research* 27, no. 1, 1994, 11–15.

Bhattacharya, Sanjoy. "World Health Organization and the Social Determinants of Health". In Sanjoy Bhattacharya, *Social Determinants of Health*, 1–10.

___, ed. *Social Determinants of Health: Assessing Theory, Policy and Practice*. New Delhi: Orient BlackSwan, 2010.

Bhatty, Muhammad Akram. "Cholera in South Asia, 1961–1966". Unpublished diss., South Asian Institute, University of Heidelberg, 1969.

Borroto, R. J., and R. Martinez-Piedra. "Geographical Patterns of Cholera in Mexico, 1991–96". *International Journal of Epidemiology* 29, no. 4, 2000, 764–72.

Breeze, E., D. A. Jones and P. Wilkinson. "Area Deprivation, Social Class and Quality of Life among People Aged 75 Years and Over in Britain". *International Journal of Epidemiology* 34, no. 2, 2005, 276–83. doi: 10.1093/ije/dyh328 (accessed 1 March 2012).

Briscoe, J. "Technology and Child Survival: The Example of Sanitary Engineering". *Population and Development Review* 10, Suppl., 1984, 237–53.

___. "Intervention Studies and the Definition of Dominant Transmission Routes". *American Journal of Epidemiology* 120, no. 3, 1984, 449–55.

Bryden, J. L. *Vital Statistics of the Bengal Presidency. Cholera Epidemics of Recent Years Viewed in Relation to Former Epidemics: A Record of Cholera in the Bengal Presidency from 1817 to 1872*. Calcutta, 1874.

Cairncross, Sandy. "Water Supply and Sanitation: An Agenda for Research". *Journal of Tropical Medicine and Hygiene* 92, no. 5, 1989, 301–14.

Caroline, O., N. Moser, Alicia J. Herbert and Roza E. Makonnen. "Urban Poverty in the Context of Structural Adjustment: Recent Evidence and Policy Responses". TWU Discussion Paper No. 4, Urban Development Division, World Bank, Washington D.C., 1993.

Census of India. Provisional Population Totals. New Delhi: Registrar General's Office, 2001.

Chakraborty, A. K., and J. C. Das. "Comparative Study of Incidence of Diarrhoea among Children in Two Different Environmental Situations in Kolkata". *Indian Pediatrics* 20, no. 12, 1983, 907–13.

Chuttani, C. S. "Epidemiological and Clinical Characteristics of Cholera in Delhi". *Indian Journal of Medical Research* 55, no. 8, 1966, 815–24.

Cohen, D. A., K. Mason, A. Bedimo, R. Scribner, V. Basalo and T. Farley. "Neighborhood Conditions and Health". *American Journal of Public Health* 93, no. 3, 2003, 467–71.

CPCB (Central Pollution Control Board). *Management of Municipal Solid Waste in Delhi and Suggested Action Plan*. http://www.cpcb.nic.in/Highlights/2005/Municipalsolidwastemanagement[1].pdf (accessed 12 December 2010).

___. *Status of Solid Waste Generation, Collection, Treatment and Disposal in Metrocities*. New Delhi: CPCB, 2000.

Das, Shukla, and Sunil Gupta. "Diversity of *Vibrio cholerae* Strains Isolated in Delhi, India during 1992–2000". *Journal of Health, Population and Nutrition* 23, no. 1, 2005, 44–51.

Das, Shukla, Rumpa Saha and Iqbal R. Kaur. "Trend of Antibiotic Resistance of *Vibrio cholerae* Strains from East Delhi". *Indian Journal of Medical Research* 127, no. 5, 2008, 478–82.

Dasgupta, P. "Valuing Health Damages from Water Pollution in Urban Delhi, India: A Health Production Function Approach". *Environment and Development Economics* 9, no. 1, 2004, 83–106.

Dasgupta, P., and R. Dasgupta. "Economic Value of Safe Water for the Infrastructurally Disadvantaged Urban Household: A Case Study in Delhi in India". *Water Resources Research* 40, 2004, W11401.

Dasgupta, R. "District Health Profile Series-I, 24-Parganas (South), West Bengal 1992–93", Working Paper Series No. 1, Jawaharlal Nehru University, New Delhi, 1995.

___. "Cholera Outbreak in Garhi". Proceedings of the Conference of the Indian Association of Epidemiologists, New Delhi, 19–21 November 1995.

___. "Mapping Cholera in Delhi: Looking at Micro and Macro Solutions". Proceedings of the Fifth All India People's Technology Congress, Kolkata, 18–20 February 2005.

___. "Exploring Intra-household Factors in Diarrhoeal Diseases: A Study in Slums of Delhi, India". *Journal of Water and Health* 6, no. 2, 2007, 289–99.

___. "Mapping Cholera Vulnerability in Delhi: An Ecosocial Perspective". *Asian Journal of Water, Environment and Pollution* 7, no. 1, 2010, 19–26.

DDA (Delhi Development Authority). *Master Plan for Delhi, 1990*. New Delhi: DDA, 1990.

___. *Master Plan Delhi 2001*. New Delhi: DDA, 1999.

Delhi—Of Population. http://www.ofpopulation.co.uk/ (accessed 17 September 2007).

Department of Planning. *Economic Survey of Delhi, 2001–02*. New Delhi: Government of National Capital Territory of Delhi, 2002.

De Stavola, Bianca L., Dorothea Nitsch, Isabel dos Santos Silva, Valerie McCormack, Rebecca Hardy, Vera Mann, Tim J. Cole, Susan Morton and David A. Leon. "Statistical Issues in Life Course Epidemiology". *American Journal of Epidemiology* 163, no. 1, 2006, 84–96.

Dhar, P. "Economic Issues Relating to Water Contamination and Waste Disposal: A Case Analysis of Urban Development in Delhi". Unpublished diss., Jawaharlal Nehru University, 2000.

Dhar Chakravarti, P. G. "Delhi's Ongoing Debate on Informal Settlements and

Work Places: Issues of Environmental Jurisprudence". Paper presented at the International Workshop on Coping with Informality and Illegality in Human Settlements in Developing Cities, Leuven and Brussels, Belgium 23–26 May 2001.

Diez Roux, A. V. "Estimating and Understanding Area Health Effects". *International Journal of Epidemiology* 34, no. 2, 2005, 284–85. doi: 10.1093/ije/dyi020: 1-2 (accessed 1 March 2012).

Diez Roux, A. V., C. I. Kiefe, D. R. Jacobs Jr, M. Haan, S. A. Jackson, F. J. Nieto, C. C. Paton and R. Schulz. "Area Characteristics and Individual-Level Socioeconomic Position Indicators in Three Population Based Epidemiologic Studies". *Annals of Epidemiology*, 11, no. 6, 2001, 395–405.

Directorate of Economics and Statistics. *Delhi Statistical Handbook, 2000*. New Delhi: Government of Delhi, 2000.

____. *Delhi Statistical Handbook, 2002*. New Delhi: Government of Delhi, 2002.

____. *Delhi Statistical Handbook, 2008*. New Delhi: Government of Delhi, 2008.

Dupont, Veronique. "Slum Demolitions in Delhi since the 1990s: An Appraisal". *Economic and Political Weekly* 43, no. 28, 2008, 79–87.

Dutta, K. K., S. Bandyopadhyay, K. K. Khanna and K. Banerjee. "Epidemiological Features of Cholera Outbreak in Delhi in 1998". *Journal of Communicable Diseases* 25, no. 2, 1993, 57–61.

Dutta, Pranati. "Push-Pull Factors of Undocumented Migration from Bangladesh to West Bengal: A Perception Study". *Qualitative Report* 9, no. 2, 2004, 335–58.

____. "Urbanisation in India". Paper presented at the European Population Conference, Liverpool, 21–24 June 2006. http://www.scribd.com/doc/27348441/Urbanization-in-India (accessed 21 August 2009).

Edelman, Brent, and Arup Mitra. "Slum Dwellers' Access to Basic Amenities: The Role of Political Contacts, Its Determinants and Adverse Effects". *Review of Urban and Regional Development* Studies 18, no. 1, 2006, 25–40.

Editorial. "Delhi: Regulating a City". *Economic and Political Weekly* 46, no. 39, 2006, 4097.

Editorial. "Delhi Master Plan: Good on Paper". *Economic and Political Weekly* 42, no. 11, 2007, 900–901.

Editorial. "The Sanitation Challenge". *Economic and Political Weekly* 44, no. 4, 2009, 6.

Esrey, S. A., R. G. Feachem and J. M. Hughes. "Interventions for the Control of Diarrhoeal Diseases among Young Children: Improving Water Supplies and Excretion Disposal Facilities". *Bulletin of the World Health Organization* 63, no. 4, 1985, 757–72.

Feachem, R. G. "Interventions for the Control of Diarrhoeal Diseases among Young Children: Promotion of Personal and Domestic Hygiene". *Bulletin of the World Health Organization* 62, no. 3, 1984, 467–76.

Fewtrell, L., and J. Colford. "Water, Sanitation and Hygiene: Interventions and Diarrhoea—A Systemic Review and Metaanalysis". Health, Nutrition, and Population Family of the World Bank Human Development Network. http://www1.worldbank.org/hnp/Pubs_Discussion/Fewtrell & ColfordJuly2004.pdf. (accessed 12 December 2005).

Frontline. "Privatisation Not Just for the Sake of It". *Frontline* 19, no. 10, 2002. http://www.hinduonnet.com/fline/fl1910/19100920.htm (accessed 22 December 2009).

Frost, Wade Hampton. "Epidemiology". In Frost, *Papers of Wade Hampton Frost*, 493–542.

___. *Papers of Wade Hampton Frost*, ed. M. D. K. E. Maxcy. New York: The Commonwealth Fund, 1941.

Fry, A. B. "Cholera in Bengal: Past and Present". *Indian Medical Gazette*, 60, 1925, 301.

Gandy, Matthew. "Rethinking Urban Metabolism: Water, Space and the Modern City". *City* 8, no. 3, 2004, 363–79.

Ghertner, Asher D. "Analysis of New Legal Discourse behind Delhi's Slum Demolitions". *Economic and Political Weekly* 43, no. 20, 2008, 57–66.

Ghosh, S., P. G. Sengupta, S. K. Mondal, M. K. Basu, D. N. Gupta and B. K. Sircar. "Risk Behavioural Practices of Rural Mothers as Determinants of Childhood Diarrhoea". *Journal of Communicable Diseases* 29, no. 1, 1997, 7–14.

Glass, R. I., A. M. Svennerholm, B. J. Stoll, M. R. Khan, K. M. B. Hossain, M. I. Haq and J. Holmgren. "Protection against Cholera in Breast-Fed Children by Antibodies in Breast Milk". *New England Journal of Medicine* 308, no. 23, 1983, 1392–98.

Gordis, Leon. *Epidemiology*. Philadelphia: Saunders, 2009.

Greenberg, Raymond S., Stephen R. Daniels, W. Dana Flanders, John William Eley and John R. Borging III. *Medical Epidemiology*. 3rd ed. New York: Mc Graw Hill, 2001.

Gugler, Josef. "Over-Urbanisation Reconsidered". *Economic Development and Cultural Change* 31, no. 1, 1982, 173–89.

Gupta, Madhvi, and Pushkar. "Ethnic Diversity and the Demand for Public Goods: Interpreting the Evidence from Delhi". *Economic and Political Weekly* 45, no. 43, 2010, 64–72.

Gupta, Narayani. "Military Security and Urban Development: A Case Study of Delhi 1857–1912". *Modern Asian Studies* 5, no. 1, 1971, 61–77.

___. *Delhi between the Two Empires, 1803–1931: Society, Government and Urban Growth*. Delhi: Oxford University Press, 1981.

Gupta, Shalu, and M. M. A. Faridi. "Cholera Pattern in Children of Delhi". *Indian Pediatrics* 42, no. 2, 2005, 90–91.

Hansen, Niles M. "Development Pole Theory in a Regional Context". *International Review for Social Sciences* 20, no. 4, 2007, 709–27.

Hardoy, Jorge E., and David Satterthwaite. "Shelter, Infrastructure and Services in Third World Cities". *Habitat International* 10, no. 3, 1986, 245–84.

Harris, W. S. "The Effect of Pipe Water Supplies in the Reduction of Cholera in Urban Areas". *Tropical Diseases Bulletin* 3, 1913, 486.

Harrison, Mark. *Public Health in British India: Anglo-Indian Preventive Medicine 1859–1914*. London: Cambridge University Press, 1994.

Hart, K. "Informal Income Opportunities and Urban Employment in Ghana". *Journal of Modern African Studies* 11, no. 1, 1973, 61–89.

Henry, F. J., and Z. Rahim. "Transmission of Diarrhoea in Two Crowded Areas with Different Sanitary Facilities in Dhaka, Bangladesh". *Journal of Tropical Medicine and Hygiene* 93, no. 2, 1990, 121–26.

Independent. "Cholera Kills 12 in South Russia". 11 August 1994.

Indian Express. "Panel Set Up to Decide Development Charges". 18 January 2011. http://www.indianexpress.com/news/panel-set-up-to-decide-development-charges/738856/ (accessed 18 January 2011).

Jabeen, K., and R. Hasan. "Re-emergence of *Vibrio cholerae* O139 in Pakistan: Report from a Tertiary Care Hospital". *Journal of Pakistan Medical Association* 53, no. 8, 2003, 335–38.

Jagmohan. *Rebuilding Shahjahanabad*. New Delhi: Vikas, 1975.

Jalgaonkar, S. V., and R. P. Fule. "Cholera Outbreak Due to *Vibrio cholerae* Serogroup O139 in Yavatmal (Maharashtra) in March–July, 1993". *Indian Journal of Medical Research* 99, 1994, 101–2.

Jesudasan, M. V., and T. Jacob John. "The Appearance and Spread of *Vibrio cholerae* O139 in India". *Indian Journal of Medical Research* 99, 1994, 97–100.

Kass, Philip H., and Ellen B. Gold. "Modern Epidemiologic Study Designs". In Ahrens and Pigeot, *Handbook of Epidemiology*, 322–23.

Khanna, K. K., Ashok Dhanvijay, L. W. Riley, Sarabjit Sehgal and S. Kumari. "Cholera Outbreak in Delhi in 1988". *Journal of Communicable Diseases* 22, no. 1, 1990, 35–38.

Koo, D., A. Aragona, V. Moscosoa, M. Gudiela, L. Biettia, N. Carrilloa, J. Chojoja, B. Gordilloa, F. Canoa, D. N. Camerona, J. G. Wells, N. H. Beana and R. V. Tauxea. "Epidemic Cholera in Guatemala, 1993: Transmission of a Newly

Introduced Epidemic Strain by Street Vendors". *Epidemiology and Infection* 116, no. 2, 1996, 121–26.

Krieger, Nancy. "Epidemiology and the Web of Causation: Has Anyone Seen the Spider?" *Social Science & Medicine* 39, no. 7, 1994, 887–903.

———. "Theories for Social Epidemiology in the 21st Century: An Ecosocial Perspective". *International Journal of Epidemiology* 30, no. 4, 2001, 668–77.

———. "Proximal, Distal and the Politics of Causation: What's Level Got to Do With It?" *American Journal of Public Health* 98, no. 2, 2008, 221–30.

Krieger, N., and S. Zierler. "What Explains the Public's Health? A Call for Epidemiologic Theory". *Epidemiology* 7, no. 1, 1995, 107–9.

Kumar, Ashok. "Condoning Unplanned Development: Reviewing the Khanna Committee Report". *Economic and Political Weekly* 41, no. 39, 2006, 4105–8.

Kumar, Avdesh, Nina Gulati, C. S. Aggarwal, S. K. Rasania and Kusum Sahgal. "An Epidemiological Profile of Gastro-enteritis Deaths in Delhi State". *Journal of Communicable Diseases* 26, no. 2, 1995, 92–99.

Kumar, P., and C. R. Babu. "Valuation of Ecological Functions and Benefits: A Case Study of Wetlands Ecosystem along the Yamuna River Corridors of Delhi Region". Mimeograph, Institute of Economic Growth, Delhi, 2001.

Kumar, Prem. "Declining Number of Slums: Nature of Urban Growth". *Economic and Political Weekly* 45, no. 41, 2008, 75–77.

Kundu, A. "Urban Development, Infrastructure Financing and Emerging System of Governance in India: A Perspective". *Social and Human Sciences* 4, no. 15, 2001. http://digital-library.unesco.org (accessed 7 January 2004).

Kundu, Amitabh. "Exclusionary Urbanisation in Asia: A Macro Overview". *Economic and Political Weekly* 44, no. 48, 2009, 48–58.

Kundu, Nitai. "The Case of Kolkata, India". 2003. http://www.ucl.ac.uk/dpu-projects/Global_Report/pdfs/Kolkata.pdf (accessed 12 August 2004).

Kuznets, Simon. "Modern Economic Growth: Findings and Reflections". *American Economic Review* 63, no. 3, 1973, 247–58.

Lahlou, Michael Z. *Water Quality in Distribution Systems*. http://www.nesc.wvu.edu (accessed 12 April 2010).

Lal, R. B. "Fairs and Festivals in India". *Indian Medical Gazette* 72, 1937, 96.

Lan, R., and P. R. Reeves. "Pandemic Spread of Cholera: Genetic Diversity and Relationships within the Seventh Pandemic Clone of *Vibrio cholerae* Determined by Amplified Fragment Length Polymorphism". *Journal of Clinical Microbiology* 40, no. 1, 2002, 172–81.

Lantagne, D. S., R. Quick and M. D. Eri. "Household Water Treatment and Safe Storage Options in Developing Countries: A Review of Current Implementation Practices", 2005. http://www.wilsoncenter.org/water (accessed 7 July 2006).

Legg, Stephen. *Spaces of Colonialism: Delhi's Urban Governmentalities*. Oxford: Wiley Blackwell, 2007.

Lilienfeld, David E., and Paul D. Stolley. *Foundations of Epidemiology*. 3rd ed. New York: Oxford University Press, 1994.

Mackay, D. M. "Cholera: The Present World Situation". *Transactions of the Royal Society of Tropical Medicine and Hygiene* 73, no. 1, 1979, 1–2.

Madhiwalla, Neha. "Healthcare in Urban Slums in India". *National Medical Journal of India* 20, no. 3, 2007, 113–14.

Mahadevia, Darshini. "NURM and the Poor in Globalising Mega Cities". *Economic and Political Weekly* 41, no. 31, 2006, 3399–403.

Mahalanabis, D., A. S. Faruque, M. J. Albert, M. A. Salam and S. S. Hoque. "An Epidemic of Cholera Due to *Vibrio cholerae* O139 in Dhaka, Bangladesh: Clinical and Epidemiological Features". *Epidemiology and Infection*, 112, no. 3, 1994, 463–71.

Malhotra, R., P. Lal, S. K. Prakash and Jugal Kishore. "Evaluation of a Health Education Intervention on Knowledge and Attitudes of Food Handlers Working in a Medical College in Delhi, India". *Asia Pacific Journal of Public Health* 20, no. 4, 2008, 277–86.

Masley, W. H. "Principles and Practice of Cholera Control". Public Health Papers No. 40, World Health Organization, Geneva, 1970.

Mazumdar, Indrani. *Unorganised Workers of Delhi and the Seven Day Strike of 1988*. http://www.indialabourarchives.org (accessed 6 March 2010).

MCD (Municipal Corporation of Delhi). *Civic Guide*. New Delhi: MCD, 1995.

Mehrotra, Ritu Priya. *The Gastroenteritis Outbreak and Its Control in Sunder Nagri: An Assessment at Community Level*. New Delhi: Jawaharlal Nehru University, 1988.

Ministry of Environment and Forests, Government of India, and Planning Department, Government of the National Capital Territory of Delhi. *Delhi 21: Delhi Urban Environment and Infrastructure Improvement Project (DUEIIP)*. Delhi: Government of India and Government of NCT of Delhi, 2001. http://delhiplanning.nic.in/Reports/Delhi21/Delhi-21.pdf (accessed 4 March 2012).

Ministry of Housing and Urban Poverty Alleviation. *National Urban Housing and Habitat Policy*. New Delhi: Government of India, 2007.

___. "Report of the Committee on Slum Statistics/Census", National Buildings Organisation, Government of India, New Delhi, 2007.

Ministry of Urban Development. *Report of the National Commission on Urbanisation*. New Delhi: Government of India, 1988.

___. "Report of the Expert Committee on Lal Dora (ECLD) and Extended La

Dora in Delhi". Government of India, New Delhi, 2007. http://urbanindia.nic.in/programme/dd/laldora.pdf (accessed 12 March 2012).

___. *National Urban Sanitation Policy, 2008*. New Delhi: Government of India, 2008. http://www.indiaurbanportal.in (accessed 28 July 2009).

___. "Whither Indian Cities: Urban Reforms". Report of the National Consultation on Jawaharlal Nehru Urban Renewal Mission, Government of India. http://www.hazardscentre.in/hazards_publications/urban_governance_resistance.html (accessed 11 September 2008).

___. "Rank of Cities on Sanitation 2009–2010: National Urban Sanitation Policy". Government of India, New Delhi. http://pib.nic.in/archieve/others/2010/may/d2010051103.pdf (accessed 17 October 2010).

Mitra, Arup. "Women in the Informal Sector: Perpetuation of Meagre Earnings". *Development and Change* 36, no. 2, 2005, 291–316.

Mitra, Arup, and Mayumi Murayama. "Rural to Urban Migration: A District Level Analysis for India", 2008. http://ideas.repec.org/p/jet/dpaper/dpaper137.html (accessed 11 June 2010).

Mittal, M. C., E. M. Beckett and M. S. Pathak. "An Epidemiological Study of Gastroenteritis (Cholera El tor) Outbreak in Indore City, 1968". *Journal of Communicable Diseases* 1, no. 1, 1969, 54–59.

Mohanty, Srujuna. "Seasonality and Antimicrobial Resistance Pattern of *Vibrio cholerae* in a Tertiary Care Hospital of North India". *Tropical Doctor* 24, no. 4, 2004, 249–51.

Mølbak K., N. Højlyng, S. Jepsen and K. Gaarslev. "Bacterial Contamination of Stored Water and Stored Food: A Potential Source of Diarrhoeal Diseases in West Africa". *Epidemiology and Infection* 102, no. 2, 1989, 309–16.

Molla, Azizur R. *Pond Water Contamination and Incidence of Disease in Rural Bangladesh*. http://paa2005.princeton.edu/download.aspx?submissionid=51339 (accessed 19 February 2006).

Morbidity and Mortality Weekly Report 40, no. 13, 1991, 225–27.

Mukherji, Shekhar. "Linkage between Migration, Urbanisation and Regional Disparities in India: Required Planning Strategies". IIPS Research Monograph, International Institute for Population Sciences, Mumbai, 2001.

Mukhopadhyay, Partha. "Whither Urban Renewal?" *Economic and Political Weekly* 41, no. 10, 2006, 879–84.

Munasinghe, M. "The Economist's Approach to Sustainable Development". In Serageldin and Steer, *Making Development Sustainable: From Concepts to Action*, 13–16.

Münch, R. "Review: On the Shoulders of Giants, Robert Koch". *Microbes and Infections* 5, no. 1, 2003, 69–74.

Napier, L. E. "Cholera". In *The Principles and Practice of Tropical Medicine*. New York: Macmillan, 1946.

Narang, P., D. K. Mendiratta, V. S. Deotale and R. Narang. "Changing Patterns of Vibrio cholerae in Sevagram between 1990 and 2005". *Indian Journal of Medical Microbiology* 26, no. 1, 2008, 40–44.

Nath, V. "Planning for Delhi and National Capital Region: Review of Plan Formulation and Implementation". *Economic and Political Weekly* 30, no. 35, 1995, 2194–202.

Page, Melvin E., and Penny M. Sonnenburg. *Colonialism: An International, Social, Cultural and Political Encyclopaedia*. Santa Barbara: ABC-CLIO, 2003.

Pal, S. C. "A Review of the Studies on Cholera and Gastroenteritis Carried Out at the National Institute of Communicable Diseases, Delhi, 1965–72". *Journal of Communicable Diseases* 4, no. 2, 1972, 219–27.

Pal, S. C., and B. S. Misra. "Laboratory Investigation of Cholera Epidemics in Delhi and Rajasthan during 1968". *Journal of Communicable Diseases* 1, no. 1, 1969, 14–17.

Pal, S. C., et al. "Cholera El Tor in Baroda". *Journal of Communicable Diseases* 4, nos 2–3, 1972, 140–49.

Pappas, G., I. J. Kiriaze and M. E. Falagas. "Insights into Infectious Disease in the Era of Hippocrates". *International Journal of Infectious Diseases* 12, no. 4, 2008, 347–50.

Patnaik, K. C., and P. N. Kapoor. *Statistical Review of Cholera Problem in India with Particular Reference to Endemicity*. New Delhi: Central Bureau of Health Intelligence, 1967.

Patnaik, Utsa. "Trends in Urban Poverty under Economic Reforms: 1993–94 to 2004–05". *Economic and Political Weekly* 45, no. 4, 2010, 42–53.

Pearce, N. "Traditional Epidemiology, Modern Epidemiology, and Public Health". *American Journal of Public Health* 86, no. 5, 1996, 678–83.

Peck, Amie, and Adam Tickell. "Neoliberalizing Space". *Antipode* 34, no. 3, 2002 380–404.

Planning Commission. *Report of the Committee on India Vision 2020*. New Delhi Government of India, 2002.

Pollitzer, R. "Cholera Studies". *Bulletin of the World Health Organization* 10, no. 3, 1954, 421–61.

___. *Cholera*. Geneva: World Health Organization, 1959.

Powell, Walter W., and Laurel Smith-Doerr. "Networks and Economic Life". In Smelser and Swedberg, *The Handbook of Economic Sociology*, 368–402.

Prabhakar, H., M. Lal and H. Kaur, "Outbreak of Gastroenteritis Due to a New

Strain of Non O Group 1 *Vibrio cholerae*, in Ludhiana in May–August 1993". *Indian Journal of Medical Research* 99, 1994, 107–8.

Priya, Ritu. "Mr. Pitroda Goes to Sunder Nagari". *Seminar* 354, 1989, 1–4.

___. "Town Planning, Public Health and Urban Poor: Some Exploration from Delhi". *Economic and Political Weekly* 28, no. 17, 1993, 824–34.

Priya, R., A. Sagar, R. Dasgupta and S. Acharya. "Operationalising the CMP". *Economic and Political Weekly* 39, no. 27, 2004, 2971–74.

Pruss, A., D. Kay, L. Fewtrell and J. Bartram. "Estimating the Burden of Disease from Water, Sanitation and Hygiene at a Global Level". *Environmental Health Perspectives* 110, no. 5, 2002, 537–42.

Quick, R. E., L. V. Venczel, E. D. Mintz, L. Soleto, J. Apariocio, M. Gironaz, L. Hutwagner, K. Greene, C. Bopp, K. Maloney, D. Chavez, M. Sobsey and R. V. Tauxe. "Diarrhoea Prevention in Bolivia through Point-of-Use Water Treatment and Safe Storage: A Promising New Strategy". *Epidemiology and Infection* 122, no. 1, 1999, 83–90.

Rajeshwari, K., Ashish Gupta, A. P. Dubey, Beena Uppal and M. M. Singh. "Diarrhoeal Outbreak of *Vibrio cholerae* O1 Inaba in Delhi". *Tropical Doctor* 28, no. 2, 2008, 105–7.

Ramachandran, R. *Urbanisation and Urban Systems in India*. Delhi: Oxford University Press, 2001.

Ramamurthy, T., S. Garg, R. Sharma, S. K. Bhattacharya, G. B. Nair, T. Shimada, T. Takeda, T. Karasawa, H. Kurazano and A. Pal. "Emergence of Novel Strain of *Vibrio cholerae* with Epidemic Potential in Southern and Eastern India". *Lancet* 341, no. 8846, 1993, 703–4.

Rao, V. K. R. V., and P. B. Desai. "Greater Delhi: A Study in Urbanisation 1940–57", Planning Commission, Government of India, New Delhi, 1965.

Risbud, Neelima. "The Case of Mumbai, India". http://www.ucl.ac.uk/dpu-projects/Global_Report/pdfs/Mumbai.pdf (accessed 4 March 2012).

___. "Typology of Slums and Land Tenure in Indian Cities", National Workshop on Land Tenure Issues in Slum Free Planning. http://www.ucl.ac.uk/dpu-projects/Global_Report/pdfs/Mumbai.pdf (accessed 4 March 2012).

Rogers, L. "The Incidence and Spread of Cholera in India: Forecasting and Control of Epidemics". *Indian Medical Research Memoirs*, no. 9, 1928.

Rose, G. D. "Community-Based Technologies for Domestic Wastewater Treatment and Reuse: Options for Urban Agriculture". CFP Report Series, Report 27, NC Division of Pollution Prevention and Environmental Assistance, North Carolina, 1999.

Rothman, Kenneth J., and Sander Greenland. *Modern Epidemiology*. 2nd ed. Hagerstown: Lippincott-Raven Publishers, 1988.

Roy, Subarna, Basabjit Dutta, Asit Ranjan Ghosh, A. P. Sugunan, Ranjan Kumar Nandy, Sujit Kumar Bhattacharya and Subhash C. Sehgal. "Molecular Tracking of the Lineage of Strains of Vibrio cholerae O1 Biotype El Tor Associated with a Cholera Outbreak in Andaman and Nicobar Islands, India". *Tropical Medicine and International Health* 10, no. 6, 2005, 604–11.

Russell, A. J. H. "Statistical Studies in the Epidemiology of Cholera", *Transactions of the Seventh Congress of the Far Eastern Association of Tropical Medicine, 1927*. Vol. 2. Calcutta, 1929.

Russell, A. J. H., and E. R. Sundararajan. "The Epidemiology of Cholera in India". *Indian Medical Research Memoirs*, no. 12, 1928.

Sabherwal, U., and Rama Sikka. "Emergence of *Vibrio cholerae* Serogroup O139 in Haryana in May–June 1993". *Indian Journal of Medical Research* 99, 1994, 105–6.

Sachdeva, Vibha, K. K. Khanna, M. Singh, J. Singh, S. Kumari and T. Verghese. "Widespread Emergence of *Vibrio cholerae* O139 in India". *Southeast Asian Journal of Tropical Medicine and Public Health* 26, no. 2, 1995, 342–46.

Safa, Helen I. *Towards a Political Economy of Ubanisation in Third World Countries* Delhi: Oxford University Press, 1982.

Saha, Renuka, Anita Nath, Nandini Sharma, S. K. Bardhan and G. K. Ingle. "Changing Profile of Disease Contributing to Mortality in a Resettlement Colony of Delhi". *National Medical Journal of India* 20, no. 3, 2007, 125–27.

Sankar, U., and O. P. Mathur, eds. *Economic Instruments for Environment Sustainability*. New Delhi: National Institute of Public Finance and Policy and Madras School of Economics, 1998.

Saran, Awadhendra. "In the City, Out of Place: Environment and Modernity, Delhi 1860s to 1960s". *Economic and Political Weekly* 47, no. 25, 2006, 4905–11.

Saxena, P. K., B. G. Prasad and J. J. Bhatnagar. "A Study of Cholera Cases (El tor) among the Cases of Gastroenteritis Admitted to Infectious Diseases Hospital, Lucknow during 1969". *Journal of Communicable Diseases* 2, nos 1–4, 1970, 162–80.

Sen Gupta, S. K., and P. N. Kapoor. "Trends in Incidence of Cholera in India". *Journal of Communicable Diseases* 1, 1969, 3–4.

Sen Gupta, S. K., M. P. Bansal, P. Mitra and K. P. Ganguli. "Epidemiological and Clinical Profile of Cholera in Aurangabad Town during 1972". *Journal of Communicable Diseases* 6, no. 1, 1972, 4–10.

Serageldin, I., and A. Steer, eds. *Making Development Sustainable: From Concepts to Action*. Environmentally Sustainable Development Occasional Paper Series No. 2. Washington, D.C.: World Bank, 1994.

Shankar, P. S. Vijay, Himanshu Kulkarni and Sunderrajan Krishnan. "India's

Groundwater Challenge and the Way Forward". *Economic and Political Weekly* 66, no. 2, 2011, 37–45.

Sharholy, Mufeed, Kafeel Ahmad, Gauhar Mahmood and R. C. Trivedi. "Municipal Solid Waste Management in Indian Cities: A Review". *Waste Management* 28, no. 2, 2008, 459–67.

Sharma, M. I. D. "Problem of Cholera in India". *Journal of Communicable Diseases* 7, no. 2, 1975, 79–83.

Sharma, N. C., P. K. Mandal, Rohini Dhillon and Madhu Jain. "Changing Profile of *Vibrio cholerae* O1, O139 in Delhi and Its Periphery (2003–2005)". *Indian Journal of Medical Research* 125, no. 5, 2007, 633–40.

Sheikh, A., A. Khan, T. Malik and S. P. Fischer-Hoch. "Cholera in a Developing Megacity: Karachi, Pakistan". *Epidemiology and Infection* 119, no. 3, 1997, 287–92.

Singh, J., D. Bora, V. Sachdeva, R. S. Sharma and T. Verghese. "Prescribing Pattern by Doctors for Acute Diarrhoea in Children in Delhi, India". *Journal of Diarrhoeal Diseases Research* 13, no. 4, 1995, 229–31.

Singh, J., K. K. Khanna, A. C. Dhariwal, J. Bhattacharjee, M. Singh, D. C. Jain and K. K. Datta. "Unusual Occurrence of Cholera in Delhi during January 1994: Epidemiological Investigations". *Journal of Diarrhoeal Diseases Research* 14, no. 2, 1996, 107–9.

Singh, Jagvir, D. Bora, K. K. Khanna, D. C. Jain, V. Sachdeva, R. S. Sharma and T. Verghese. "Epidemiology and Transmission of *V. cholerae* O1 and *V. cholerae* O139 Infections in Delhi in 1993". *Journal of Diarrheal Diseases Research* 14, no. 3, 1996, 182–86.

Singh, Jagvir, D. Bora, V. Sachdeva, R. S. Sharma and T. Verghese. "*Vibrio cholerae* O1 and O139 in Less Than 5 Years Old Children Hospitalised for Watery Diarrhoea in Delhi, 1993". *Journal of Diarrheal Diseases Research* 15, no. 1, 1997, 3–6.

Singh, Jagvir, Vibha Sachdeva, Rajesh Bhatia, D. Bora, D. C. Jain and Jotna Sokhey. "Endemic Cholera in Delhi, 1995: Analysis of Data from a Sentinel Centre". *Journal of Diarrhoeal Diseases Research* 16, no. 2, 1998, 66–73.

Smelser, Neil J., and Richard Swedberg, eds. *The Handbook of Economic Sociology*. Princeton: Princeton University Press, 1994.

Smith, George Davey, and Shah Ebrahim. "Epidemiology—Is It Time to Call It a Day?" Editorial. *International Journal of Epidemiology* 30, no. 1, 2001, 1–11.

Smith, J. C. "The Basic Sciences of Public Health: The Theory and Practice of Modern Epidemiology and the Population Perspective on Health and Diseases", Centre of Social Medicine and Community Health, School of Social Sciences, Jawaharlal Nehru University, New Delhi, 1996.

Snow, John. "On the Pathology and Mode of Communication of Cholera". *London Medical Gazette* 44, 1849, 745–52 and 923–29.

Souza, R., and V. Tokman. "The Informal Urban Sector in Latin America". *International Labour Review* 114, no. 3, 1976, 355–66.

Subrahmanyan, K. "Note on the Importance of Environmental Sanitation in the Campaign against Cholera". Unpublished working document, WHO/Cholera/12, World Health Organization, Geneva, 1951.

Sundaram, K. "Agriculture-Industry Interrelations: Issues of Migration". In *The Balance between Industry and Agriculture in Economic Development*, Proceedings of the Eighth World Congress of the International Economic Association, Delhi, India, vol. 3: *Manpower and Transfers*, ed. S. Chakravarty, 177–206. London, Macmillan, 1989.

Susser, M., and E. Susser. "Choosing a Future for Epidemiology—Parts I and II". *American Journal of Public Health*, 86, no. 5, 1996, 668–77.

Swaroop, S. "Endemicity of Cholera in India". *Indian Journal of Medical Research*, 39, no. 2, 1951, 141–83.

Tabibzadeh, I., A. Rossi-Espagnet and R. Maxwell. "Spotlight on the Cities: Improving Urban Health in Developing Countries", World Health Organization, Geneva, 1989.

TERI (Tata Energy Research Institute). *Tata Energy Data Directory and Yearbook (TEDDY) 1999/2000*. New Delhi: TERI, 1999.

The Groundwater UP Project. http://www.groundwaterup.com/?page_id=112 (accessed 14 January 2011).

Tilak, V. W., R. Bhalwar and J. S. Ratti. "Epidemiological Study of an Outbreak of Cholera in Delhi Cantonment". *Indian Journal of Public Health* 41, no. 2, 1997, 61–67.

Trevett, A. F., R. C. Carter and S. F. Tyrrel. "The Importance of Domestic Water Quality Management in the Context of Faecal-Oral Disease Transmission". *Journal of Water and Health* 3, no. 3, 2005, 259–70.

UNESCO (United Nations Educational, Scientific and Cultural Organization). "2003: International Year of Freshwater". http://www.wateryear2003.org/en/ev.php-URL_ID=5970&URL_DO=DO_TOPIC&URL_SECTION=201.html (accessed 7 October 2006).

UN-HABITAT (United Nations Centre for Human Settlements). *Cities in a Globalizing World: Global Report on Human Settlements 2001*. London: Earthscan, 2001.

United Nations. *World Urbanization Prospects: The 2009 Revision*. New York: United Nations Department of Economic and Social Affairs, 2010.

Vathanophas, K., T. Indrasukhsri, P. Bunyaratabandhu, O. Suthienkul and W.

Varavithya. "The Study of Socioeconomic, Behavioural and Environmental Factors Related to Diarrhoeal Diseases in Children under 5 in Congested Areas of Bangkok Metropolis". *Journal of Medical Association of Thailand* 69, Suppl. 2, 1986, 156–62.

VHAI (Voluntary Health Association of India). *Civic Neglect and Ill-Health*. Delhi: VHAI, 1988.

___. *Report of the Independent Commission on Health in India*. New Delhi: VHAI, 1997.

Weber, J. T., E. D. Mintz, R. Cañizares, A. Semiglia, I. Gomez, R. Sempértegui, A. Dávila, K. D. Greene, N. D. Puhr and D. N. Cameron. "Epidemic Cholera in Ecuador: Multidrug Resistance and Transmission by Water and Seafood". *Epidemiology and Infection* 112, no. 1, 1994, 1–11.

Whitcombe, E. "Famine Mortality". *Economic and Political Weekly* 28, no. 23, 1993, 1169–79.

WHO (World Health Organization). *Our Planet, Our Health: Report of the WHO Commission on Health and Environment*. Geneva: WHO, 1992.

___. *WHO Chronicle No. 31*. Geneva: WHO, 1997.

___. *Guidelines for Drinking-Water Quality*. 2nd ed., vol. 3. Geneva: WHO, 1997.

___. "Diarrhoeal Disease Factsheet N330". World Health Organization, 2009. http://www.who.int/mediacentre/factsheets/fs330/en/index.html (accessed 4 April 2010).

WHO CSDH (World Health Organization Commission on Social Determinants of Health). *Closing the Gap in a Generation: Health Equity through Action on the Social Determinants of Health*. Final Report of the CSDH. Geneva: WHO, 2008.

World Bank. *World Development Report 1990*. New York: Oxford University Press, 1990.

___. "Urban Policy and Economic Development: An Agenda for the 1990s". World Bank Policy Paper, World Bank, Washington, D.C., 1991.

Wratten, Ellen. "Conceptualising Urban Poverty". *Environment and Urbanization* 7, no. 1, 1995, 11–36.

Yacob, M. "Epidemiology of Cholera in the Punjab". *Indian Medical Gazette* 79, 1944, 383.

Yapa, Lakshman. "What Causes Poverty? A Postmodern View". *Annals of the Association of American Geographers* 86, no. 4, 1996, 707–28.

Zerah, Marie-Helene. "Household Strategies for Coping with Unreliable Water Supplies: The Case of Delhi". *Habitat International* 24, no. 3, 2000, 295–307.

___. "Middle Class Neighbourhood Associations as Political Players in Mumbai". *Economic and Political Weekly* 42, no. 47, 2007, 61–68.

Zurbrigg, S. "Hunger and Epidemic Malaria in Punjab, 1868–1940". *Economic and Political Weekly* 25, no. 1, 1992, 2–26.

Index